Recent Progress in Anesthesiology

Recent Progress in Anesthesiology

Edited by Quentin Hardy

hayle
medical

New York

Hayle Medical,
750 Third Avenue, 9th Floor,
New York, NY 10017, USA

Visit us on the World Wide Web at:
www.haylemedical.com

ISBN: 978-1-63241-780-0

Cataloging-in-Publication Data

Recent progress in anesthesiology / edited by Quentin Hardy.
    p. cm.
Includes bibliographical references and index.
ISBN 978-1-63241-780-0
1. Anesthesiology. 2. Anesthesia. 3. Surgery. I. Hardy, Quentin.
RD81 .R43 2019
617.96--dc23

Table of Contents

Preface

I am honored to present to you this unique book which encompasses the most up-to-date data in the field. I was extremely pleased to get this opportunity of editing the work of experts from across the globe. I have also written papers in this field and researched the various aspects revolving around the progress of the discipline. I have tried to unify my knowledge along with that of stalwarts from every corner of the world, to produce a text which not only benefits the readers but also facilitates the growth of the field.

The medical study and application of anesthesia is known as anesthesiology. A physician trained in this specialty is called an anesthesiologist. The chief responsibility of an anesthesiologist is ensuring adequate pain relief at every stage of a surgical procedure, from the operative period to full recovery. An understanding of operative risk and complications, the methods to mitigate such risks and the management of the illness is crucial to the practice of anesthesiology. Anesthesiologists work in major trauma, airway management and resuscitation and care for patients who have clinical emergencies that pose an immediate threat to life. In recent years, the role of anesthesiologists has extended into the identification of high-risk patients and optimization of their fitness, improvement of safety during the surgery and promotion of recovery. This book covers in detail some existing theories and innovative concepts revolving around anesthesiology. From theories to research to practical applications, case studies related to all contemporary topics of relevance to this field have been included herein. Coherent flow of topics, student-friendly language and extensive use of examples make this book an invaluable source of knowledge.

Finally, I would like to thank all the contributing authors for their valuable time and contributions. This book would not have been possible without their efforts. I would also like to thank my friends and family for their constant support.

Editor

Unusual Perioperative Cardiac Emergency in a Healthy Young Woman

**Pragati Ganjoo,[1] Vijay K. Pandey,[1] Hukum Singh,[2]
Monica S. Tandon,[1] and Daljit Singh[2]**

[1] Department of Anaesthesiology and Intensive Care, GB Pant Hospital, Maulana Azad Medical College,
   New Delhi 110002, India
[2] Department of Neurosurgery, GB Pant Hospital, Maulana Azad Medical College, New Delhi 110002, India

Correspondence should be addressed to Pragati Ganjoo, pganjoo@gmail.com

Academic Editors: J. J. Derose, L. Hebbar, and P.-H. Tan

Serious cardiac complications occurring during noncardiac surgery in a young and otherwise normal person can be quite alarming for the anesthesiologist. We report here the case of a young, healthy woman who immediately after an uncomplicated spinal surgery developed a clinical picture suggestive of an acute myocardial infarction (MI) with positive relevant investigations. However, she had an abrupt and full clinical recovery and complete normalization of her cardiac investigations within a few days of this event and thereafter continued to lead a normal, symptom-free life unlike the usual course in an MI; her coronary angiography was also normal. A diagnosis of perioperative stress-induced cardiomyopathy or Takotsubo cardiomyopathy was subsequently made. This condition is characterized by a rapid, severe, but reversible, cardiac dysfunction triggered by physical or mental stress. Awareness of this entity should help anesthesiologists manage better this infrequent, but potentially life-threatening, perioperative complication.

1. Introduction

Life-threatening cardiac complications during noncardiac surgery are not unexpected in patients at risk for, or with, proven coronary artery disease (CAD). The anesthesiologist usually anticipates and prepares in advance to handle these cases. However, the same occurring in an otherwise normal young adult during a low-risk surgery can be alarming. Acute myocardial infarction (MI) in young adults is well known. Another relatively uncommon condition mimicking an acute MI is Takotsubo cardiomyopathy (TCM) that can present as an unexpected serious perioperative cardiac complication in apparently normal individuals [1–4]. It is characterized by rapid, severe, but reversible, cardiac dysfunction triggered by intense emotional or physical stress, including surgery. Familiarity with this unusual condition is thus important for its appropriate perioperative management. We report here the occurrence of this transient cardiac syndrome in a healthy young woman following an uneventful spinal surgery and briefly discuss the relevant medical literature.

2. Case Report

A 25-year-old female patient, ASA grade I, underwent laminectomy and excision of an L2-L3 intradural tumor under general anesthesia. Her intraoperative course was largely uneventful and she was awake and hemodynamically stable on transfer to the postoperative area. However, within 30 min, she complained of uneasiness and vomited once. Her blood pressure (BP) decreased to 74/52 mmHg and oxygen saturation to 74%, and her heart rate increased to 128/min. She did not have chest pain, dyspnea, arrhythmias, or cyanosis. Chest auscultation revealed bilateral rales and normal heart sounds. Invasive monitoring was established which revealed a central venous pressure of 10 mmHg, hypoxia, severe metabolic acidosis, and normal electrolytes on arterial blood gas analysis. She was treated with oxygen, soda bicarbonate, furosemide, and dopamine infusion at 7 µg/kg/min. Her ECG showed ST depression in diffuse leads and chest X-ray showed bilateral lung haziness. A 2-D echocardiography revealed regional wall motion abnormalities (RWMA), namely, hypokinesia of basal and mid-septal and mid and apical anterior walls with moderate left ventricular dysfunction (ejection fraction ~30–35%). Troponin-T test done twice, 5 hours apart, was positive (0.16 µg/L and 0.34 µg/L, respectively, normal range at our lab ~0.0–0.1 µg/L). Acute MI was suspected and the patient further treated in the coronary care unit. Percutaneous coronary intervention was considered here but consent for the procedure could not be obtained. She continued to have hypotension (systolic BP ~80–85 mmHg) over the next 2 days despite adequate inotropic support. However, on the 4th postoperative day, her condition improved abruptly and within the next 24 hours she had completely recovered with normal vital parameters and ECG; dopamine was discontinued. Her remaining hospital stay was uneventful and she was discharged after 10 days on beta-adrenergic blocker, angiotensin-converting enzyme inhibitor, and statin therapy and put on regular cardiac followup. Her evaluation after 3 weeks revealed no cardiac manifestations and a normal ECG and echocardiography (no RWMA, ejection fraction ~60%); her cardiac drugs were withdrawn. She subsequently underwent a stress echocardiography which was negative for inducible ischemia. This was followed by a computed tomography (CT) coronary angiography which revealed the coronaries to be normal in origin, caliber, and outline with no evidence of any plaque or stenosis and a normal cardiac function (ejection fraction ~69%, end-diastolic volume ~64.83 mL, end-systolic volume ~44.81 mL, and cardiac output ~4.12 L/min). In her year-long followup until now, she continues to be totally symptom-free and has a normal echocardiography despite resuming all routine work.

3. Discussion

The perioperative cardiac events in this patient were completely unexpected. Though her initial presentation was suggestive of an acute MI, her young age and apparently normal prior health made us first think of pulmonary embolism, aspiration, and pneumothorax as the probable causes; these were soon ruled out. Though rare, acute MI is known in young adults [5]. Its causative factors include coronary artery aneurysm and dissection, anomalous origin of coronary arteries, coronary vasospasm due to illicit substances misuse, premature atherosclerotic CAD, and thrombotic occlusion of coronaries in hyper-coagulable conditions like systemic lupus erythematosis, hyperhomocysteinemia, and hormonal contraceptive pill use. Perioperative MI usually occurs during emergence from anesthesia and may be clinically silent, manifesting only as ST-segment depression on ECG and raised troponin levels, as was evident in our patient also. However, the abrupt and complete normalization of her hemodynamic status, ECG, and echocardiography within a few days was inconsistent with an MI where abnormal cardiac changes are expected to persist because of irreversible

myocardial damage. This patient's typical clinical picture, highlighted by significant, but short-lived cardiac destabilization followed by full recovery and continued normal symptom-free life, a normal stress echocardiography, and no obvious abnormality seen on CT coronary angiography, is very indicative of TCM, also known as stress-induced cardiomyopathy or broken-heart syndrome [6, 7]. Normalization of cardiac function within days to a few weeks is the cardinal feature of this condition. TCM is often mistakenly diagnosed as an acute MI as both have similar clinical manifestations; 2% of suspected MI patients were subsequently seen to have TCM [8]. The modified Mayo Clinic criteria for diagnosing TCM include (a) transient hypokinesis, dyskinesis, or akinesis of the left ventricular mid-segments with or without apical involvement, the RWMA extending beyond a single epicardial vascular distribution, and presence of a stressful trigger often, but not always; (b) absence of angiographic evidence of obstructive CAD or of acute plaque rupture; (c) new ECG abnormalities (ST segment and/or T-wave changes) or modest elevation in cardiac troponin level; (d) absence of pheochromocytoma, myocarditis, or hypertrophic cardiomyopathy [9]. Several variant forms of TCM with different patterns of clinical presentation and cardiac wall motion abnormalities have also been reported [10]. Though more commonly seen in postmenopausal women aged 62–75 years, TCM is also reported in younger patients [6, 10]. Unlike CAD, it has no known risk factors like hyperlipidemia, smoking, positive family history, hypertension, and diabetes. Some of the proposed etiologies for TCM include excess catecholamine-induced myocardial stunning, multivessel coronary artery spasm, transient epicardial coronary thrombosis, impaired cardiac microvascular function, and dynamic left ventricular outflow tract obstruction. The initial management of TCM is similar to that of an MI. Close cardiac followup and serial echocardiograms are recommended till complete cardiac recovery and beta-adrenergic blocker therapy may be beneficial [6, 7]. Though TCM has an excellent prognosis, life-threatening complications like congestive cardiac failure (44–57% of cases), cardiogenic shock (15–45%), pulmonary edema, dysrhythmias, thromboembolism, left ventricular wall rupture, and death have been reported [8, 10].

Although infrequently encountered, perioperative TCM is a well-established clinical syndrome reported in a variety of surgeries, particularly following emergence from anesthesia [1–4]. For anesthesiologists, however, many vital issues regarding TCM still remain unresolved like preoperative identification of susceptible patients and high-risk surgeries, identifying the various triggers, the best anesthesia technique to help prevent onset, and the optimal therapy in the acute phase. To understand these concerns better, large population cohort studies and perioperative patient registries have been suggested [10].

This case highlights the importance of TCM as a potential cause of severe perioperative hemodynamic instability and emphasizes the need for adequate preparedness to manage serious cardiac complications in all surgical patients, irrespective of their age and preoperative state. More frequent diagnosis and improved management of perioperative TCM are likely with its increased awareness and reporting among anesthesiologists.

References

[1] A. Kogan, P. Ghosh, E. Schwammenthal, and E. Raanani, "Takotsubo syndrome after cardiac surgery," *Annals of Thoracic Surgery*, vol. 85, no. 4, pp. 1439–1441, 2008.

[2] L. Meng and C. Wells, "Takotsubo cardiomyopathy during emergence from general anaesthesia," *Anaesth Intensive Care*, vol. 37, no. 5, pp. 836–839, 2009.

[3] N. Takayama, Y. Iwase, S. Ohtsu, and H. Sakio, ""Takotsubo" cardiomyopathy developed in the postoperative period in a patient with amyotrophic lateral sclerosis," *Japanese Journal of Anesthesiology*, vol. 53, no. 4, pp. 403–406, 2004.

[4] B. Bradbury and F. Cohen, "Early postoperative takotsubo cardiomyopathy: a case report," *AANA Journal*, vol. 79, no. 3, pp. 181–188, 2011.

[5] S. Osula, G. M. Bell, and R. S. Hornung, "Acute myocardial infarction in young adults: causes and management," *Postgraduate Medical Journal*, vol. 78, no. 915, pp. 27–30, 2002.

[6] S. Buchholz and G. Rudan, "Tako-tsubo syndrome on the rise: a review of the current literature," *Postgraduate Medical Journal*, vol. 83, no. 978, pp. 261–264, 2007.

[7] T. M. Pilgrim and T. R. Wyss, "Takotsubo cardiomyopathy or transient left ventricular apical ballooning syndrome: a systematic review," *International Journal of Cardiology*, vol. 124, no. 3, pp. 283–292, 2008.

[8] E. B. Tomich, E. Merchant, and C. S. Kang, "Takotsubo cardiomyopathy," Emedicine, 2011, http://emedicine.medscape.com/article/1513631- overview.

[9] A. Prasad, "Apical ballooning syndrome: an important differential diagnosis of acute myocardial infarction," *Circulation*, vol. 115, no. 5, pp. e56–e59, 2007.

[10] E. A. Hessel and M. J. London, "Takotsubo (stress) cardiomyopathy and the anesthesiologist: enough case reports. Let's try to answer some specific questions!," *Anesthesia and Analgesia*, vol. 110, no. 3, pp. 674–679, 2010.

X-Ray of One-Sided "White Lung" after Central Venous Catheterization

Michel Casanova and Wolfgang Ummenhofer

Department for Anesthesia, Surgical Intensive Care, Prehospital Emergency Medicine and Pain Therapy, University Hospital of Basel, Spitalstrasse 21, 4031 Basel, Switzerland

Correspondence should be addressed to Michel Casanova; michel.casanova@usb.ch

Academic Editors: S. Faenza, T. Ho, D. Lee, and C.-S. Sung

Complications during insertion of a subclavian central venous line are rare but potentially serious. This case report describes the radiological abnormality of a one-sided pleural effusion during a routine control directly after a difficult central venous catheterization. We illustrate the findings, the initial emergency management, and our procedure to rule out an iatrogenic hemothorax. Possible differential diagnoses and strategies for management of a suspected complication are discussed.

1. Introduction

For patients in the United States, as many as five million central venous lines are placed annually.

Perforation of the subclavian artery occurs in about 0.1–1% of cases, leading to hemothorax (1%) and rarely quadriplegia. Perforation of the aorta and cardiac tamponade can occur if the cannula-site perforation is within the pericardial reflection. This complication is associated with a death rate of 90% [1, 2]. Compulsory radiological control of central venous access is debated but is still routinely performed in our institution.

2. Case Description

An 88-year-old woman was initially admitted for correction of poorly controlled diabetes mellitus. During her hospitalization, she developed peripheral catheter-associated *Staphylococcus aureus* thrombophlebitis in her left cubital region. The patient was on IV antibiotics for four days. Initially, trimethoprim/sulfamethoxazole had been used. After 2 days, this was followed by ceftriaxone due to antibiotic resistance. After deciding on long-term antibiotic treatment with IV cefazolin and due to bad peripheral venous conditions, the patient was scheduled for central venous catheterization.

Relevant diagnoses of the patient were (i) known hypertensive cardiac disease (transthoracic echocardiography 6 months before had shown a LV-EF of 54% and a light mitral and tricuspid insufficiency) and (ii) liver cirrhosis with portal hypertension.

A recent CT scan showed signs of liver cirrhosis with ascites and splenomegaly, and abdominal sonography 2 months ago supposed the findings to be due to a steatohepatitis. Liver serologies were negative for a lack or deficiency of alpha-1 antitrypsin. Ceruloplasmin and alpha-fetoprotein were normal. No signs of active viral hepatitis were found, and the patient's carcinoembryonic antigen value was within the normal range. Finally, cytological screens of the ascites showed no signs of malignancy.

Besides the antibiotics, medical therapy at the time of consultation included torsemide, spironolactone, and sitagliptin.

Laboratory examination revealed thrombocytopenia ($78,000/\mu L$) and a spontaneous international normalized ratio INR of 1.2. The thrombocytopenia was assumed to be due to splenomegaly (Table 1).

Clinically, the patient breathed normally and had a normal heart rate and blood pressure when arriving for the intervention. For comfort reasons of the patient, we decided to perform cannulation of the right subclavian vein. Cannulation of the vein was successful upon the first attempt, but we

TABLE 1: Summary of important laboratory values.

	Measured	Normal value
Hematology		
Hemoglobin (g/L)	120	140–180
Hematocrit (%)	34	40–52
Thrombocytes ($\times 10^9$/L)	78	136–380
Chemistry		
INR	1.2	0.8–1.2
Creatinine (Nmol/L)	164	81–133
Albumin (g/L)	23	35–53
Bilirubin total (Nmol/L)	11	5.0–18.0
CRP (mg/L)	27.5	<5.0
ASAT (U/L)	40	11.0–34.0
ALAT (U/L) 45 8–63	24	8.0–41.0
Alkaline phosphatase (U/L)	168	<104
GGT (U/L)	278	6.0–40.0
Total protein (g/L)	62	64–83
LDH (U/L)	209	135–214
Pleural punctate		
Total protein (g/L)	16	
LDH (U/L)	50	
Bacterial growth	No aerobic- or anaerobic bacterial growth	
Gram staining	No bacteria	
Mycobacterium-tuberculosis complex PCR	Negative	

ALAT: alanine transaminase; ASAT: aspartate transaminase; CRP: C-reactive protein; GGT: gamma-glutamyltransferase; INR: international normalized ratio; LDH: lactate dehydrogenase.

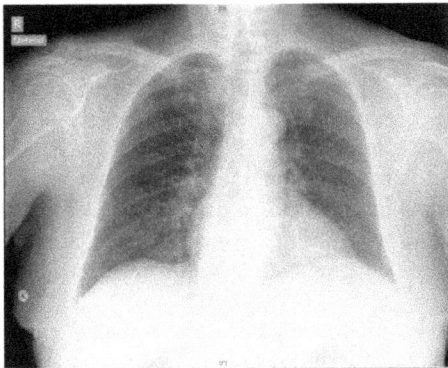

FIGURE 1: Chest X-ray anteroposterior at admission (sitting).

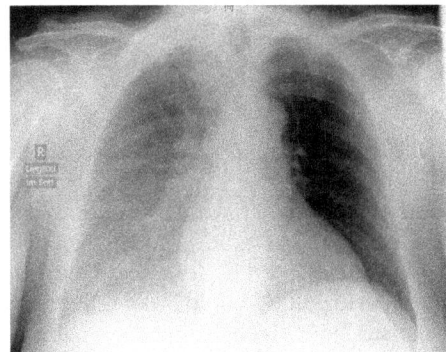

FIGURE 2: Chest X-ray anteroposterior after puncture (lying).

were twice unable to advance the guide wire. Consequently, we changed to an ultrasound-controlled puncture of the right internal jugular vein, which worked well on the first attempt. The catheter was placed without problem. According to our internal guidelines, a chest X-ray was taken on the patient's return to the ward.

Surprisingly, when controlling the radiographic finding one hour after the procedure, the X-ray showed a one-sided "white lung." Comparison of the chest X-ray from the day of admission showed no effusion or cardiac decompensation (Figure 1), whereas the current image clearly depicted what we believed to be a pleural effusion on the right side, which

was the puncture site for the subclavian as well as the internal jugular vein (Figure 2).

We were suspicious of an iatrogenic lesion of the right subclavian artery or vein with consecutive hematothorax and immediately saw the patient at the ward.

Contrary to our apprehension, we found the patient to be hemodynamically stable and without dyspnea. Auscultation of the right chest revealed breath sounds but percussion of the right hemithorax an obvious dullness. In addition, a bedside HemoCue measurement showed a lowered hemoglobin value of 96 g/L compared with 130 g/L the day before.

We took specimens for type and screening, blood cell count, and emergency chemistry and reflected on reasonable

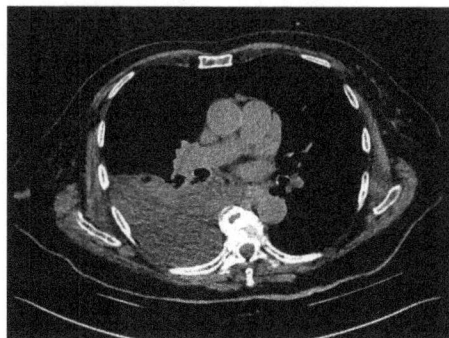

FIGURE 3: CT scan (MDCT, arterial with 40 mL Ultravist 370 and 5 min p.i. DLP 335 mGycm) of the thorax.

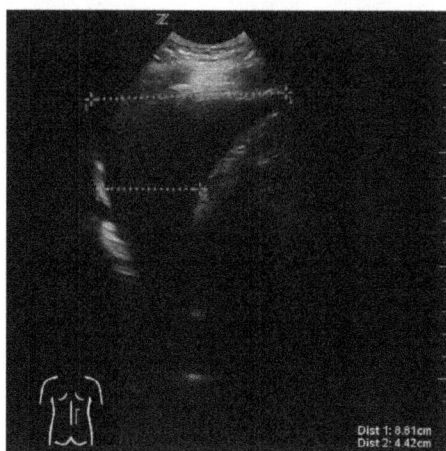

FIGURE 4: Ultrasound of lower thorax.

TABLE 2: Light's criteria [3].

Pleural fluid is an exudate if one or more of the following criteria are met
(i) Pleural fluid protein divided by serum protein is > 0.5
(ii) Pleural fluid lactate dehydrogenase (LDH) divided by serum LDH is > 0.6
(iii) Pleural fluid LDH > 0.6 or is 2/3 times the normal upper limit for serum

The evaluation of the laboratory values of the puncture liquid showed a transudate according to Light's criteria (Table 2) [3]. No signs of mycobacteria could be found.

We received the above-mentioned emergency laboratory (Table 1), which showed a hemoglobin value of 120 g/L in comparison to 130 g/L the day before. Retrospectively, the HemoCue bedside value seemed to be an inaccurately low determination.

The conclusive diagnosis for our patient was a right-sided pleural effusion due to a nonalcoholic steatohepatitis (NASH)-mediated liver cirrhosis. The patient had already suffered a right-sided pleural effusion five months earlier, which was unknown to both us and the treating physician at the ward at the time our intervention. Treatment for the ascites was adjusted. Spironolactone and torsemide were augmented, and lactulose was added.

3. Discussion

Routine chest X-ray following central venous catheterization revealed a white chest on the puncture side. The position of the catheter tip was radiologically correct. However, the puncture process with unsuccessful attempt for subclavian vein access (impossibility to insert the guide wire and a second puncture site at the internal jugular vein of the same side) aroused suspicion for a perforation complication and a subsequent hemothorax. Since a chest X-ray few days before our intervention had been normal, we were even more concerned.

However, immediate clinical examination could exclude acute hemodynamic and respiratory compromise. Interdisciplinary discussion of options with radiology and pneumology consultants offered a reasonable strategy for an eventually unexpected explanation.

Besides a hemothorax, there are more than 50 recognized causes of one-sided pleural liquid accumulation. Pleural effusions are a common medical problem resulting from diseases local to the pleura or underlying lung, systemic conditions, organ dysfunction, and drugs [4]. In addition, different etiologies can produce one-sided effusions more frequently than others.

In cardiac insufficiency, bilateral effusions are present in 81%, right-sided in 12%, and left-sided in 7% of all cases [5]. Hepatic hydrothorax is a rare but important cause of—usually unilateral—pleural effusion. About 85–90% of the cases are isolated right-sided effusions [6]. Hepatic hydrothorax can be observed as a complication of portal hypertension in <10%

next steps and possible options. Of course, a chest drain would have relieved possible hemothorax, but the lack of hemodynamic or respiratory compromise did not require immediate action. With strong suspicion of arterial or venous perforation, we felt that a CT scan could be helpful and that additional perfusion CT could be an important asset for localization of the potential bleeding site. Internal stenting and/or surgical repair would probably benefit from radiological identification of the possible iatrogenic injury.

We involved the CT consultant on call, who confirmed the plausibility of the indication and initiated a plain and subsequent contrast medium CT scan (MDCT, arterial with 40 mL Ultravist 370 and 5 min pi; DLP 335 mGycm). Fortunately, no arterial or venous leakage with active bleeding could be found. In addition and even more surprisingly, calculation of density revealed that a hemothorax was unlikely to be the source of the white chest X-ray. The Hounsfield scale value of 0 HU native of the liquid was consistent for an effusion (Figure 3), and the preliminary CT diagnosis was a right pleural effusion 6 cm long.

A pleural sonograph (Figure 4) showed an estimated 900 mL of homogenic anechogenic pleural effusion. The subsequent ultrasound-guided puncture extracted clear liquid, and the hematothorax could be definitively ruled out.

of patients with ascites secondary to advanced liver cirrhosis. The underlying pathophysiological mechanism seems to be a direct movement of fluid from the peritoneal cavity into the pleural space through diaphragmatic defects [7]. In rare cases, complete translocation of fluid into the pleural space without ascites can be observed [8, 9].

Acknowledgments

Unfortunately, the patient died three months later due to reasons unrelated to the intervention described herein. The authors wish to thank the patient's daughter who kindly gave written consent for publication of this case report. We would like to thank Allison Dwileski for her expert editorial assistance.

References

[1] M. Carr and A. Jagannath, "Hemopericardium resulting from attempted internal jugular vein catheterization: a case report and review of complications of central venous catheterization," *CardioVascular and Interventional Radiology*, vol. 9, no. 4, pp. 214–218, 1986.

[2] P. Fangio, E. Mourgeon, A. Romelaer, J.-P. Goarin, P. Coriat, and J.-J. Rouby, "Aortic injury and cardiac tamponade as a complication of subclavian venous catheterization," *Anesthesiology*, vol. 96, no. 6, pp. 1520–1522, 2002.

[3] R. W. Light, M. I. Macgregor, P. C. Luchsinger, and W. C. Ball Jr., "Pleural effusions: the diagnostic separation of transudates and exudates," *Annals of Internal Medicine*, vol. 77, no. 4, pp. 507–513, 1972.

[4] S. A. Sahn and J. E. Heffner, "Pleural fluid analysis," in *Textbook of Pleural Diseases*, R. W. Light and Y. C. G. Lee, Eds., pp. 209–226, Arnold Press, London, UK, 2nd edition, 2008.

[5] Pleural Effusion: Mediastinal and Pleural Disorders: Merck Manual Professional.

[6] G. T. Kinasewitz and J. I. Keddissi, "Hepatic hydrothorax," *Current Opinion in Pulmonary Medicine*, vol. 9, no. 4, pp. 261–265, 2003.

[7] T. Zenda, S. Miyamoto, S. Murata, and H. Mabuchi, "Detection of diaphragmatic defect as the cause of severe hepatic hydrothorax with magnetic resonance imaging," *American Journal of Gastroenterology*, vol. 93, no. 11, pp. 2288–2289, 1998.

[8] A. F. G. Von Bierbrauer, M. Dilger, P. Weissenbach, and J. Walle, "Hepatic hydrothorax—a rare cause of pleural effusion that is difficult to manage," *Pneumologie*, vol. 62, no. 1, pp. 40–43, 2008.

[9] C. M. Kirsch, D. W. Chui, G. G. Yenokida, W. A. Jensen, and P. B. Bascom, "Case report: hepatic hydrothorax without ascites," *American Journal of the Medical Sciences*, vol. 302, no. 2, pp. 103–106, 1991.

Transient Left-Sided Paralysis following Robotic-Assisted Laparoscopic Uteropexy

Jasmina Kurdija and Jan G. Jakobsson

*Department of Anaesthesia & Intensive Care, Institution for Clinical Science, Karolinska Institutet,
Danderyds Hospital, 182 88 Stockholm, Sweden*

Correspondence should be addressed to Jan G. Jakobsson; jan.jakobsson@ki.se

Academic Editor: Maria Jose C. Carmona

We describe a case report of a 47-year-old ASA 2 female patient who exhibits severe headache and hemineurology during awakening following robotic pelvic prolapse surgery. The symptoms resolved spontaneously during the first postoperative day. We could not find any explicit root cause. Robotic surgery associated adverse events are discussed.

1. Introduction

Robotic surgery is increasingly adopted. Robotic technique is increasingly used for urology and gynecoligical surgery [1, 2]. A number of procedures are nowadays conducted with robotic technique improving the surgical outcome. Robotic surgery demands however an adequate anaesthesia strategy. Procedures such as prostatectomy and prolapse surgery demand furthermore that the patient is placed in Trendelenburg position and CO_2 gas is insufflated creating a surgical field. Gas insufflations have a number of effects reducing venous return, in combination with head-down moving diaphragm, and subsequently impairing ventilation perfusion matching and further increasing intracranial pressure. Vascular gas entrainment causing intravascular gas emboli is also a well-known risk associated with surgery requiring CO_2 insufflation. Thus robotic surgery is associated with risks and the benefit versus risk must be acknowledged [3]. We describe a patient complaining of severe headache and hemiparesis after awakening from robotic surgery. The symptoms resolved spontaneously during the first 24 postoperative hours. Side effects and complications associated with robotic surgery and CO_2 insufflation are discussed.

2. Case Report

The patient has given informed consent to present this case report. A 47-year-old woman with uterus prolapse was admitted for elective robotic prolapse surgery. The patient had a BMI 32 but was otherwise healthy. She had previously been examined with transthoracic echocardiography (TTE) and 24 h Holter EKG because of subjective symptoms of arrhythmia. Nothing pathologic was found except for sparse supraventricular extrasystoles. She has also had an asthma attack 2 years prior to this. She had no current medication.

She underwent selective standard robotic-assisted laparoscopic uteropexy. The operation was performed in general anaesthesia. Anaesthesia was induced with intravenous propofol 200 mg and target controlled remifentanil infusion. The patient was muscle-relaxed with rocuronium 40 mg and intubated. Anaesthesia was maintained with target controlled remifentanil infusion and sevoflurane. She was monitored with EKG, pulse oximetry, and capnography, and the blood pressure (BP) was monitored with an arterial line in the left radial artery. Immediately after the start of anaesthesia patient's BP dropped to 90–100/50 mmHg and remained that way during the preoperative preparations until start of surgery. During the operation that lasted approximately 2.5 h, the patient was in Trendelenburg position (27 degrees head down). She was respiratory and circulatory stable during the operation with a BP around 115/70 and heart rate of 60–75 beats per minute. SpO_2 was 99% with FiO_2 0.35–0.5, $EtCO_2$ 4.3–5.2, and peak pressure in the ventilator was 17–30 cmH_2O.

During emergence from anaesthesia the patient woke up and was moving all four extremities. She was taken to the postoperative ward where she initially was sleeping. She woke up after two hours with anxiety, severe headache, and complaint of loss of sensation in the left side of the body. She could move her right arm and leg. She was able to do minor movements in left leg and arm but was not able to lift left arm or leg from the surface of the bed. There was a sensory impairment on the left side compared to the right, with lowered sensation for pain and touch. A neurologic examination showed no other abnormities.

The patient underwent an acute computed tomography (CT) of the brain and CT-angiography of the arteries in the neck and brain. Both examinations were normal with no detected haemorrhage, infarction, or expansive process/oedema in the brain. There was no thrombosis, occlusion, or stenosis in the arteries.

The patient was discharged from the recovery room and admitted to a neurologic ward. During the night the patient's symptoms improved and within 24 hours she was fully restored. All symptoms resolved spontaneously, and no interventions were undertaken. All follow-up examinations including MRI of the brain, blood tests, and lumbar puncture were normal. She was discharged home after three days without any neurological sequelae.

We were not able to make conclusive diagnosis for the patient's transient left-sided paralysis. There are several potential causes: positioning injury, gas embolism, migraine, and transient ischemic attack.

3. Positioning Injury

There is a known risk for perioperative positioning injuries. With the not uncommonly extreme positioning head-down tilt positioning of patients undergoing robotic-assisted surgery (RAS) that risk may be increased. Some authors report Trendelenburg position of even 45 degrees [4]. Examples of such injuries specific to RAS are compartment syndrome, rhabdomyolysis, ischemic optic neuropathy, and upper or lower extremity peripheral neuropathies [5]. Mild-to-severe stretching or compression of a specific nerve or nerve plexus is thought to be the cause of the nerve damage in these cases. Mills et al. [6] looked specifically at nerve damage associated with robotic-assisted urological surgery and found that the factors significantly associated with injury were long operative time (>328 min), in room time and ASA classes 2–4. Time required to recover from these injuries varies with the severity of the injury [7, 8]. Our patient was positioned on a vacuum mattress containing beans with her arms at the side. Pads for shoulder support were fixated on the operating table. Her legs were put in leg braces so that she could be put in a lithotomy position if needed. She underwent a normal length surgery (146 minutes), in room time being 253 minutes, and is ASA 2. Directly after the finish of surgery she was examined for pressure damage and none was found. Her symptoms are unlikely related to peripheral neuropathy since she experienced paralysis in both her arm and her leg, which together with severe headache suggest a central cause.

4. Gas Embolism

Venous gas embolism can cause acute symptoms such as tachycardia, cardiac arrhythmias, hypotension, desaturation, or EKG changes. Studies have been performed using transesophageal echocardiography (TEE) to detect gas embolism in the right atrium. Incidences of embolism with or without cardiorespiratory symptoms have been reported in up to 100% of cases during total laparoscopic hysterectomy, 69% during laparoscopic cholecystectomy, 76% during neurosurgery in the sitting position, and 69–100% during laparoscopic hepatic resection [9–12]. Symptomatic gas emboli are however infrequent. There are unfortunately no firm incident data available. It is hardly possible to gain an incident from study data and there is no gas emboli register that could help compile data for statistical analysis. Hong et al. [13] interestingly found that incidence of venous gas embolism during robotic-assisted laparoscopic radical prostatectomy was 38% in comparison with 80% during radical retropubic prostatectomy. Paradoxical CO_2 embolism, gas emboli in the arterial circulation, during laparoscopic surgery is most rare event. Arterial gas emboli can of course result in serious consequences such as neurologic injury. Systemic gas emboli are thought to be right to left shunting of venous gas embolism, either intracardiac due to patent foramen ovale (PFO) or extracardiac via transpulmonary air passage [14, 15]. Huang et al. [15] described a case report with presumed extracardiac paradoxical CO_2 embolism, which resulted in neurologic deficit and weakness of all four limbs. In this case TEE showed acute gas embolism in both left and right side of the heart with no embolism detected on CT of MRI of the brain. We did not perform an acute TEE on our patient. TTE performed before the surgery did not however show any signs of left to right heart wall defects. No special maneuvers were performed in order to identify PFO (e.g., injecting contrast material into the bloodstream or applying positive pressure to the airway). Thus we cannot explicitly exclude the possibility that the patient has an undetected PFO. Extracardiac paradoxical gas embolism cannot be excluded either. The delay in onset makes gas emboli less likely. Carbon dioxide gas entrainment is generally seen only during gas insufflation and increase in pressure.

5. Migraine and Transitory Ischemic Attack

Migraine may be associated with neurology however uncommon. Our patient had no history of migraine. The headache was intense and bilateral; still a vascular "migraine" equivalent cannot be excluded. A first migraine attack in age of 50 associated with surgery seems however less likely. Transitory ischemic attack (TIA) generally defined as a neurologic deficit lasting less than 24 hours could be a plausible cause. Our patient had a BMI of 32, thus by definition being obese, but she had no history of cardiovascular disease or arthrosclerosis. CT-angiography showed no stenosis in her carotid arteries. One could speculate whether a relative cerebral ischemia following reversal of the head-down positioning during surgery and possibly mild hypotension following awakening and reduced stress may have caused a transient cerebral hypoperfusion and ischemia.

We are not able to provide any firm explanation to our patients' symptoms. The increased use of robotic surgery calls however for a vigilant awareness around side effects to avoid putting patients at risk. Maintenance of blood pressure, safe positioning, periodically checking, vigilance for the risk of CO_2 emboli, cautious observation of $EtCO_2$, and possibly added echocardiography in cases of suspicion is of great value to prevent possible complications.

References

[1] A. Sivaraman, R. Sanchez-Salas, D. Prapotnich et al., "Robotics in urological surgery: evolution, current status and future perspectives," *Actas Urológicas Españolas*, 2015.

[2] K. P. Sajadi and H. B. Goldman, "Robotic pelvic organ prolapse surgery," *Nature Reviews Urology*, vol. 12, no. 4, pp. 216–224, 2015.

[3] A. Khajuria, "Robotics and surgery: a sustainable relationship?" *World Journal of Clinical Cases*, vol. 3, no. 3, pp. 265–269, 2015.

[4] T. Sukhu and T. L. Krupski, "Patient positioning and prevention of injuries in patients undergoing laparoscopic and robot-assisted urologic procedures," *Current Urology Reports*, vol. 15, no. 4, article 398, 2014.

[5] J. Song, "Severe brachial plexus injury after retropubic radical prostatectomy—a case report," *Korean Journal of Anesthesiology*, vol. 63, no. 1, pp. 68–71, 2012.

[6] J. T. Mills, M. B. Burris, D. J. Warburton, M. R. Conaway, N. S. Schenkman, and T. L. Krupski, "Positioning injuries associated with robotic assisted urological surgery," *Journal of Urology*, vol. 190, no. 2, pp. 580–584, 2013.

[7] C. J. Winfree and D. G. Kline, "Intraoperative positioning nerve injuries," *Surgical Neurology*, vol. 63, no. 1, pp. 5–18, 2005.

[8] D. Shveiky, J. N. Aseff, and C. B. Iglesia, "Brachial plexus injury after laparoscopic and robotic surgery," *Journal of Minimally Invasive Gynecology*, vol. 17, no. 4, pp. 414–420, 2010.

[9] C. S. Kim, J. Y. Kim, J.-Y. Kwon et al., "Venous air embolism during total laparoscopic hysterectomy: comparison to total abdominal hysterectomy," *Anesthesiology*, vol. 111, no. 1, pp. 50–54, 2009.

[10] M. Derouin, P. Couture, D. Boudreault, D. Girard, and D. Gravel, "Detection of gas embolism by transesophageal echocardiography during laparoscopic cholecystectomy," *Anesthesia and Analgesia*, vol. 82, no. 1, pp. 119–124, 1996.

[11] H. J. Schmitt and T. M. Hemmerling, "Venous air emboli occur during release of positive end-expiratory pressure and repositioning after sitting position surgery," *Anesthesia & Analgesia*, vol. 94, no. 2, pp. 400–403, 2002.

[12] T. C. Schmandra, S. Mierdl, H. Bauer, C. Gutt, and E. Hanisch, "Transoesophageal echocardiography shows high risk of gas embolism during laparoscopic hepatic resection under carbon dioxide pneumoperitoneum," *British Journal of Surgery*, vol. 89, no. 7, pp. 870–876, 2002.

[13] J. Y. Hong, J. Y. Kim, Y. D. Choi, K. H. Rha, S. J. Yoon, and H. K. Kil, "Incidence of venous gas embolism during robotic-assisted laparoscopic radical prostatectomy is lower than that during radical retropubic prostatectomy," *British Journal of Anaesthesia*, vol. 105, no. 6, pp. 777–781, 2010.

[14] E. A. Bedell, K. H. Berge, and T. J. Losasso, "Paradoxic air embolism during venous air embolism: transesophageal echocardiographic evidence of transpulmonary air passage," *Anesthesiology*, vol. 80, no. 4, pp. 947–950, 1994.

[15] Y.-Y. Huang, H.-L. Wu, M.-Y. Tsou et al., "Paradoxical carbon dioxide embolism during pneumoperitoneum in laparoscopic surgery for a huge renal angiomyolipoma," *Journal of the Chinese Medical Association*, vol. 71, no. 4, pp. 214–217, 2008.

Anesthetic Management of Direct Laryngoscopy and Dilatation of Subglottic Stenosis in a Patient with Severe Myasthenia Gravis

Hesham A. Elsharkawy and Ursula Galway

Department of General Anesthesiology and Outcomes Research, Anesthesiology Institute, Cleveland Clinic,
9500 Euclid Avenue, Cleveland, OH 44195, USA

Correspondence should be addressed to Hesham A. Elsharkawy, elsharh@ccf.org

Academic Editor: U. Buyukkocak

We describe the anesthetic management of a patient with severe myasthenia gravis and tracheal stenosis; the patient was scheduled for direct laryngoscopy and dilatation. The combination of myasthenia gravis and tracheal obstruction presents several difficulties for anesthetic management. The airway is shared; therefore, any complications are also shared by the anesthesiologist and bronchoscopists. The potential for respiratory compromise in patients undergoing the two procedures requires that anesthesiologists be familiar with the underlying disease state, as well as the interaction of anesthetic and nonanesthetic drugs in a case involving myasthenia gravis. We reviewed the literature and report our experience in this case. There is no strong evidence for choosing one approach to general anesthesia over another for bronchoscopy. Careful preoperative planning and experience in airway management and jet ventilation are crucial to prevent an adverse outcome and obtain favorable results.

1. Introduction

We present the anesthetic management of a patient with severe myasthenia gravis (MG) and tracheal stenosis she was scheduled for direct laryngoscopy and dilatation. Institutional review board (IRB) approval is not required by our institution for single case reports; therefore, written patient permission was not obtained.

The combination of myasthenia gravis and tracheal stenosis presents several challenges for the anesthesiologist. Therefore, preoperative evaluation of the MG patient should include a review of the severity of the patient's disease and the treatment regimen. The case should therefore be reviewed with the surgeon before formulating the anesthesia plan. Specific attention should be paid to voluntary and respiratory muscle strength. The patient's ability to protect and maintain a patent airway postoperatively may be compromised if any bulbar involvement exists preoperatively. Respiratory muscle strength can be quantified by pulmonary function tests. Finally, it is critical to evaluate the severity of the subglottic stenosis and the difficulty of the intubation.

2. Case Presentation

The patient was a 24-year-old female with a past medical history of myasthenia gravis (MG) and asthma. Her history included nine days of orotracheal intubation for myasthenia exacerbation. She needed five plasma phoresis exchanges and high doses of corticosteroids and azathioprine. Afterwards, the patient was discharged home in stable condition.

At home, the MG was treated with oral pyridostigmine 60 mg, 3 times per day; prednisone 20 mg daily in the morning; oral azathioprine 75 mg twice per day. Later, she experienced about two weeks of progressive shortness of breath and stridor, which worsened with a nonproductive cough.

She was admitted for difficulty in breathing and examined by an the ear, nose, and throat (ENT) team on arrival at the emergency department. She was found to have severe subglottic stenosis. A computerized tomography (CT) scan of the neck on admission showed that severe subglottic stenosis has developed with minimal cross-sectional diameters of 4×5 mm at the narrowest point (0.3^2 cm) approximately 75% narrowing of her trachea. Stenosis extended over a craniocaudal distance of 15 mm. Beyond the stenosis, the trachea and central airways were normal. This hourglass configuration of the stenosis is very characteristic of endotracheal intubation injury.

She was scheduled for microdirect laryngoscopy and tracheostomy with tracheal and subglottic dilation, injection of Depo-Medrol, and placement of mitomycin-C. The preoperative vital signs were BP 111/63; pulse 67; temperature 35.8°C (axillary); respiratory rate 20; weight 67.586 kg; SpO2 97% on room air. Airway assessment: Mallampati Score (MP) 1; neck full ROM; Airway evaluation: showed no significant abnormalities. Her voice was mildly hoarse, with mild biphasic stridor during sitting and supine position. Lung fields were clear to auscultation. Results of the neurologic and musculoskeletal examination were normal, and no bulbar weakness was evident.

After detailed discussion with the surgeon regarding the planned surgical procedure with a patient whose recent history included MG exacerbation, we decided not use muscle relaxants. After application of the standard American Society of Anesthesiologist (ASA) monitors, we preoxygenated with 100% oxygen. General anesthesia was induced intravenously (i.v.) with midazolam 1 mg, lidocaine 60 mg, propofol 200 mg. We verified easy mask ventilation with bag and mask. General anesthesia was maintained with propofol/remifentanil infusion, and titrated with the degree of surgical stimulation and the patient's hemodynamic response. We started with propofol 300 mcg/kg/min (IV) and remifentanil 0.5 mcg/kg/min. Hydrocortisone 100 mg was given to decrease airway edema. No neuromuscular blockers were given during the surgery.

The surgeon started with suspension laryngoscopy, sprayed lidocaine, passed the vocal cords, then completed a rigid bronchoscopy. We ventilated the lungs using jet ventilation through the ventilating bronchoscope. Initially, we started at 20 pounds per square inch (PSI). However, this was insufficient to generate a good chest rise, although oxygen saturation was in the 90s. We, therefore, decided to gradually increase the PSI to 40, with a respiratory rate of 14–18 jets per minute, allowing adequate time for exhalation. We monitored chest rise and oxygen saturation. We were able to maintain oxygen saturation between 94% and 99%.

The patient's larynx was examined and found to be normal. Advancement of the scope to separate the true vocal folds showed good exposure of the subglottis and trachea. There was an approximately 2.5 cm stenosis about 1 cm distal to the glottis, and having 2 areas of focal webs. Her trachea was approximately 60% to 70% stenosed, which matched the preoperative CT scan. At the point, Depo-Medrol 40 mg/ML was injected into the 2 webs. Then a knife was used to make radial cuts in these 2 webs. Next, the 10–12 mm balloon was placed into the stenotic area under apnea. The patient's saturation never dropped during this time. Afterward, she was jet-ventilated without difficulty. Since we used jet ventilation during the entire procedure, we were concerned that subcutaneous emphysema would develop; but there were no clinical signs of it.

A small mucosal tear was observed within the trachea in the posterolateral position, but it was less than 1 cm; we

therefore believed it would have little effect on the patient's airway. The patient's lungs were ventilated back with bag and mask without difficulty. Surgery lasted one hour and the estimated blood loss was 20 mL. Throughout the procedure, the patient received 1 liter of crystalloid. Blood pressure was maintained with mean blood pressure (MBP) between 70 and 80 mmHg. Finally, the airway was suctioned and the patient became fully awake in the operating room. She was then transferred to the postanesthesia care unit for observation. Postoperatively, she remained in stable condition and the stridor resolved. The patient was discharged home 2 days later.

3. Discussion

Myasthenia gravis (MG) is an autoimmune disease characterized by weakness and fatigability of skeletal muscles, with improvement following rest. It may be localized to specific muscle groups or generalized. It has an estimated prevalence of 1 in 20,000 [1], and affects females more than males. MG is caused by a decrease in the number of postsynaptic acetylcholine receptors at the neuromuscular junction; this decrease in turn reduces the capacity of the neuromuscular end-plate to transmit the nerve signal. Initially, in response to a stimulus resulting in depolarization, acetylcholine is released presynaptically. In MG, the number of activated postsynaptic receptors may be insufficient to trigger a muscle action potential [1].

Some clinicians choose not to administer anticholinesterase on the morning of surgery, in order to minimize the need for muscle relaxants whereas others administer it for psychological support of the patient. If the patient is poorly controlled, a course of plasmapheresis may be beneficial in the preoperative period [2].

The steroid-dependent patient will require perioperative coverage. Anxiolytic, sedative, and opioid premedications are rarely given to patients who may have little respiratory reserve. However, if the patient has primarily ocular symptoms, a small dose of benzodiazepine is acceptable [3].

Several general anesthetic techniques have been proposed, although none have been demonstrated as superior to the others. Some anesthesiologists prefer to avoid muscle relaxants, instead using potent inhaled agents both for facilitating tracheal intubation and providing relaxation for surgery. These agents allow neuromuscular transmission to recover, and the agents are rapidly eliminated at the end of surgery. In theory, desflurane and sevoflurane may offer some advantages, due to their low blood solubility. Sevoflurane is probably more effective than desflurane, due to its lower incidence of excitatory airway reflexes during inhalational induction [3].

It was very challenging to keep the patient relaxed without muscle relaxants when the suspension laryngoscope was introduced and airway manipulations were stimulated. When required, small doses (10–25% of ED 95) of intermediate-acting relaxants are titrated to the evoked MMG or EMG for both intubation and surgical relaxation. Whether or not to reverse residual neuromuscular blockade at the end of surgery is controversial.

Response to muscle relaxants is unpredictable. Patients may be resistant to succinylcholine due to a diminished number of available receptors but sensitive to nondepolarizing agents. Therefore, muscle relaxants should be avoided, and shorter-acting drugs chosen and closely monitored.

Some argue that anticholinesterases and antimuscarinics militate against efforts to differentiate weakness due to inadequate neuromuscular transmission from cholinergic crisis in the recovery room. They, therefore, prefer spontaneous recovery and extubation when the patient has demonstrated adequate parameters for extubation (e.g., head life, tongue protrusion) [4, 5]. Total intravenous anesthesia (TIVA) for the management of myasthenic patients has been reported. The use of remifentanil as part of TIVA may alleviate some hemodynamic instability. When feasible, many clinicians prefer to utilize regional or local anesthetic techniques [6]. Regional techniques may reduce or eliminate the need for muscle relaxant in abdominal surgery. However, jet ventilation carries its own risks, such as damage to tracheal mucosa, subcutaneous emphysema, pneumomediastinum, and pneumothorax [3].

References

[1] M. Naguib, A. A. el Dawlatly, M. Ashour, and E. A. Bamgboye, "Multivariate determinants of the need for postoperative ventilation in myasthenia gravis," *Canadian Journal of Anaesthesia*, vol. 43, no. 10, pp. 1006–1013, 1996.

[2] J. F. Howard, "The treatment of myasthenia gravis with plasma exchange," *Semin Neurol*, vol. 2, pp. 273–288, 1982.

[3] M. Abel and J. B. Eisenkraft, "Anesthetic implications of myasthenia gravis," *Mount Sinai Journal of Medicine*, vol. 69, no. 1-2, pp. 31–37, 2002.

[4] S. R. Leventhal, F. K. Orkin, and R. A. Hirsh, "Prediction of the need for postoperative mechanical ventilation in myasthenia gravis," *Anesthesiology*, vol. 53, no. 1, pp. 26–30, 1980.

[5] A. Baraka, S. Taha, V. Yazbeck, and P. Rizkallah, "Vecuronium block in the myasthenic patient. Influence of anticholinesterase therapy," *Anaesthesia*, vol. 48, no. 7, pp. 588–590, 1993.

[6] D. O'Flaherty, J. H. Pennant, K. Rao, and A. H. Giesecke, "Total intravenous anesthesia with propofol for transsternal thymectomy in myasthenia gravis," *Journal of Clinical Anesthesia*, vol. 4, no. 3, pp. 241–244, 1992.

5

A Novel Anaesthetical Approach to Patients with Brugada Syndrome in Neurosurgery

Pietro Paolo Martorano,[1] Edoardo Barboni,[2] Giovanni Buscema,[3] and Alessandro Di Rienzo[4]

[1] *Head of Neuroanesthesia Unit, Ospedali Riuniti, Via Conca 71 - 60126 Ancona, Italy*
[2] *Clinic of Anesthesia and Intensive Care Unit, Department of Emergency, Ospedali Riuniti, Via Conca 71 - 60126 Ancona, Italy*
[3] *Anesthesia and Intensive Care Unit, AOU G. Rodolico, Via S. Sofia 78 - 95123 Catania, Italy*
[4] *Department of Neurosurgery, Università Politecnica delle Marche, Ospedali Riuniti, Via Conca 71 - 60126 Ancona, Italy*

Correspondence should be addressed to Pietro Paolo Martorano; p.martorano@tin.it

Academic Editors: A. Apan, M. R. Chakravarthy, and A. Trikha

Brugada syndrome (BrS) is one of the most common causes of sudden death in young people. It usually presents with life-threatening arrhythmias in subjects without remarkable medical history. The need for surgical treatment may unmask BrS in otherwise asymptomatic patients. The best anaesthesiological treatment in such cases is matter of debate. We report a case of neurosurgical treatment of cerebello pontine angle (CPA) tumor in a BrS patient, performed under total intravenous anesthesia (TIVA) with target controlled infusion (TCI) modalities, using midazolam plus remifentanil and rocuronium, without recordings of intraoperative ECG alterations in the intraoperative period and postoperative complications.

1. Introduction

BrS is a rare dominant autosomal disease with incomplete penetrance, first described in 1992 by P. Brugada and J. Brugada [1]. More common in men than in women, it is typically diagnosed during the fourth decade of life, and it is caused by a genetic mutation affecting the ion channels of the cardiac conduction system. The typical clinical correlate is a coved ST segment elevation in the right precordial leads that can occur with or without an incomplete right bundle branch block.

Owing to its phenotypic variability, clinical manifestations of BrS are protean, including syncope or spontaneous ventricular arrhythmias that can lead to a sudden death [2, 3], which all may be elicited in such peculiar situations (vagal tone increase, fever, and electrolytes disorder) or by peculiar drugs administration including some anaesthetics [4]. There is still no consense on which the golden standard should be in case of general anaesthesia in these cases, especially because of the low prevalence of BrS, the absence of

large prospective study, and the different anaesthesiological needs according to different surgical specialties. Existing guidelines derives from theoretical model based on the pathophysiological mechanism of BrS and from case series regarding a small number of patients. As regards the use of intravenous anesthetics in patients with BrS, propofol, and midazolam wase successfully used in different procedures [5, 6]. Propofol is a short acting, intravenous hypnotic, that ensures fast onset and rapid recovery of anesthesia, reducing PONV (postoperative nausea and vomiting). It represents the hypnotic of choice for TIVA/TCI use in neurosurgery, due to his low impact on CBF and the ability to mantain cerebral autoregulation, however, allowing a rapid recovery of the cognitive function at the end of the procedure. The recommendation to avoid it in patient with BrS is based on it is potential to expose patients to the risk of developing malignant arrhythmias like ventricular tachycardia (VT) or fibrillation followed by death [7, 8] and the acquired Brugada-like electrocardiographic (ECG) changes following high-dose propofol infusion over prolonged periods of time [9].

Midazolam is a short-acting benzodiazepine (BZD) [10] commonly used for sedation or induction in anesthesia, that appears to be safe in patient with BrS. It has a low metabolic, hemodynamic impact, and recent evidences of neuroprotective effects [11]. Its pharmacokinetics change significantly during continuous infusion [12], resulting in prolonged duration of action and delayed recovery. In this setting it could be worthwhile to use a target controlled infusion (TCI) system, like navigator suite GE, to provide a better dosage adjustments on an real time basis to maintain adequate hypnosis and rapid recovery especially during neurosurgery procedure.

We report our experience with the intraoperative use of midazolam in a BrS patient undergoing a neurosurgery procedure for the removal of a large tumor of the cerebello-pontine angle (CPA).

2. Case Presentation

A 44-year-old male patient, BMI 23.45, ASA score 2, was scheduled for the removal of a cerebellopontine angle tumor. At neurological examination he presented with incomplete left VIIth cranial nerve deficit (House Brackmann grade II), dysphagia, lateral left gaze diplopia. MRI examination evidenced a 4 cm diameter tumor of the left cerebellopontine angle, with brainstem compression/dislocation, suspect for a meningioma. The patient reported a recent history of severe cardiac symptoms (arrhythmias and cardiac arrest) with full recovery and a diagnosis of Brugada syndrome based on the ECG pattern (type 1).

Previously had undergone appendectomy, without report of cardiological complication.

Preoperative blood analysis and serum electrolytes were normal.

3. Intraoperative Anaesthesiological Management

Peripheral venous access was obtained by a 18 Ga needle, then a 0.9% NaCl infusion was started. Before induction, adhesive plaques connected to a biphasic defibrillator with pacemaker (PM) features were applied to the patient. During surgery, electrocardiography, invasive blood pressure, pulse oximetry, body temperature, and neuromuscular blockade degree were continuously recorded, and the depth of anaesthesia was monitored by entropy (GE Healthcare, Finland) [13].

Total intravenous anaesthesia was administered using a Fresenius Orchestra Base Primea (Fresenius Kabi, France) linked to a multimodal navigator suite GE (GE Healthcare Finland).

General anesthesia was induced by intravenous midazolam (0.2 mg/kg) plus remifentanil (1 μg/kg) followed by rocuronium (0.9 mg/kg), before intubation. Mechanical ventilation (tidal volume 6 mL/kg; FiO$_2$ O$_2$ 50%) was started and settled to an EtCO$_2$ of 30–35 mmHg. The anaesthesiological plan was maintained by infusion of midazolam (Effect Site concentration: Ce 0.68 ± 2.25 ng/mL) and remifentanil (effect

TABLE 1: The average values of the concentrations of the drugs infused in target controlled infusion (TCI), the average values of Entropy and heart rate and mean arterial pressure.

	Mean ± St. dev.
Remifentanil Ce induction (ng/mL)	5.78 ± 0.00
Remifentanil Ce intraoperative (ng/mL)	5.60 ± 1.23
Midazolam Ce induction (μg/mL)	1.23 ± 0.00
Midazolam Ce intraoperative (μg/mL)	0.68 ± 2.25
State entropy (SE) intraoperative	45.51 ± 9.98
Response entropy (RE) intraoperative	49.29 ± 12.16
Heart rate (bpm)	79.13 ± 5.41
Mean arterial pressure (mmHg)	67.34 ± 14.90

Values are presented as mean ± standard deviation.

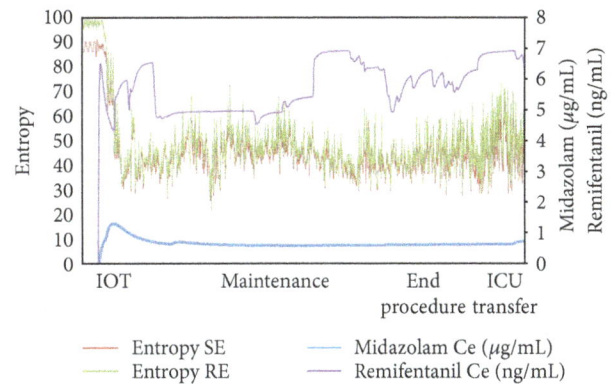

FIGURE 1: This figure represents the trend of the concentrations of hypnotic (midazolam) and opioid (remifentanil) and their correlation with the adequacy of the anesthesia plan obtained by entropy (state entropy (SE), response entropy (RE)).

site concentration: Ce 5.60 ± 1.23 ng/mL) in order to maintain state entropy <55 (SE) (Table 1) (Figure 1).

Data were collected every 10 seconds by a dedicated software (S5 collect GE Healthcare, Finland) and stored in Excel files.

Crystalloids were infused at a speed of 6 mL/kg/h. Surgery lasted approximately 240 min. No shiver episodes, psychomotor agitation, respiratory crises, or any cardiovascular issue or were observed either at induction and during maintenance. At the end of surgery the patient was transferred to the ICU, and the following postoperative course was uneventful.

4. Discussion

BrS patients are at elevated risk of death, this condition being considered the most prevalent cause of sudden cardiac death in a young population [3]. Such disorder raises specific concerns as anesthesiologists routinely administer drugs that interact with cardiac ion channels, potentially triggering the development of malignant arrhythmias. Previous surgeries performed under uneventful general anaesthesia do not lower risks of subsequent adverse events, so that an accurate preoperative evaluation of symptoms and a multidisciplinary approach are required for a well-planned management. There is a lack of evidence in the literature about the most suitable drugs and their side effects during anaesthesiological treatment of BrS.

Absence of prospective studies combined with low prevalence of BrS hinder exact guidelines creation and recommendations are derived exclusively from theoretical models based on disease pathophysiology and direct observations from case reports and short series [7].

Propofol, a phenol derived drug, represents the choice hypnotic for TIVA/TCI use in neurosurgery, due to his low impact on CBF, fast offset, and low PONV. Unfortunately, it is burdened from the potential to alter ion channel function inducing Brugada-like ECG abnormalities, which implies an increased risk of malignant arrhythmias in BrS patients [4, 5]. The literature supports the recommendation to avoid propofol administration either during induction or continuous infusions in BrS patients.

Midazolam is a largely diffused benzodiazepine with no adverse cardiac effects. Nonetheless, its use is penalized by a trend toward accumulation and by the following unpredictable recovery. In the case reported, such difficulty was to be overcome by using a TIVA/TCI midazolam/remifentanil pump (pharmacokinetic/pharmacodynamic (PK/PD) model) coupled with monitoring of hypnosis depth by spectral entropy. This allowed a closer titration of drug administration based on calculation of the predicted synergistic effects of the two drugs and on the feedback of brain electrical activity. Factors that might exacerbate ST segment elevations and lead to dysrhythmias, as hyperthermia, bradycardia, electrolyte imbalances, hyper/hypokalemia, and hypercalcemia, could be rapidly identified and corrected, as well as autonomic imbalance and fast postural changes.

Current recommendations about patients diagnosed with a hereditary arrhythmogenic syndrome, mostly derive from expert's opinions [5], a careful evaluation before operation, and close intraoperative hemodynamic monitoring are advised. The specific anaesthesiological implications and prompt therapeutic interventions required in these cases make the perioperative management of these patients a challenge for the anesthesiologist.

Adequate anaesthesia and analgesia, propofol avoidance, maintenance of homeostasis and continuous monitoring in the postoperative period for at least 24 h are strongly recommended.

More studies about anaesthetic drugs and molecular biology are necessary to choose the optimal drugs and anaesthesiological management in these patients. A multidisciplinary approach is recommended for a well-planned perioperative management tailored to individual patient's needs. In this context we believe that the use of anaesthesia multimodality systems ensures better intraoperative conditions while offering assurances of safety and efficacy.

References

[1] P. Brugada and J. Brugada, "Right bundle branch block, persistent ST segment elevation and sudden cardiac death: a distinct clinical and electrocardiographic syndrome. A multicenter report," *Journal of the American College of Cardiology*, vol. 20, no. 6, pp. 1391–1396, 1992.

[2] H. Morita, D. P. Zipes, and J. Wu, "Brugada syndrome: insights of ST elevation, arrhythmogenicity, and risk stratification from experimental observations," *Heart Rhythm*, vol. 6, no. 11, pp. S34–S43, 2009.

[3] C. Antzelevitch, P. Brugada, M. Borggrefe et al., "Brugada syndrome: report of the second consensus conference," *Circulation*, vol. 111, no. 5, pp. 659–670, 2005.

[4] P. Brugada, J. Brugada, and R. Brugada, "Arrhythmia induction by antiarrhythmic drugs," *Pacing and Clinical Electrophysiology*, vol. 23, no. 3, pp. 291–292, 2000.

[5] P. G. Postema, C. Wolpert, A. S. Amin et al., "Drugs and Brugada syndrome patients: review of the literature, recommendations, and an up-to-date website (www.brugadadrugs.org)," *Heart Rhythm*, vol. 6, no. 9, pp. 1335–1341, 2009.

[6] C. Staikou*, K. Chondrogiannis, and A. Mani, "Perioperative management of hereditary arrhythmogenic syndromes," *The British Journal of Anaesthesia*, vol. 108, no. 5, pp. 730–44, 2012.

[7] I. Riezzo, F. Centini, M. Neri et al., "Brugada-like EKG pattern and myocardial effects in a chronic propofol abuser," *Clinical Toxicology*, vol. 47, no. 4, pp. 358–363, 2009.

[8] J. B. Weiner, E. V. Haddad, and S. R. Raj, "Recovery following propofol-associated brugada electrocardiogram," *Pacing and Clinical Electrophysiology*, vol. 33, no. 4, pp. e39–e42, 2010.

[9] B. Kloesel, M. J. Ackerman, J. Sprung, B. J. Narr, and T. N. Weingarten, "Anesthetic management of patients with Brugada syndrome: a case series and literature review," *Canadian Journal of Anesthesia*, vol. 58, no. 9, pp. 824–836, 2011.

[10] D. J. Greenblatt, B. L. Ehrenberg, K. E. Culm et al., "Kinetics and EEG effects of midazolam during and after 1-minute, 1-hour, and 3-hour intravenous infusions," *Journal of Clinical Pharmacology*, vol. 44, no. 6, pp. 605–611, 2004.

[11] I. S. Kass, B. Lei, S. Popp, and J. E. Cottrell, "Effects of midazolam on brain injury after transient focal cerebral ischemia in rats," *Journal of Neurosurgical Anesthesiology*, vol. 21, no. 2, pp. 131–139, 2009.

[12] FragenRJ, "Pharmacokinetics and pharmacodynamics of midazolam given via continuous intravenous infusion in intensive care units," *Clinical Therapeutics*, vol. 19, no. 3, pp. 405–419, 1997.

[13] H. Viertiö-Oja, V. Maja, M. Särkelä et al., "Description of the Entropy algorithm as applied in the Datex-Ohmeda 5/5 entropy module," *Acta Anaesthesiologica Scandinavica*, vol. 48, no. 2, pp. 154–161, 2004.

Administration of Anesthesia in a Patient with Allgrove Syndrome

Ayse B. Ozer, Omer L. Erhan, Cevdet Sumer, and Ozden Yildizhan

Anaesthesiology and Reanimation Department, Faculty of Medicine, Firat University, 23119 Elazig, Turkey

Correspondence should be addressed to Ayse B. Ozer, abelinozer@gmail.com

Academic Editors: U. Buyukkocak and D. A. Story

The aim of the present paper is to report the anesthesia administration to a patient who was planned to undergo Heller myotomy for achalasia. There wasnot property in the patient whom allgrove syndrome was excepted any steroid treatment in preoperative period. The night before the operation 18 mg of prednisolone was administered intravenously. Induction of anesthesia was performed with thiopental sodium, vecuronium and fentanyl and the patient received endotracheal intubation. Eyes were taped closed and protected with ointment during surgery. Maintenance of anesthesia was achieved with 2% sevoflurane concentration in 50% O_2-50% N_2O. 25 mg of prednisolone was infused preoperatively, and intervention with insulin treatment was initiated when blood glucose level rose to 18 mmol/L at 2 hours. Safe anesthesia can be achieved by observing the preoperative development of tracheal aspiration, adrenal insufficiency and, autonomic dysfunction carefully and maintaining eye protection.

1. Introduction

Allgrove syndrome (AS), which isolates adrenal insufficiency, achalasia of the esophageal cardia, and reduction in eye-tear production, and deficient tear production, was first described by Allgrove and his colleagues in 1978 [1]. The disease, also known as triple A or 4A syndrome, is an autosomal recessive disorder associated with autonomic dysfunction, adrenal insufficiency due to ACHT, alacrima, and achalasia [2]. The disease has been supposed to be in relation to ALADIN and AAAS genes, in the vicinity of the type 2 keratin gene clusters, during localization of 12q13 chromosome [3, 4].

Allgrove syndrome generally initiates with the classic findings of primary adrenal insufficiency such as hypoglycemic seizures and shock. Some nonspecific symptoms such as muscle weakness, dizziness and, slow weight loss may also accompany the clinical manifestation [5, 6]. Patients are admitted to hospital with complaints of recurrent vomiting, dysphagia, and growth retardation due to achalasia, besides crying without tears, keratoconjunctivitis sicca, optic atrophy and pupil anomalies associated with alacrima [7–9]. Neurological influences are in relation to peripheral, central and autonomic nervous systems. Microcephaly, mental retardation and learning difficulties may be observed during early life stages. Patients may display progression to bulbospinal amyotrophy, dysarthria, ataxia, muscle weakness, myoclonus, hyperreflexia, and polyneuropathy in the course of time. Autonomic dysfunction may progress with reduction or lack of sweating, postural hypotension, deterioration of cardiac reflexes, change in the reaction of the skin to histamine, and abnormal methacholine test [10].

The aim of the present study was to discuss the application of general anesthesia to a patient with a diagnosis of AS who was planned to undergo Heller myotomy.

2. Case Report

A nine-year-old girl who had complaint of vomiting following eating and growth retardation after birth had been diagnosed with achalasia at the age of one. Endoscopic balloon dilation for achalasia had been performed for three times. The patient was one year old when she underwent the first endoscopic trial. No complications emerged during the endoscopic procedures. Allgrove syndrome was diagnosed in the patient due to adrenal insufficiency, developed nearly a year ago; consequently, hydrocortisone therapy was initiated.

The typical facial appearance of Allgrove syndrome including long philtrum, narrow upper lip, and fish mouth was observed during the preoperative assessment. At the same time retardation of growth and development, hypernasal speech, alacrima and adrenal insufficiency were observed. Her weight are only fifteen kilograms, hypernasal speech, alacrima, and adrenal insufficiency were observed. Oral hydrocortisone was also used due to adrenal insufficiency. Physical examination and interpretation of laboratory tests were defined normal (fasting blood glucose: 6,6 mmol/L, Na: 143 mEq/L, and K: 3,5 mEq/L). Postural tests were performed to assess autonomic dysfunction. We observed a decrease of approximately 15 mmHg in systolic artery pressure and an increase about 10 mm Hg in diastolic artery pressure. We concluded that autonomic dysfunction did not exist. The doses of steroids to be applied during the postoperative and preoperative periods were determined in the pediatric clinic. The patient, assessed in ASA risk group III, was given no premedication before anesthesia. Prednisolone 18 mg was administered intravenously on the night before surgery. The preoperative blood glucose level was recorded as 11 mmol/L.

The ECG, noninvasive blood pressure and SpO_2 of the patient who was transferred onto the operating table, were monitored; infusion fluid which includes NaCl (4,5 g/l) and glucose (25 g/l) was started at the speed of 125 mL/h, because preoperative fluid deficit was given before. The patient was intubated with a 4 mm ID cuffed endotracheal tube after the anesthesia was induced by 75 mg of thiopental sodium, 1 mg of vecuronium, and 20 μcg fentanyl. For protective purposes topical polymyxin ophthalmic ointment was used an the eyes before they were covered. Anesthesia was maintained with 2% sevoflurane in concentration of 50% O_2 and 50% N_2O. Mechanical ventilation was continued to be $ETCO_2$ 30–40 mmHg. Prednisolone 25 mg was infused preoperatively. Monitoring of blood glucose was performed hourly.

In perioperative and postoperative period, we did not observe a condition that requires the intervention at HR, SAP and SpO_2 (Table 1).

In intraoperative period, blood glucose was measured 12 mmol/L was at the first hour and 18 mmol/L at the second hour. Then, vascular access was opened and 0.9% NaCl infusion was started at 100 mL/h. 50 U regular insulin in 50 mL of 0.9% NaCl solution was prepared and it started infusion at 1,5 mL/h. Fluid infusion rate was reduced from 125 mL/h to 50 mL/h, and 15 mEq KCl was added. The operation is completed at 135 minutes in other words 15 minutes after the start of insulin infusion. Blood glucose was measured 13 mmol/L at postoperative 30th minute and insulin infusion rate was reduced to 0.7 mL/h. Because blood glucose decreased to 10 at postoperative first hour, insulin infusion was stopped.

Tramadol 30 mg is administrated by intravenous route as postoperative analgesic. There were no problems at extubation nor recovery from anesthesia. Consciousness, HR, SAP, SpO_2, and respiration rate and pattern were normal. Blood glucose, Na, and K levels were measured 200, 148, and 3.2, respectively, at postoperative twelve hour, respectively.

The patient did not have any preoperative or postoperative anesthetic problems except a rise in the blood glucose

TABLE 1: Hemodynamic changes.

	HR (beat/minute)	SAP (mmHg)	SpO_2 (%)
Preinduction	90	120	97
Induction	120	100	100
Postinduction	110	110	99
10 minutes	100	95	99
20 minutes	95	95	99
30 minutes	80	90	99
40 minutes	80	90	99
50 minutes	85	90	99
60 minutes	85	90	99
70 minutes	85	95	99
80 minutes	80	95	99
90 minutes	85	100	99
100 minutes	85	100	98
110 minutes	85	95	99
120 minutes	85	95	99
130 minutes	95	125	99
Recovery	120	130	98
Postop 10 Minutes	115	105	98
Postop 20 Minutes	100	95	97
Postop 30 minutes	100	100	98

level. The patient was discharged from the hospital on postoperative day 5.

3. Discussion

Allgrove syndrome is a multisystem disease associated with ACTH-resistant adrenal insufficiency, alacrima, achalasia, and autonomic dysfunction. Approach to endoscopic balloon dilatation or indication for surgical treatment is required in patients with Allgrove syndrome due to preexisting achalasia. Undefined or inadequately treated adrenal insufficiency at the preoperative period may cause preoperative adrenal crisis consisting of shock, hyponatremia, hyperkalemia, or hypoglycemia. Cushing syndrome may develop also in these patients with the excessive use of glucocorticoids [11]. They may cause life-threatening conditions such as severe hypoglycemia which may result in an incognizable coma [12, 13]. Therefore, the stress-dose steroids should be used cautiously during the application of anesthesia [11]. Glycemic control should be closely monitored due to the contribution of the administered steroid doses to hyperglycemia induced by anesthesia and surgery. If necessary, insulin involvement should be applied. Serum electrolytes did not change significantly. Blood glucose had risen which requires insulin therapy in the patient.

Autonomic, motor, and sensory neuropathies, cerebellar ataxia, progressive spastic tetraparesis, increased nerve conduction time, and development of mental retardation are quite frequent in these patients. Regurgitation- and aspiration-associated gastroparesis may develop intraoperatively and postoperatively besides autonomic-neuropathy-associated heart rate variations, orthostatic hypotension, and differences in response to the deep respiration and Valsalva maneuvers. Since the influences of the hemodynamic state may emerge especially during position changes, they should be performed slowly, delicately, and cautiously [13, 14]. We thought originate from which autonomic dysfunction has not yet begun in the patients the reason why hemodynamic impairment have not saw at perioperative period.

Swallowing difficulty and vomiting associated with achalasia are accompanied by regurgitation, aspiration, and associated conditions as well. Pneumonia and respiratory failure associated with regurgitation and aspiration may increase [15, 16]. Consequently, the risk for aspiration in patients with Allgrove syndrome should be observed especially during the induction phase and rapid sequence intubation should be performed. Cuffed endotracheal tubes should be preferred to prevent another aspiration in these patients with high aspiration risk.

Another noteworthy point in our 9-year-old subject was the application of intubation using an endotracheal tube whose inner diameter was 4 mm. Although diameter of the tube was calculated as small according to patient's age, it provided effective breathing. This situation was thought associated with the present retardation in growth and development. We believe that loss of weight associated with achalasia and adrenal insufficiency in patients especially with late diagnosis and inadequate therapy may cause retardation in growth and development.

Disappearance of protective corneal reflexes, reduced tear production, and the loss of pain sensation during general anesthesia application result in the development of ocular complications. Protection of eyes under general anesthesia comes into question when the ocular influences such as alacrima-associated keratopathy and ulceration are also combined with the above situation in patients with AS [7, 9], [17]. In our case, because of the taken measures to protect the eyes, there was no symptoms associated with the patient's visual at postoperative period.

AS specializes application of anesthesia owing to its present components. We should feel alerted for a possible diagnosis of AS in patients with achalasia. The presence of adrenal insufficiency, appropriate therapy, and regulation of additional steroid doses should be assessed as well as the evaluation of achalasia-associated respiratory problems, retardation of growth and development, and autonomic and ophthalmic influences. We suggest caution for the application of steroids, because the risk of aspiration during anesthesia. We believe that a safe anesthesia can be achieved with very careful preoperative examination, application of steroids, control of glycemia, consideration of risk aspiration, and protection of the eyes.

References

[1] J. Allgrove, G. S. Clayden, D. B. Grant, and J. C. Macaulay, "Familial glucocorticoid deficiency with achalasia of the cardia and deficient tear production," *The Lancet*, vol. 1, no. 8077, pp. 1284–1286, 1978.

[2] M. Gazarian, C. T. Cowell, M. Bonney, and W. G. Grigor, "The "4A" syndrome: adrenocortical insufficiency associated with achalasia, alacrima, autonomic and other neurological abnormalities," *European Journal of Pediatrics*, vol. 154, no. 1, pp. 18–23, 1995.

[3] A. Weber, T. Wienker, M. Jung et al., "Linkage of the gene for the triple A syndrome to chromosome 12q13 near the type II keratin gene cluster," *Human Molecular Genetics*, vol. 5, no. 12, pp. 2061–2066, 1996.

[4] M. Salehi, H. Houlden, A. Sheikh, and L. Poretsky, "The diagnosis of adrenal insufficiency in a patient with Allgrove syndrome and a novel mutation in the ALADIN gene," *Metabolism*, vol. 54, no. 2, pp. 200–205, 2005.

[5] P. A. Kasar, V. V. Khadilkar, and V. N. Tibrewala, "Allgrove syndrome," *Indian Journal of Pediatrics*, vol. 74, no. 10, pp. 959–961, 2007.

[6] E. A. Ismail, A. Tulliot-Pelet, A. M. Mohsen, and Q. Al-Saleh, "Allgrove syndrome with features of familial dysautonomia: a novel mutation in the AAAS gene," *Acta Paediatrica, International Journal of Paediatrics*, vol. 95, no. 9, pp. 1140–1143, 2006.

[7] K. Babu, K. R. Murthy, N. Babu, and S. Ramesh, "Triple A syndrome with ophthalmic manifestations in two siblings," *Indian Journal of Ophthalmology*, vol. 55, no. 4, pp. 304–306, 2007.

[8] A. Shah and A. Shah, "Esophageal achalasia and alacrima in siblings," *Indian Pediatrics*, vol. 43, no. 2, pp. 161–163, 2006.

[9] C. Villanueva-Mendoza, O. Martínez-Guzmán, D. Rivera-Parra, and J. C. Zenteno, "Triple A or Allgrove syndrome. A case report with ophthalmic abnormalities and a novel mutation in the AAAS gene," *Ophthalmic Genetics*, vol. 30, no. 1, pp. 45–49, 2009.

[10] D. B. Grant, N. D. Barnes, M. Dumic et al., "Neurological and adrenal dysfunction in the adrenal insufficiency/alacrima/achalasia (3A) syndrome," *Archives of Disease in Childhood*, vol. 68, no. 6, pp. 779–782, 1993.

[11] M. F. Roizen and L. A. Fleisher, "Anesthetic implications of concurrent diseases," in *Miller's Anesthesia*, R. D. Miller, Ed., pp. 1017–1051, Elsevier, Philadelphia, Pa, USA, 5th edition, 2005.

[12] S. K. Fernbach and A. K. Poznanski, "Pediatric case of the day. Triple A syndrome: achalasia, alacrima and ACTH insensitivity," *Radiographics*, vol. 9, no. 3, pp. 563–564, 1989.

[13] M. Etemadyfar and R. Khodabandehlou, "Neurological manifestations of Allgrove syndrome," *Archives of Iranian Medicine*, vol. 7, no. 3, pp. 225–227, 2004.

[14] D. Bishop, "Autonomic neuropathy in anaesthesia," University of Kwazulu-Natal, Department of Anaesthetics, 2009, http://anaesthetics.ukzn.ac.za/Libraries/FMM_R_B_2009/Autonomic_Neuropathy_in_Anaesthesia_Dr_D_Bishop.sflb.ashx.

[15] H. A. Ali, G. Murali, and B. Mukhtar, "Respiratory failure due to achalasia cardia," *Respiratory Medicine CME*, vol. 2, no. 1, pp. 40–43, 2009.

[16] S. Teramoto, H. Yamamoto, Y. Yamaguchi et al., "Diffuse aspiration bronchiolitis due to achalasia," *Chest*, vol. 125, no. 1, pp. 349–350, 2004.

[17] R. K. Stoelting and R. D. Miller, *Basics of Anesthesia*, Churchill-Livingstone, Philadelphia, Pa, USA, 2007.

A New Biplane Ultrasound Probe for Real-Time Visualization and Cannulation of the Internal Jugular Vein

Jeremy Kaplowitz and Paul Bigeleisen

Department of Anesthesiology, University of Maryland School of Medicine, 22 S. Greene Street S11C00, Baltimore, MD 21201, USA

Correspondence should be addressed to Jeremy Kaplowitz; jkaplowitz@anes.umm.edu

Academic Editors: U. Deveci, S. K. Dube, and J. Malek

Ultrasound guidance is recommended for cannulation of the internal jugular vein. Use of ultrasound allows you to identify relevant anatomy and possible anatomical anomalies. The most common approach is performed while visualizing the vein transversely and inserting the needle out of plane to the probe. With this approach needle tip visualization may be difficult. We report the use of a new biplane ultrasound probe which allows the user to simultaneously view the internal jugular vein in transverse and longitudinal views in real time. Use of this probe enhances needle visualization during venous cannulation.

1. Introduction

Ultrasound (US) guidance is recommended for cannulation of the internal jugular vein (IJ) [1–3]. A recent meta-analysis found that US guided central venous access may lead to decreased risks of hematoma, arterial puncture, or pneumothorax [4]. Use of US in real time allows you to identify the relevant anatomy and any possible anatomical anomalies and visualize the path of your needle. US guided central venous access is primarily performed while visualizing the vein transversely and inserting the needle out of plane to the US probe. One major limitation of this approach is that visualization of the needle tip can be difficult. Failure to visualize your needle tip can lead to inadvertent arterial puncture or pneumothorax. We report the use of a new dual plane 4–10 megahertz US probe (BK 8824, BK Medical USA; Peabody, MA) which allows the user to simultaneously view the carotid artery (CA) and IJ in transverse and longitudinal views in real time (Figure 1). This provides the user with the familiar transverse view while being able to more clearly visualize your needle in the longitudinal view.

2. Case Presentation

After positive initial experiences using this probe with a phantom (Blue Phantom, CAE Healthcare Sarasota, FL; Figure 2), we were able to cannulate the right IJ in a patient requiring central venous cannulation for surgery.

A 60-year-old, 78 kg, female with a past medical history significant for coronary artery disease, hypertension, diabetes type II, and hyperlipidemia was scheduled to undergo coronary bypass surgery. The patient was placed in a slight trendelenburg position and her head turned leftwards. A US scan was performed and we were able to identify the IJ and CA in both views. Her right IJ was cannulated using a 70 mm VascularSono cannula (Pajunk USA, Norcross, GA). A drawing of the probe and its intended positioning is shown in Figure 3. A transverse transducer and a longitudinal transducer sit over the CA and IJ, allowing you to simultaneously view the IJ in transverse and longitudinal views.

Ultrasound images of the CA, IJ, and guidewire are shown in transverse section in Figure 4(A). The IJ and guide wire are shown in longitudinal section in Figure 4(B). The user must manipulate the probe to find the best combination of transverse and longitudinal images.

3. Discussion

Numerous methods have been evaluated to enhance needle visualization during US guided vascular central venous access. These include use of needle guides [5], needle tracking

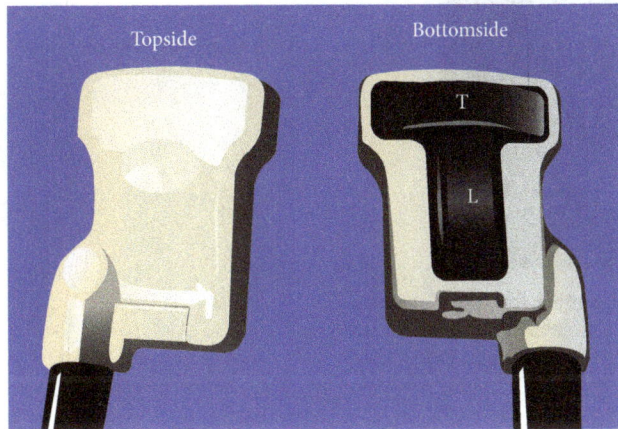

FIGURE 1: A pictorial depiction of the BK 8824 US probe showing the configuration of the transverse and longitudinal transducers. T: transverse transducers; L: longitudinal transducer.

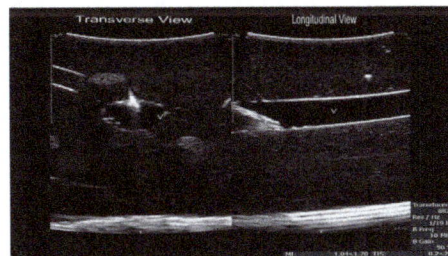

FIGURE 2: Images from our use in a Blue Phantom training phantom with an 18 gauge 40 millimeter VascularSono cannula (Pajunk USA, Norcross, GA). This is the ideal view that can be obtained with this probe. You can clearly see the needle entering the simulated vein in both views, and the tip is clearly in the lumen in the longitudinal view. V: simulated vein.

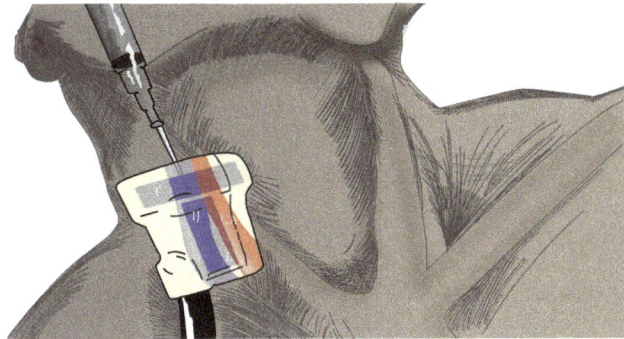

FIGURE 3: A depiction of the intended probe position over the IJ. In this orientation the transverse transducer is cephalad. T: transverse transducer; L: longitudinal transducer; IJ: internal jugular vein; CA: carotid artery.

devices [6], and using the long axis approach [7]. This is the first report describing the use of simultaneous biplane ultrasonography to enhance needle visualization while performing US guided central venous access. We found use of this probe to be helpful in the performance of US guided central venous cannulation. It required minimal effort to learn and it enhanced needle visualization. We did discover that the best orientation of the probe would be opposite of how it is depicted in Figure 2. By reversing the orientation of the probe by 180° the longitudinal probe would be cephalad.

This helps ensure that you see the needle tip during the cannulation of the IJ. Further studies are planned to formally evaluate the benefits of real-time biplane ultrasonography for central venous cannulation.

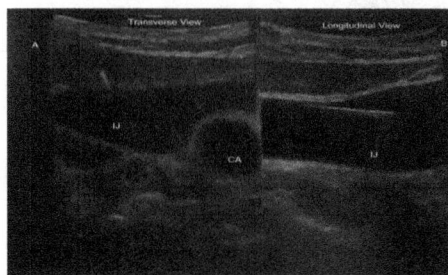

FIGURE 4: Real-time biplane view of the guide wire during central venous cannulation in our patient. The guidewire is visible in the lumen of the IJ in both views. IJ: internal jugular vein; CA: carotid artery.

Acknowledgments

The patient granted permission to publish this case report. The authors would like to acknowledge Evan Norris for his help with production of the medical illustrations in this paper.

References

[1] B. R. Ray, V. K. Mohan, L. Kashyap, D. Shende, V. M. Darlong, and R. K. Pandey, "Internal jugular vein cannulation: a comparison of three techniques," *Journal of Anaesthesiology Clinical Pharmacology*, vol. 29, no. 3, pp. 367–371, 2013.

[2] N. Mehta, W. W. Valesky, A. Guy, and R. Sinert, "Systematic review: is real-time ultrasonic-guided central line placement by ED physicians more successful than the traditional landmark approach?" *Emergency Medicine Journal*, vol. 30, no. 5, pp. 355–359, 2013.

[3] M. Dowling, H. A. Jlala, J. G. Hardman, and N. M. Bedforth, "Real-time three-dimensional ultrasound-guided central venous catheter placement," *Anesthesia and Analgesia*, vol. 112, no. 2, pp. 378–381, 2011.

[4] S. Y. Wu, Q. Ling, L. H. Cao, J. Wang, M. X. Xu, and W. A. Zeng, "Real-time two-dimensional ultrasound guidance for central venous cannulation: a meta-analysis," *Anesthesiology*, vol. 118, pp. 361–375, 2013.

[5] R. D. Ball, N. E. Scouras, S. Orebaugh, J. Wilde, and T. Sakai, "Randomized, prospective, observational simulation study comparing residents needle-guided vs free-hand ultrasound techniques for central venous catheter access," *British Journal of Anaesthesia*, vol. 108, no. 1, pp. 72–79, 2012.

[6] D. S. Kopac, J. Chen, R. Tang, A. Sawka, and H. Vaghadia, "Comparison of a novel real-time SonixGPS needle-tracking ultrasound technique with traditional ultrasound for vascular access in a phantom gel model," *Journal of Vascular Surgery*, vol. 58, no. 3, pp. 735–741, 2013.

[7] M. B. Stone, C. Moon, D. Sutijono, and M. Blaivas, "Needle tip visualization during ultrasound-guided vascular access: short-axis vs long-axis approach," *American Journal of Emergency Medicine*, vol. 28, no. 3, pp. 343–347, 2010.

A Case of Prolonged Delayed Postdural Puncture Headache in a Patient with Multiple Sclerosis Exacerbated by Air Travel

Jahan Porhomayon,[1,2] **Gino Zadeii,**[3] **Alireza Yarahamadi,**[4] **and Nader D. Nader**[5]

[1] VA Western New York Healthcare System, Division of Critical Care and Pain Medicine, Department of Anesthesiology, School of Medicine and Biomedical Sciences, State University of New York at Buffalo, Buffalo, NY, USA
[2] VA Medical Center, Rm 203C, 3495 Bailey Ave, Buffalo, NY 14215, USA
[3] Mason City Cardiology Clinic, University of Iowa, Mason City, IA 50401, USA
[4] Mason City Neurology Clinic, University of Iowa, Mason City, IA 50401, USA
[5] VA Western New York Healthcare System, Division of Cardiothoracic Anesthesia and Pain Medicine, Department of Anesthesiology, School of Medicine and Biomedical Sciences, State University of New York at Buffalo, Buffalo, NY 14215, USA

Correspondence should be addressed to Jahan Porhomayon; jahanpor@buffalo.edu

Academic Editors: E. Farag, D. Lee, I.-O. Lee, and J.-J. Yang

The developments of new spinal needles and needle tip designs have reduced the incidence of postdural puncture headache (PDPH). Although it is clear that reducing the loss of CSF leak from dural puncture reduces the headache, there are areas regarding the pathogenesis, treatment, and prevention of PDPH that remain controversial. Air travel by itself may impose physiological alteration in central nervous system that may be detrimental to patients with PDPH. This case report highlights a case of a young female patient who suffered from a severe incapacitating PDPH headache during high-altitude flight with a commercial jet.

1. Introduction

The first case report of postdural puncture headache (PDPH) was described in about 100 years ago by Bier and his assistant [1]. It was later postulated that PDPH is triggered by leakage of cerebrospinal fluid through the dural rent, but the cause of the pain is probably due to intracranial arterial and venous dilatation [2]. PDPH remains one of the major complications of spinal tap performed for diagnostic purposes. Other adverse events after lumbar puncture include dysesthesia, backache, nerve palsies, infectious processes, and bleeding disorders [3]. The patterns of development of PDPH depend on a number of procedure and nonprocedure-related risk factors. Knowledge of procedure-related factors supports interventions designed to reduce the incidence of PDPH. Despite the best preventive efforts, PDPH may still occur and be associated with significant morbidity [4, 5]. The potential risks for developing PDPH include female gender [6], young adults, repeated attempt with multiple dural punctures, and the size/type and orientation of the needle [7]. Gender is believed to be an independent risk factor for the development of PDPH as demonstrated by the recent meta-analysis by Wu et al. [6]. Clinical presentation of the PDPH or "spinal headache" is usually described as a severe, dull pain, usually frontal occipital, which is irritated in the upright position and decreased in the supine position. It may or may not be accompanied by nausea, vomiting, and visual/auditory disturbances. The onset of PDPH is between 2 to 72 hours, and latency period of up to 15 days has generally been described in the literature [8, 9].

2. Case Report

This is unique case of a young 23 years old middle Eastern female who developed an acute unilateral eye pain and generalized headache with visual disturbances associated with fatigue and weakness in lower extremities for two days. She presented to a local community hospital and was examined by a neurologist. Physical examination revealed an exaggerated deep tendon reflexes and sustained clonus of extensor plantar responses. Ophthalmologic examination was normal. A spinal tap was performed in the neurologist office with a 22 gauge Quincke spinal needle between the third and fourth lumbar spaces after the first attempt with free flow of clear cerebral spinal fluid (CSF). This fluid was analyzed for IgG, albumin, and oligoclonal banding to confirm the diagnosis of multiple sclerosis (MS), and a magnetic resonance imaging (MRI) of the brain was also obtained. All laboratory tests confirmed the diagnosis of MS. Patient returned home with follow-up appointment in 2 days. She later developed severe headache 10 hours after returning home. Headache was more localized to the back of the head and worsened with ambulation. Patient returned to the neurologist office the next day and was prescribed acetaminophen with bed rest. Nevertheless, she continued with severe headache on ambulation. In addition, she experienced dizziness and neck stiffness for the next 7 days. Follow-up evolutions and repeat physical examination revealed similar findings. Patient family remained concerned and decided to travel to the USA for additional treatment and consultation. She completed an 18 hours flight from her home town to the USA in a sitting position. At the completion of her journey, she experienced severe occipital and frontal headache associated with nausea/vomiting with neck stiffness and back pain. The pain intensity increased particularly during aircraft takeoff. Upon landing at airport, she had to be transported by a wheel chair to her car. She was seen the next day by another neurologist in the USA and after a complete examination was diagnosed with PDPH and repeated MRI of brain was completed at the same day (Figure 1). She was prescribed complete bed rest, oral analgesics, caffeine 300 mg orally. She was seen again in 72 hours with similar complain of occipital headache worse on ambulation and was referred to a pain clinic for epidural blood patch. An appointment was scheduled for her with an anesthesiologist 4 weeks later after obtaining insurance coverage. An epidural blood patch was performed by withdrawing 20 mL of blood from the right antecubital vein under aseptic condition. At the same, the epidural space was identified between the third and fourth lumbar vertebrate space using the loss of resistance technique. Subsequently, 20 mL of blood was injected into the epidural space. She had an immediate relief of her headache and was able to ambulate to her car without difficulty.

3. Discussion

Here we report a case of PDPH from spinal tab for the evaluation of MS that lasted up to 6 weeks after procedure and was exacerbated by air travel and prolong sitting position. There is scarce data on prolonged case of PDPH and the physiologic impact of air travel on regional spinal and intracranial pressures following dural puncture.

Despite the current recommendations for the use of atraumatic and smaller size spinal catheters for diagnostic spinal puncture [10], we continue to see reported cases of PDPH in the literatures worldwide [11]. Pedersen reported 42% incidence of PDPH with a 22 Quincke needle in patient undergoing diagnostic lumbar punctures [12]. The study

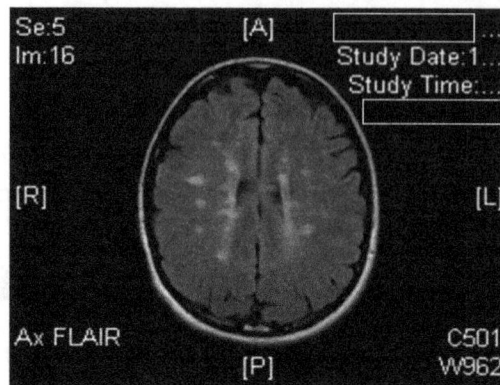

(a)

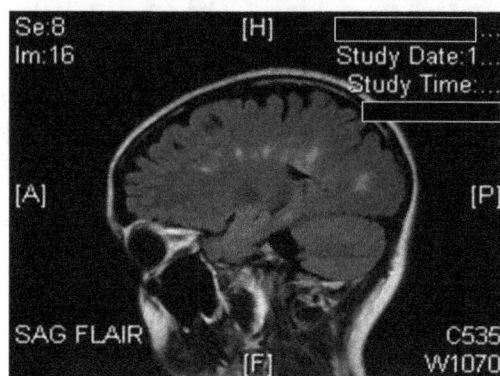

(b)

FIGURE 1: R: imaging demonstrates periventricular high signal intensity lesions, which exhibit a typical distribution for multiple sclerosis (Dawson's fingers). A: it shows corpus callosal hyperintensities suggestive of a demyelinating process. Patient does not have evidence of brain stem sagging, dilatation of vein or dural sinuses, and effacement of hemispheric cortical sulci. Absence of any of these signs does not preclude the diagnosis of postdural puncture headache.

by Hammond et al. reported the incidence of PDPH at 30 percents with the use of traumatic 20 and 22 gauges Quincke spinal needles [7]. Geurts et al. reported an incidence of 25% PDPH in a prospective study of 80 patients less than 40 years of age, given spinal anesthesia through a 0.52 mm (25 gauge) needle [13]. The incidence of PDPH after lumbar puncture can be reduced from 36% to 0–9% with the use of an atraumatic needle size 24 gauge (G)/0.56 mm rather than a traumatic needle size 22 G/0.7 mm [11]. As a result, selection of a spinal needle played a major role for developing PDPH. Additionally, air travel probably contributed to exacerbation of her symptoms. There is only one previously published case report of prolonged PDPH after air travel [14]. Vacanti reported a case of an 18-year-old soldier who developed PDPH after a knee surgery. He had increased headache with air travel 7 days after operation. The headache intensified particularly during takeoff and subsided several days later [15]. Mulroy reported an unintentional dural puncture postepidural anesthesia that was treated with epidural blood patch twice. His patient developed PDPH after air travel that lasted up to six weeks and relieved with epidural blood patch [14]. Likewise, Panadero et al. reported a case of a healthy 42-year-old adult male who underwent arthroscopy with spinal anesthesia and was completely asymptomatic. Thirty-six hours after procedure and 10 minutes after aircraft took off, he complained of severe headache and nausea. Symptoms subsided after landing and resolved few days later [16]. It was postulated that rapid decompression during aircraft taking off may have altered the relationship of epidural and dural pressures and resulted in increased CSF leak during landing or taking off. Additionally, autoregulatory changes of CSF pressure at high altitudes may have been impaired [17]. In 1962 Safar and Tenicela also reported increased incidence of PDPH at higher altitudes when anesthesiologist performed spinal anesthesia [18]. Data available from Singh et al. looking invasively at the lumbar CSF pressures in 34 Indian soldiers transported rapidly via helicopter from sea level to altitude of 5867 meters recorded elevated pressures of 6–20 cm H_2O compared to baseline suggesting impaired CSF pressure regulation with rapid ascend [19]. Other investigators have reported rise in intracranial pressure secondary to hypoxia rise in intracranial pressure secondary to hypoxia [20, 21]. Therefore, in our patient a combination of factors may have contributed to severe PDPH. Not only size and type of needle played an important role in developing PDPH but also air travel, high altitude, hypoxia, changes in CSF and intracranial pressure, and prolonged sitting position may have all contributed to worsening of her symptoms.

Our current knowledge regarding air travel and physiologic changes related to spinal and epidural pressures is very limited. Moreover, autoregulatory mechanisms for maintaining CSF pressures are disturbed during high-altitude flights. Further studies are needed to provide the clinicians with recommendations and management of PDPH on long-range intercontinental flights after dural puncture or central neuraxial anesthesia.

References

[1] A. Bier, "Versuche uber cocainisirung des ruckenmarkes," Deutsche Zeitschrift fur Chirurgie, vol. 51, no. 3-4, pp. 361–369, 1899 (German).

[2] E. Fernandez, "Headaches associated with low spinal fluid pressure," Headache, vol. 30, no. 3, pp. 122–128, 1990.

[3] C. Chordas, "Post-dural puncture headache and other complications after lumbar puncture," Journal of Pediatric Oncology Nursing, vol. 18, no. 6, pp. 244–259, 2001.

[4] D. Bezov, S. Ashina, and R. Lipton, "Post-dural puncture headache: part II—prevention, management, and prognosis," Headache, vol. 50, no. 9, pp. 1482–1498, 2010.

[5] D. Bezov, R. B. Lipton, and S. Ashina, "Post-dural puncture headache: part i diagnosis, epidemiology, etiology, and pathophysiology," Headache, vol. 50, no. 7, pp. 1144–1152, 2010.

[6] C. L. Wu, A. J. Rowlingson, S. R. Cohen et al., "Gender and post-dural puncture headache," Anesthesiology, vol. 105, no. 3, pp. 613–618, 2006.

[7] E. R. Hammond, Z. Wang, N. Bhulani, J. C. McArthur, and M. Levy, "Needle type and the risk of post-lumbar puncture headache in the outpatient neurology clinic," Journal of the Neurological Sciences, vol. 306, no. 1-2, pp. 24–28, 2011.

[8] J. A. Amorim, M. V. Gomes de Barros, and M. M. Valenca, "Post-dural (post-lumbar) puncture headache: risk factors and clinical features," Cephalalgia, vol. 32, no. 12, pp. 916–923, 2012.

[9] K. B. Alstadhaug, F. Odeh, F. K. Baloch, D. H. Berg, and R. Salvesen, "Post-lumbar puncture headache," Tidsskr Nor Laegeforen, vol. 132, no. 7, pp. 818–821, 2012.

[10] Y. Dakka, N. Warra, R. J. Albadareen, M. Jankowski, and B. Silver, "Headache rate and cost of care following lumbar puncture at a single tertiary care hospital," Neurology, vol. 77, no. 1, pp. 71–74, 2011.

[11] L. Stendell, J. S. Fomsgaard, and K. S. Olsen, "There is room for improvement in the prevention and treatment of headache after lumbar puncture," Danish Medical Journal, vol. 59, no. 7, article A4483, 2012.

[12] O. N. Pedersen, "Use of a 22-gauge Whitacre needle to reduce the incidence of side effects after lumbar myelography: a prospective randomised study comparing Whitacre and Quincke spinal needles," European Radiology, vol. 6, no. 2, pp. 184–187, 1996.

[13] J. W. Geurts, M. C. Haanschoten, R. M. van Wijk, H. Kraak, and T. C. Besse, "Post-dural puncture headache in young patients. A comparative study between the use of 0.52 mm (25-gauge) and 0.33 mm (29-gauge) spinal needles," Acta Anaesthesiologica Scandinavica, vol. 34, no. 5, pp. 350–353, 1990.

[14] M. F. Mulroy, "Spinal headache and air travel," Anesthesiology, vol. 51, no. 5, p. 479, 1979.

[15] J. J. Vacanti, "Post-spinal headache and air travel," Anesthesiology, vol. 37, no. 3, pp. 358–359, 1972.

[16] A. Panadero, P. Bravo, and F. Garcia-Pedrajas, "Postdural puncture headache and air travel after spinal anesthesia with a 24-gauge Sprotte needle," Regional Anesthesia, vol. 20, no. 5, pp. 463–464, 1995.

[17] W. W. Zuurmond, E. Lagerweij, and L. Deen, "Changes in the spinal fluid pressure due to spinal anaesthesia in the sheep (author's transl)," Anaesthesist, vol. 29, no. 4, pp. 27–30, 1980.

[18] P. Safar and R. Tenicela, "High altitude physiology in relation to anesthesia and inhalation therapy," Anesthesiology, vol. 25, pp. 515–531, 1964.

[19] I. Singh, P. K. Khanna, M. C. Srivastava, M. Lal, S. B. Roy, and C. S. Subramanyam, "Acute mountain sickness," The New England Journal of Medicine, vol. 280, no. 4, pp. 175–184, 1969.

[20] M. A. Gendreau and C. Dejohn, "Responding to medical events during commercial airline flights," New England Journal of Medicine, vol. 346, no. 14, pp. 1067–1073, 2002.

[21] J. J. Cottrell, "Altitude exposures during aircraft flight. Flying higher," Chest, vol. 93, no. 1, pp. 81–84, 1988.

Hemodynamic Instability Induced by Superselective Angiography of the Ophthalmic Artery

Stephan Klumpp,[1] Lydia M. Jorge,[1] and Mohammed Ali Aziz-Sultan[2]

[1] Department of Clinical Anesthesia, Jackson Memorial Hospital, University of Miami, Miami, FL 33136, USA
[2] Department of Clinical Neurologic Surgery, 201 Pope Life Center, University of Miami, Miami, FL 33136, USA

Correspondence should be addressed to Lydia M. Jorge; ljorge@med.miami.edu

Academic Editors: M. Dauri, I.-O. Lee, P. Michalek, and J.-J. Yang

Retinoblastoma is one of the most common ophthalmic neoplasms affecting children worldwide. Since its recent introduction, superselective ophthalmic artery injection of chemotherapy with melphalan has significantly reduced the need for enucleation in patients with advanced disease and also shown to have minimal adverse effects on visual acuity as compared to the conventional therapy. Although no severe complications resulting in strokes or deaths have been reported, this treatment modality is not without difficulties. In this case discussion, we describe an event that has occurred to several pediatric patients undergoing superselective angiography of the ophthalmic artery that may be due to an oculopulmonary type reflex causing significant hemodynamic instability and hypoxemia.

1. Introduction

Intra-arterial chemotherapy infusion of the ophthalmic artery is a relatively new endovascular procedure for the treatment of retinoblastoma and is always performed under general anesthesia [1, 2]. We describe a cardiovascular reflex in the pediatric retinoblastoma population during superselective angiography of the ophthalmic artery.

2. Case Presentation

This is an account of a typical response noted in multiple cases.

A two-year-old boy was diagnosed with retinoblastoma involving the right eye. Following consultation with the pediatric oncology and ophthalmology oncology services, the patient was referred for intra-arterial chemotherapy infusion of Melphalan to the right ophthalmic artery. General anesthesia was induced with Propofol 3 mg/kg, Midazolam 0.2 mg/kg, and Rocuronium 0.6 mg/kg. After induction, the patient was successfully intubated with a 4.5 cuffed endotracheal tube and pressure controlled ventilation was initiated. Sevoflurane (1.6 Vol%), oxygen (0.5 L/min), and air (1.5 L/min) were administered for maintenance of general anesthesia.

Femoral access was obtained and a 4-French sheath was placed and perfused with heparinized saline. A 4-French Terumo angle glide catheter was navigated to the right internal carotid where cerebral angiograms were obtained. Under magnified roadmap guidance, a microcatheter was navigated into distal supraclinoid carotid. The microwire was withdrawn into the lumen of the microcatheter, and the microcatheter was slowly withdrawn within the carotid, thus selecting the ostium of the ophthalmic artery. Superselective angiography was performed demonstrating successful ophthalmic catheterization. Two minutes later, the patient's end tidal CO_2 (EtCO_2) decreased from 35 mmHg to 21 mmHg (normal 33–40 mmHg) followed by a subsequent deterioration in the oxygen saturation(SpO_2) to 40% (normal 97%–100%). The microcatheter was withdrawn and ventilation with aFiO_2 of 100% was initiated. On auscultation of the lungs, no abnormalities such as wheezing or rhonchi were appreciated. Within 4 minutes, the SpO_2 and EtCO_2 returned to baseline of 100% and 34–36 mmHg, respectively; however, the patient became hypotensive (Figure 1) requiring

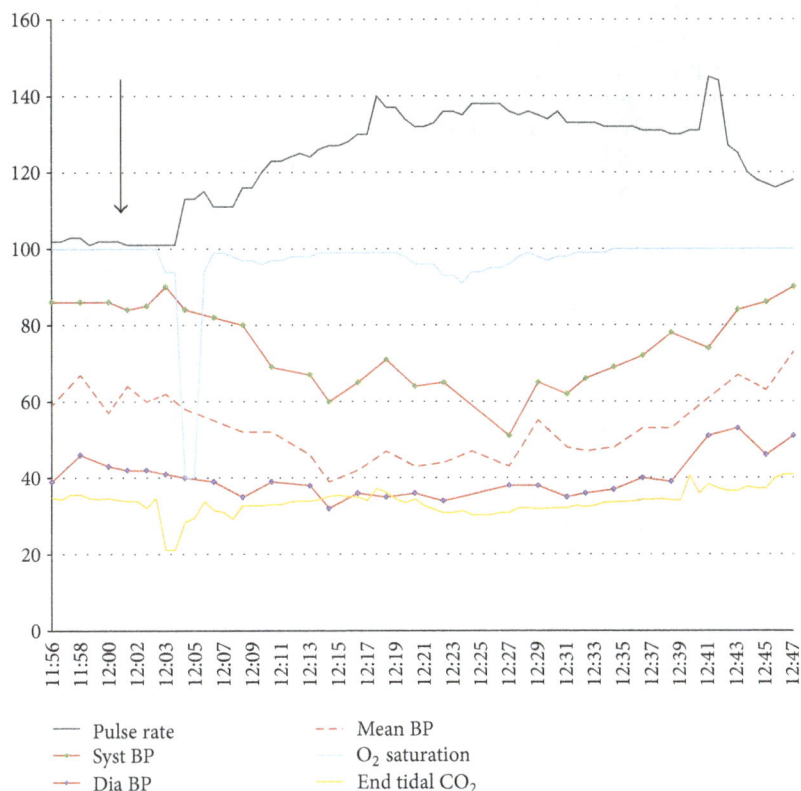

FIGURE 1: Vital signs recorded after stimulus occurred at 12:00.

vasopressor support with Phenylephrine (2 mcg/kg) and fluid bolus for the next 30 minutes.

After stabilization, the procedure was resumed, the microcatheter was again navigated to the ophthalmic artery, and superselective angiography was performed. No further clinical changes were experienced. Manual micropulse infusion of chemotherapy proceeded over 30 minutes. Follow-up selective angiography demonstrated no change from baseline, and the microcatheter was removed. Final angiography demonstrated again no change from baseline, and the guide catheter was removed. After emergence from anesthesia, the patient was extubated and transported to the recovery room in stable condition. The patient was subsequently discharged home without any clinical sequela on postprocedure day 1.

3. Discussion

In our series of 30 pediatric patients with retinoblastoma, superselective ophthalmic microcatheterizations were performed 50 times under general anesthesia. We have experienced physiologic responses similar to those described in this case report on 8 distinct occasions. When elicited, the reflex unfolds as a characteristic and predictable sequence of events, which may vary in degree of magnitude. Severe manifestations of this phenomenon are observed as a temporary decrease in EtCO$_2$ (mean decrease of EtCO$_2$: 15.13 mmHg, range: 22 mmHg, and median: 13 mmHg) with profound hypoxia (mean decrease of SpO$_2$: 24.8 percentage points,

range: 37 points, and median: 9.5 points) followed by prolonged hemodynamic instability with a decrease in blood pressure of over 50% from baseline. The mean time of the prolonged instability was 13 minutes (min) with a range of 37 min and median of 13 min. Milder forms are characterized by a decrease in EtCO$_2$ with a concomitant decrease in SpO$_2$ and minimal hemodynamic changes lasting less than 5 minutes.

This response is often accompanied by tachycardia. Bradycardia was never observed. The symptoms are triggered by one of two types of mechanical stimulation involving the ophthalmic artery: selective ophthalmic microcatheterization (the advancement of the catheter in the ophthalmic artery) or superselective ophthalmic angiography (the administration of contrast into the ophthalmic artery after catheter positioning). When elicited, the reaction occurs predictably within minutes after the stimulus. We have never seen the reflex start more than 5 minutes after the stimulus. Elicitation of the response appears isolated to the initial instance of offending mechanical stimulus. That is, if the reflex is not triggered by the initial microcatheterization or the initial selective angiography, in our experience, the reflex will not occur during the remainder of the procedure. Further, the reflex displays tachyphylaxis and has never occurred more than once during the same treatment session. These observations suggest a possible habituation mechanism. Three of the patients experienced the response on follow-up treatments (2 in the first month and 1 in the second month period). However, the magnitude of the response may vary.

In our series, no patient demonstrating the reflex experienced subsequent morbidity. In all instances, the patients were successfully stabilized and the procedures were resumed and carried to completion. All patients returned to baseline, and we have not experienced the need to alter routine postoperative management prescribed in the treatment protocol. When this phenomenon is experienced, the family is informed of the event.

The specific eliciting stimuli, predictable onset, stereotypical sequence of physiologic changes, and the possibility of habituation may suggest a reflex mechanism which may lead to an acute increase of pulmonary arterial pressure and of pulmonary vascular resistance. The ensuing elevation of the right ventricular afterload may lead to a decrease of right ventricular stroke volume and a decrease in cardiac output and blood pressure. The observed deterioration in lung compliance combined with the decrease in cardiac output results in the decreased $EtCO_2$ and SpO_2 due to decreased minute ventilation and an increased right to left pulmonary shunt. The precise nature of the physiologic process that triggers the described reflex is unclear.

An allergic reaction must be considered in any patients experiencing hypotension after injection of contrast media [3]. The incidence of acute allergic type reaction to nonionic iodinated contrast material has been documented approximately 0.18% in the pediatric population [4]. Anaphylaxis or anaphylactoid reaction appears unlikely, since the contrast media were given prior to and after entering the ophthalmic artery and in subsequent treatments without eliciting any reactions. In one patient, the reflex was elicited by mechanical stimulation during advancement of the catheter into the ophthalmic artery without the administration of contrast at this time.

The oculocardiac reflex has been well known in the literature for over 50 years [5]. More recently, the reflex has been identified as occurring during select endovascular procedures [6]. We described an activation of a similar reflex in the pediatric retinoblastoma population during selective angiography of the ophthalmic artery. However, the patients in our series did not show the typical bradycardia of the oculocardiac reflex.

4. Conclusion

The symptoms described may represent an acute onset of pulmonary hypertension mediated by release of vasoactive hormones or secondary to a vagal response triggered by stimulation of the ophthalmic artery. However, further investigations are needed to improve the understanding of the manifestations, management, and clinical significance of the described oculopulmonary reflex.

References

[1] L. M. Vajzovic, T. G. Murray, M. A. Aziz-Sultan et al., "Supraselective intra-arterial chemotherapy: evaluation of treatment-related complications in advanced retinoblastoma," *Clinical Ophthalmology*, vol. 5, no. 1, pp. 171–176, 2011.

[2] C. L. Shields, A. Ramasubramanian, R. Rosenwasser, and J. A. Shields, "Superselective catheterization of the ophthalmic artery for intraarterial chemotherapy for retinoblastoma," *Retina*, vol. 29, no. 8, pp. 1207–1209, 2009.

[3] J. Singh and A. Daftary, "Iodinated contrast media and their adverse reactions," *Journal of Nuclear Medicine Technology*, vol. 36, no. 2, pp. 69–74, 2008.

[4] J. R. Dillman, P. J. Strouse, J. H. Ellis, R. H. Cohan, and S. C. Jan, "Incidence and severity of acute allergic-like reactions to IV nonionic iodinated contrast material in children," *American Journal of Roentgenology*, vol. 188, no. 6, pp. 1643–1647, 2007.

[5] P. P. Bosomworth, C. H. Ziegler, and J. Jacoby, "The oculocardiac reflex in eye muscle surgery," *Anesthesiology*, vol. 19, no. 1, pp. 7–10, 1958.

[6] M. Sakamoto, T. Watanabe, and H. Inagaki, "Oculocardiac reflex induced by catheterization of the distal ophthalmic artery: case Report," *Journal of Neuroendovascular Therapy*, vol. 2, no. 1, pp. 34–37, 2008.

Open Tracheostomy after Aborted Percutaneous Approach due to Tracheoscopy Revealing Occult Tracheal Wall Ulcer

John Schweiger,[1,2] **Collin Sprenker,**[1] **Devanand Mangar,**[1] **Rachel Karlnoski,**[1,2] **Naga Pullakhandam,**[3] **and Enrico M. Camporesi**[1,2]

[1] Florida Gulf to Bay Anesthesiology Associates, LLC, Tampa, FL 33606, USA
[2] University of South Florida, Department of Surgery, Tampa, FL 33606, USA
[3] Florida Hospital, Orlando, FL 32804, USA

Correspondence should be addressed to Enrico M. Camporesi; ecamporesi@gmail.com

Academic Editors: A. Apan, A. Han, T. Ho, R. Riley, and A. Trikha

Tracheostomy is a common procedure for intensive care patients requiring prolonged mechanical ventilation. In this case report, we describe a 78-year-old female patient admitted for an aneurysm of the cerebral anterior communicating artery. Following immediate endovascular coiling, she remained ventilated and was transferred to the neurological intensive care unit. On postoperative day ten, a percutaneous tracheostomy (PCT) was requested; however, a large ulcer or possible tracheoesophageal fistula was identified on the posterior tracheal wall following bronchoscopic assessment of the trachea. Therefore, the requested PCT procedure was aborted. An open tracheostomy in the operating room was completed; however, due to the position and depth of the ulcer, a reinforced endotracheal tube (ETT) was placed via the tracheostomy. Four days later, the reinforced ETT was replaced with a Shiley distal extended tracheostomy tube to bypass the ulceration. Careful inspection and evaluation of the tracheostomy site before PCT prevented a potentially life-threatening issue in our patient.

1. Introduction

Tracheostomy is a routine procedure for critically ill patients. The percutaneous tracheostomy (PCT) approach has been shown to be safer and is the preferred method compared to the open technique [1, 2]. However, there are still some instances in which open tracheostomies are the necessary method.

The technique and equipment of PCT have significantly evolved since the first description of the percutaneous dilatational report described by Ciaglia et al. [3]. Bronchoscopic guidance with a fiberoptic endoscope during PCT allows direct visualization for tracheal tube positioning placement and control of the entire PCT [4–6]. Lower complication and infection rates with PCT procedures performed under bronchoscopic guidance versus "blind" PCT have been demonstrated [5, 7, 8]. Bronchoscopic guidance may also prevent iatrogenic damage to the posterior tracheal wall. Despite this, recent reports have concluded that routine bronchoscopy is not recommended prior to PCT [9, 10].

This case presents a sequence of altered clinical decisions after bronchoscopic visualization of the trachea revealed a large unexpected posterior wall ulcer before PCT. We aim to emphasize the importance of routine bronchoscopy before a tracheostomy, to assess the tracheal wall and to verify correct placement.

2. Case Report

A 78-year-old female with past medical history of hypertension, chronic obstructive pulmonary disease, gastroesophageal reflux disease, dyslipidemia, and panic disorder was admitted to an outside hospital after falling in her home. Cranial CT revealed an intraparenchymal hemorrhage with intraventricular extension within the right frontal segment of her brain. A subsequent CT angiogram revealed an aneurysm of the anterior communicating artery. The patient was transferred to our hospital for further care and evaluation.

The hemorrhage was categorized as world federation of neurosurgeons (WFNS) grade 2 and Fisher grade 4.

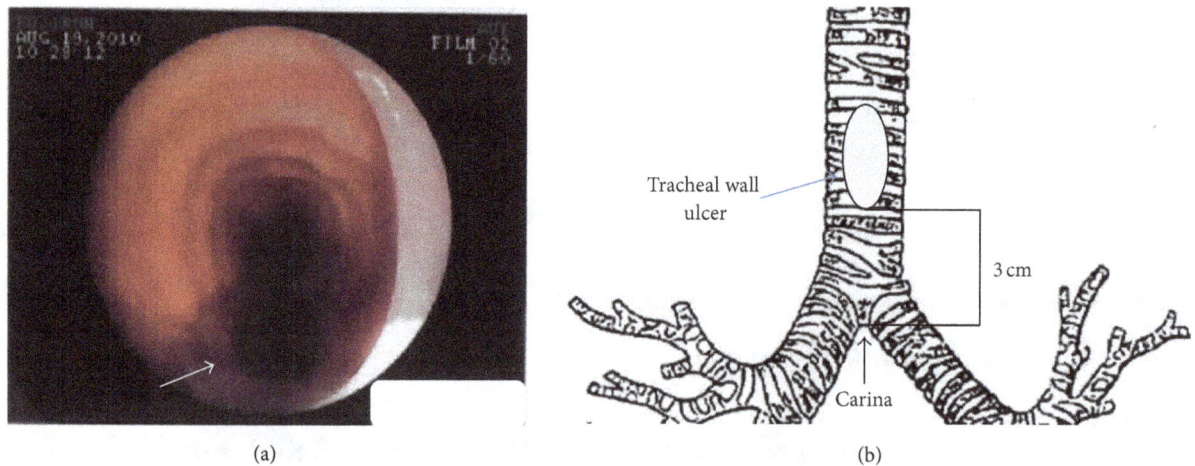

(a)   (b)

FIGURE 1: (a) Bronchoscopic visualization of the tracheal lesion (white arrow). (b) Position of posterior tracheal wall lesion in reference to the carina.

Following admission to the neurological intensive care unit (ICU), the patient underwent endovascular coiling of the aneurysm after general endotracheal anesthesia was initiated. An attempted intraoperative nasogastric tube placement was traumatic, resulting in bleeding from bilateral nasal passages and blood pooling into the oropharynx. An orogastric tube was then placed successfully. After the procedure, on post-operative day 1, the patient remained ventilated and was transferred to the ICU where the ear, nose, and throat (ENT) service repaired the oropharyngeal trauma.

Our critical care service was initially consulted on hospital admission day five for acute respiratory failure secondary to a new left lower lobe atelectasis and small left pleural effusions as indicated from a chest X-ray. Upon initial bronchoscopy inspection, the distal tip of the ETT was found to be 1 cm above the carina; therefore, the cuff was deflated, and the ETT was withdrawn 2 cm and secured in place. The bronchoscopy further revealed copious old/clotted blood in the distal hypopharynx and between the wall of the ETT tube and lining of the trachea. Additionally, mild-to-moderate tracheobronchitis in the right mainstem bronchus and the left lung was found to be nearly completely occluded with a "cast" of old blood and mucus outlining the entire length of the left bronchus.

Four days later, our service was consulted for PCT placement. After confirmation of informed consent and patient identification, the patient was medicated with 200 mcg of fentanyl, 4 mg of midazolam, and 150 mg of rocuronium. A flexible fiberoptic bronchoscope was advanced into the ETT before starting the procedure; no abnormalities were observed. The ETT cuff was deflated and slowly moved directly above the vocal chords. A second bronchoscopic view revealed mild-to-moderate persistent nonpurulent tracheobronchitis and an ulcer on the posterior tracheal wall noted 3-4 cm above the carina extending 2 cm in length and 1 cm in width (Figure 1). Due to the length of the ulcer, obtaining a proper seal with the balloon of the Shiley tracheostomy tube was expected to be difficult. Therefore, the tracheostomy

procedure was aborted, and the ENT service was consulted for evaluation. The ETT was changed to a reinforced ETT following bronchoscopic guidance. FiO_2 was weaned from 100% to 40%, oxygen saturation was kept greater than 92%, respiratory rate was reduced to maintain a $PaCO_2$ between 35 and 45 mmHg, and a bronchodilator treatment was recommended.

Later that evening the patient was transported to the operating room for an open tracheostomy by the ENT service. After the incision (approximately 2 cm below the cricoid cartilage) and dissection (superior to the thyroid isthmus), the second tracheal ring was identified. The ETT was removed just superior to the tracheal window under direct visualization with a flexible bronchoscope. The before-mentioned ulcer was identified inferior to the tracheal window and confirmed with its distal end 3 cm above the carina. Upon careful fiberoptic evaluation, the surgeon suspected the ulcer to be a tracheoesophageal (TE) fistula. At this time, the decision was made to place another reinforced ETT through the tracheal stoma, sutured to the skin, with the tip 0.5 cm above the carina and the cuff inferior to the TE fistula. The severity and location of the ulcer warranted an esophagogastroduodenoscopy to rule out a TE fistula. After evaluation with a rigid esophagoscope, a small amount of petechial type hemorrhage next to the tracheal ulcer, but no fistula, was identified.

Four days later, the ENT service replaced the reinforced ETT with a size six cuffed TracheoSoft XLT Extended-Length Tracheostomy Tube to bypass the ulceration. Over the following week, the patient was weaned from mechanical ventilation, determined stable, and discharged with the tracheostomy cannula sutured in place.

3. Discussion

The use of flexible bronchoscopy during PCT reduces the risk of procedural-related complications. Reported benefits include protection against loss of airway, submucosal flaps, improper positioning of the initial needle puncture, fractures of the anterior tracheal ring, misplacement of the tube, and discovery of tracheal stenosis and tracheomalacia [11]. Additionally, deflating the ETT cuff and withdrawing the ETT to a level above the vocal cords allow assessment of possible tracheal damage. Therefore, early recognition and treatment of a tracheal wall lesion is possible.

Intubations of one to five weeks can cause erosion and ischemic damage to the trachea, potentially yielding stenosis of the trachea or glottis, tracheomalacia, tracheoesophageal fistula, tracheal rupture, or ventilator-associated pneumonia [12]. These tracheal lesions are relatively common with the duration of intubation being the only independent risk factor [13]. ETT cuff inflation pressure greater than 30 cm H_2O or that exceeding capillary perfusion pressure is also a risk factor for tracheal lesions [12].

The subglottic positioning of the artificial airway prevents proper visualization of tracheal lesions which can be fatal if undetected. Our initial fiberoptic passage through the ETT revealed no abnormalities or injuries because the ETT tip was 1 cm above the carina, and the bronchoscopy was focused on the acute respiratory deficiency in the left lung. The large tracheal ulcer was detected four days later, with the ETT withdrawn, exposing the distal trachea to direct visualization prior to the PCT. The likely cause of the ulcer was tracheal wall ischemia from over inflation of the ETT cuff; however, intracuff pressures were not recorded via a manometer throughout the hospital stay. The traumatic placement of the NG tube is excluded as the cause because endotracheal anesthesia was already initiated for the angiogram prior to its placement. If the patient's tracheal injury remained undetected during the initial assessment, blind placement of the PCT over the ulceration could have caused an iatrogenic esophageal rupture or perforation, and the PCT would have been the blamed cause.

Possible complications have been attributed to bronchoscopy such as increased risk for hypercarbia, respiratory acidosis, intracranial pressure, and loss of airway in some cases [14–16]. Additionally, bronchoscopy was observed to be cumbersome and sometimes unfeasible due to logistic reasons [17]. Despite this, in most situations the benefits of bronchoscopy before PCT likely outweigh the disadvantages.

Paran and colleagues developed a modified PCT technique: guidance provided by the user's finger [18]. Their modified technique was evaluated in 61 patients, three experienced complications. In response, Gründling et al. proposed that bronchoscopy could have prevented these complications, [19] and Melloni et al. recognized the unnecessary exposure of patients to potentially serious complications [20].

Our presented case reveals a critical example where devastating complications with a PCT were avoided after the usage of fiberoptic bronchoscopy inspection. Because of the increased likelihood of ischemic lesions after prolonged intubation, clinicians should routinely assess the trachea with a bronchoscope for unexpected tracheal pathology in addition to a constant visual survey during the PCT. We emphasize that bronchoscopy-guided PCT provides significant benefits and should be performed regardless of initial necessity.

References

[1] L. Z. Kornblith, C. C. Burlew, E. E. Moore et al., "One thousand bedside percutaneous tracheostomies in the surgical intensive care unit: time to change the gold standard," *Journal of the American College of Surgeons*, vol. 212, no. 2, pp. 163–170, 2011.

[2] S. M. Susarla, Z. S. Peacock, and H. B. Alam, "Percutaneous dilatational tracheostomy: review of technique and evidence for its use," *Journal of Oral and Maxillofacial Surgery*, vol. 70, no. 1, pp. 74–82, 2012.

[3] P. Ciaglia, R. Firsching, and C. Syniec, "Elective percutaneous dilatational tracheostomy: a new simple bedside procedure; preliminary report," *Chest*, vol. 87, no. 6, pp. 715–719, 1985.

[4] C. A. Barba, P. B. Angood, D. R. Kauder et al., "Bronchoscopic guidance makes percutaneous tracheostomy a safe, cost-effective, and easy-to-teach procedure," *Surgery*, vol. 118, no. 5, pp. 879–883, 1995.

[5] W.-B. Winkler, R. Karnik, O. Seelmann, J. Havlicek, and J. Slany, "Bedside percutaneous dilational tracheostomy with endoscopic guidance: experience with 71 ICU patients," *Intensive Care Medicine*, vol. 20, no. 7, pp. 476–479, 1994.

[6] H. Park, J. Kent, M. Joshi et al., "Percutaneous versus open tracheostomy: comparison of procedures and surgical site infections," *Surgical Infections*, vol. 14, no. 1, pp. 21–23, 2013.

[7] L. Fernandez, S. Norwood, R. Roettger, D. Gass, and H. Wilkins III, "Bedside percutaneous tracheostomy with bronchoscopic guidance in critically ill patients," *Archives of Surgery*, vol. 131, no. 2, pp. 129–132, 1996.

[8] D. Marelli, A. Paul, S. Manolidis et al., "Endoscopic guided percutaneous tracheostomy: early results of a consecutive trial," *Journal of Trauma*, vol. 30, no. 4, pp. 433–435, 1990.

[9] L. S. M. Jackson, J. W. Davis, K. L. Kaups et al., "Percutaneous tracheostomy: to bronch or not to bronch-that is the question," *Journal of Trauma*, vol. 71, no. 6, pp. 1553–1556, 2011.

[10] B. M. Dennis, M. J. Eckert, O. L. Gunter, J. A. Morris, and A. K. May, "Safety of bedside percutaneous tracheostomy in the critically ill: evaluation of more than 3,000 procedures," *Journal of the American College of Surgeons*, vol. 216, no. 4, pp. 858–865, 2013.

[11] W. H. Marx, P. Ciaglia, and K. D. Graniero, "Some important details in the technique of percutaneous dilatational tracheostomy via the modified seldinger technique," *Chest*, vol. 110, no. 3, pp. 762–766, 1996.

[12] R. D. Seegobin and G. L. van Hasselt, "Endotracheal cuff pressure and tracheal mucosal blood flow: endoscopic study of effects of four large volume cuffs," *British Medical Journal*, vol. 288, no. 6422, pp. 965–968, 1984.

[13] L. Touat, C. Fournier, P. Ramon, J. Salleron, A. Durocher, and S. Nseir, "Intubation-related tracheal ischemic lesions: incidence, risk factors, and outcome," *Intensive Care Medicine*, vol. 39, no. 4, pp. 575–582, 2013.

[14] M. Beiderlinden, M. K. Walz, A. Sander, H. Groeben, and J. Peters, "Complications of bronchoscopically guided percutaneous dilational tracheostomy: beyond the learning curve," *Intensive Care Medicine*, vol. 28, no. 1, pp. 59–62, 2002.

[15] P. M. Reilly, R. F. Sing, F. A. Giberson et al., "Hypercarbia during tracheostomy: a comparison of percutaneous endoscopic, percutaneous Doppler, and standard surgical tracheostomy," *Intensive Care Medicine*, vol. 23, no. 8, pp. 859–864, 1997.

[16] P. M. Reilly, H. L. Anderson III, R. F. Sing, C. W. Schwab, and R. H. Bartlett, "An unrecognized phenomenon during percutaneous endoscopic tracheostomy," *Chest*, vol. 107, no. 6, pp. 1760–1763, 1995.

[17] M. M. Maddali, M. Pratap, J. Fahr, and A. W. Zarroug, "Percutaneous tracheostomy by guidewire dilating forceps technique: review of 98 patients," *Journal of Postgraduate Medicine*, vol. 47, no. 2, pp. 100–103, 2001.

[18] H. Paran, G. Butnaru, I. Hass, A. Afanasyv, and M. Gutman, "Evaluation of a modified percutaneous tracheostomy technique without bronchoscopic guidance," *Chest*, vol. 126, no. 3, pp. 868–871, 2004.

[19] M. Gründling, D. Pavlovic, S.-O. Kühn, and F. Feyerherd, "Is the method of modified percutaneous tracheostomy without bronchoscopic guidance really simple and safe?" *Chest*, vol. 128, no. 5, pp. 3774–3775, 2005.

[20] G. Melloni, L. Libretti, M. Casiraghi, P. Zannini, H. Paran, and M. Gutman, "A modified percutaneous tracheostomy technique without bronchoscopic guidance: a note of concern," *Chest*, vol. 128, no. 6, pp. 4050–4051, 2005.

11

Sensitivity to Rocuronium-Induced Neuromuscular Block and Reversibility with Sugammadex in a Patient with Myotonic Dystrophy

Akihiro Kashiwai, Takahiro Suzuki, and Setsuro Ogawa

Department of Anesthesiology, Nihon University School of Medicine, 30-1 Oyaguchi Kamimachi, Itabashi-ku, Tokyo 173-8610, Japan

Correspondence should be addressed to Takahiro Suzuki, suzukit@cd5.so-net.ne.jp

Academic Editors: J. Malek, R. Riley, and C. Seefelder

We report a patient with myotonic dystrophy who showed prolonged rocuronium-induced neuromuscular blockade, although with a fast recovery with sugammadex. During general anesthesia with propofol and remifentanil, the times to spontaneous recovery of the first twitch (T1) of train of four to 10% of control values after an intubating dose of rocuronium 1 mg/kg and an additional dose of 0.2 mg/kg were 112 min and 62 min, respectively. Despite the high sensitivity to rocuronium, sugammadex 2 mg/kg administered at a T1 of 10% safely and effectively antagonized rocuronium-induced neuromuscular block in 90 s.

1. Introduction

Myotonic dystrophy (MD), an autosomal dominant disorder, is the commonest of all myotonic syndromes, with an incidence of approximately 1 in 8000. It is characterized by progressive muscle weakness of the face, neck, pharynx, and distal limbs, with difficulty initiating movements and delayed muscle relaxation [1]. Careful anesthetic management is required for MD patients due to the likelihood of various coexisting disorders, such as cardiac conduction abnormalities, hypotension, diabetes mellitus, dysphagia, and malignant hyperthermia [2]. Changes in the sensitivity of these patients to neuromuscular blocking agents also require special consideration. In particular, the potential requirement of prolonged ventilatory support due to hypersensitivity to nondepolarizing neuromuscular blockade [3, 4], cardiac arrest provoked by succinylcholine [5], and neostigmine-induced myotonia [6] should be considered in MD patients. We present a patient with MD whose neuromuscular function was successfully managed with rocuronium and sugammadex during general anesthesia.

2. Case Presentation

A 37-year-old female patient with MD, weighing 55 kg and 154 cm tall, was scheduled for open resection of an ovarian tumor under general anesthesia combined with epidural anesthesia. Beside MD, her surgical history included retroperitoneal tumor resection under general anesthesia, although details about the surgery and the patient's perioperative condition were not known. Preoperative manual muscle tests revealed mild muscular weakness and myotonia in her upper limbs. She complained of mild difficulty in swallowing, although her respiratory efforts did not seem to be impaired. Moderate masseter muscle atrophy led us to predict difficulty with bag and mask ventilation during the induction of anesthesia. Routine preoperative blood tests were within normal ranges with no elevation of creatine kinase levels and no indication of liver or renal insufficiency. Arterial blood gas analysis at a F_IO_2 of 0.21 showed an arterial oxygen tension of 85 mmHg and carbon dioxide tension of 47 mmHg.

Premedication consisted of oral administration of 150 mg ranitidine the night before and on the morning of surgery. On arrival at the operating room, the patient was monitored with ECG, noninvasive blood pressure, and pulse oximetry. Epidural puncture and catheterization were performed at the Th12-L1 intervertebral space. General anesthesia was induced with fentanyl 2 µg/kg and a target controlled infusion of propofol 4 µg/mL (Terufusion TCI pump TE-371, Terumo, Tokyo Japan) while the patient received 100% oxygen

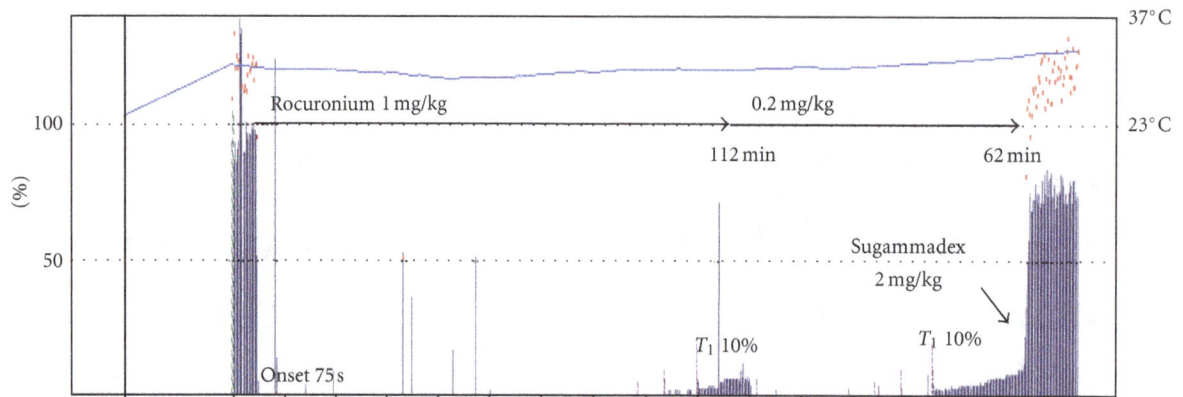

FIGURE 1: A serial recording of acceleromyography in a patient with myotonic dystrophy. Blue longitudinal bars show T1 height in the train-of-four responses, and red dots mean the train-of-four ratios. Marked prolongation in durations of rocuronium-induced neuromuscular block and rapid recovery from neuromuscular block after sugammadex administration are shown.

through an anesthesia facemask. After loss of consciousness, the left ulnar nerve was stimulated at the wrist with supra-maximal and square-wave stimuli of 0.2 ms duration, which was delivered in a train-of-four (TOF) mode at 2 Hz every 15 s. Contraction of the ipsilateral adductor pollicis muscle was measured using an acceleromyograph (TOF-Watch SX; Organon, Dublin, Ireland). Immediately after obtaining baseline levels of TOF responses, the patient received a bolus of rocuronium 1 mg/kg. Complete neuromuscular block was obtained 75 seconds after rocuronium administration, and the patient's trachea was intubated thereafter without any difficulty. Ventilation was controlled with a tidal volume of 500 mL and at a rate of 10/min. Anesthesia was maintained with propofol 2–4 μg/mL, remifentanil 0.05–0.3 μg/kg/min, and intermittent epidural injections of 0.375% ropivacaine. The first twitch (T1) of train of four recovered to 10% of control levels 112 min after administration of the intubating dose of rocuronium. At that time, rocuronium 0.2 mg/kg was administered to obtain complete neuromuscular blockade, as observed by absent TOF responses. The duration to spontaneous recovery to a T1 of 10% of control levels was also prolonged to 62 min (Figure 1). At the time of uneventful completion of the surgery, the rocuronium-induced moderate neuromuscular block was still present, and the observed TOF count was only 2. Sugammadex 2 mg/kg rapidly antagonized the neuromuscular block, such that the TOF ratio reached 0.9 in 90 s. Several minutes after discontinuation of propofol and remifentanil, the patient could breathe adequately and was extubated. Oxygen saturation measured by pulse oximetry remained at 100% while the patient received 100% oxygen via a facemask. Postanesthetic shivering that could have pre-cipitated the myotonia was avoided by ensuring adequate intraoperative warming and temperature maintenance. Adequate postoperative analgesia was provided by continuous epidural injection of 0.2% ropivacaine without the addition

of opioids. The postoperative course was also uneventful, and no respiratory complications were observed.

3. Discussion

Our patient exhibited a higher sensitivity to rocuronium-in-duced neuromuscular blockade. The time from administration of rocuronium 1 mg/kg until T1 spontaneously reached 10% of the control value was markedly longer in our patient as compared to patients with normal neuromuscular function (70 min [7]). The time taken for T1 to reach 10% in our patient (112 min) was measured during intravenous anesthesia using propofol and remifentanil, while the previous data was observed during anesthesia with sevoflurane [7], which is known to significantly prolong the duration of action of rocuronium to 1.5–2 times [8, 9]. Assuming that the values observed in the other study were potentiated by sevoflurane, the time from administration of rocuronium 1 mg/kg to the recovery of T1 to 10% of the control level observed in our MD patient seems to have been roughly doubled.

The response of MD patients to non-depolarizing neu-romuscular blocking agents is controversial. Increased sen-sitivity [3, 4], normal response [4], and even resistance [10] to non-depolarizing neuromuscular block have all been re-ported. It is likely that the degree of severity of the patho-logy may determine the sensitivity to neuromuscular block-ade [11]. To eliminate the risk of prolonged neuro-mus-cular block and avoid the need for mechanical ventilation in the post operative period in these patients, avoidan-ce of the use or reduction in the dose of neuromuscular blocking agents is recommended [4]. However, vocal cord injury is a serious concern when tracheal intubation is performed without neuromuscular blocking agents [12]. In addition, inadvertent patient movement can be trigger-ed if neuromuscular blockade during surgery is inadequate.

More importantly, our patient had dysphagia associated with dysfunction of the pharyngeal muscles and the risk of regurgitation of gastric contents [11]. Furthermore, difficulty with bag and mask ventilation during induction of anesthesia was predicted because of the masseter muscle atrophy. Therefore, rapid sequence intubation using a high dose of rocuronium was planned to avoid aspiration pneumonia and difficult ventilation, despite the risk of prolonged neuromuscular blockade. Use of cisatracurium also seemed like a logical choice because the benzylisoquinoline compound constantly undergoes pH- and temperature-dependent Hofmann elimination in plasma and tissues [13]. Although the use of neuromuscular blocking agents without reversal has been shown to be a significant risk factor for postoperative respiratory complications [14], anticholinesterases should also be avoided in these patients so as to avoid evoking myotonia, even at the potential cost of residual neuromuscular blockade postoperatively. These contraindications to the use of non-depolarizing muscle relaxants and their reversal agents and the availability of sugammadex, which can promptly antagonize rocuronium-induced neuromuscular block even in myasthenic patients [15], partly contributed to our decision to use high-dose rocuronium. In fact, reversibility of rocuronium-induced neuromuscular block with sugammadex has been proved to be adequate even in MD patients with a high sensitivity to rocuronium. In such cases, however, the dosing of rocuronium and sugammadex should be individually optimized by neuromuscular monitoring because recurarization may occur after administration of a lower dose of sugammadex [16].

Acceleromyography was very useful to evaluate the onset of and recovery from rocuronium-induced neuromuscular block in our MD patient, although it may underestimate the degree of neuromuscular block during recovery on the negative side [11]. It has been reported that T1 is still recovering from neuromuscular block even when the TOF ratio reaches 0.9 after reversal with sugammadex [17]. Therefore, when residual neuromuscular block is suspected by clinical signs of respiratory insufficiency and inadequate muscular strength, additional doses of sugammadex should be considered.

It is likely that not only rapid reversal of rocuronium-induced neuromuscular block with sugammadex but also short-acting intravenous anesthesia with propofol and remifentanil and postoperative analgesia without opioids all contributed to the rapid recovery of respiratory function seen in our patient. Given the importance of the marked susceptibility of MD patients to anesthetics, which may cause apnea and respiratory depression [18], careful titration of propofol and remifentanil by a target-controlled infusion is thought to be appropriate when anaesthetizing MD patients.

In conclusion, the combination of rocuronium and sugammadex may allow safe and effective management of neuromuscular function during general anesthesia in patients with MD. Further systematic studies are warranted to verify the safety and efficacy of perioperative use of rocuronium and sugammadex in MD patients.

References

[1] E. D. Briggs and J. R. Kirsch, "Anesthetic implications of neuromuscular disease," *Journal of Anesthesia*, vol. 17, no. 3, pp. 177–185, 2003.

[2] M. K. Urban and S. Lahlou, "Muscle disease," in *Anesthesia and Uncommon Diseases*, L. A. Fleisher, Ed., pp. 303–325, Elsevier, Philadelphia, Pa, USA, 2006.

[3] B. J. Mudge, P. B. Taylor, and A. F. L. Vanderspek, "Perioperative hazards in myotonic dystrophy," *Anaesthesia*, vol. 35, no. 5, pp. 492–495, 1980.

[4] C. Diefenbach, J. Lynch, M. Abel, and W. Buzello, "Vecuronium for muscle relaxation in patients with dystrophia myotonica," *Anesthesia & Analgesia*, vol. 76, no. 4, pp. 872–874, 1993.

[5] L. Kaufman, "Dystrophia myotonica and succinylcholine," *Anaesthesia*, vol. 55, no. 9, p. 929, 2000.

[6] W. Buzello, N. Krieg, and A. Schlickewei, "Hazards of neostigmine in patients with neuromuscular disorders: report of two cases," *British Journal of Anaesthesia*, vol. 54, no. 5, pp. 529–534, 1982.

[7] T. Suzuki, H. Mizutani, E. Miyake, N. Fukano, S. Saeki, and S. Ogawa, "Infusion requirements and reversibility of rocuronium at the corrugator supercilii and adductor pollicis muscles," *Acta Anaesthesiologica Scandinavica*, vol. 53, no. 10, pp. 1336–1340, 2009.

[8] D. W. Lowry, R. K. Mirakhur, G. J. McCarthy, M. T. Carroll, and K. C. McCourt, "Neuromuscular effects of rocuronium during sevoflurane, isoflurane, and intravenous anesthesia," *Anesthesia & Analgesia*, vol. 87, no. 4, pp. 936–940, 1998.

[9] F. S. Xue, X. Liao, S. Y. Tong, J. H. Liu, G. An, and L. K. Luo, "Dose-response and time-course of the effect of rocuronium bromide during sevoflurane anaesthesia," *Anaesthesia*, vol. 53, no. 1, pp. 25–30, 1998.

[10] K. Kodama, T. Akata, T. Sasaki, Y. Sakaguchi, and S. Takahashi, "Unexpected resistance to pancuronium in a patient with myotonic dystrophy (myotonia dystrophica)," *Journal of Anesthesia*, vol. 14, no. 3, pp. 160–163, 2000.

[11] L. E. H. Vanlinthout, L. H. D. J. Booij, J. van Egmond, and E. N. Robertson, "Comparison of mechanomyography and acceleromyography for the assessment of rocuronium induced neuromuscular block in myotonic dystrophy type 1," *Anaesthesia*, vol. 65, no. 6, pp. 601–607, 2010.

[12] T. Mencke, M. Echternach, P. K. Plinkert et al., "Does the timing of tracheal intubation based on neuromuscular monitoring decrease laryngeal injury? A randomized, prospective, controlled trial.," *Anesthesia & Analgesia*, vol. 102, no. 1, pp. 306–312, 2006.

[13] D. F. Kisor, V. D. Schmith, W. A. Wargin, C. A. Lien, E. Ornstein, and D. R. Cook, "Importance of the organ-independent elimination of cisatracurium," *Anesthesia & Analgesia*, vol. 83, no. 5, pp. 1065–1071, 1996.

[14] J. L. Sinclair and P. W. Reed, "Risk factors for perioperative adverse events in children with myotonic dystrophy," *Paediatric Anaesthesia*, vol. 19, no. 8, pp. 740–747, 2009.

[15] H. Argiriadou, K. Anastasiadis, E. Thomaidou, and D. Vasilakos, "Reversal of neuromuscular blockade with sugammadex in an obese myasthenic patient undergoing thymectomy," *Journal of Anesthesia*, vol. 25, no. 2, pp. 316–317, 2011.

[16] P. Duvaldestin, K. Kuizenga, V. Saldien et al., "A randomized, dose-response study of sugammadex given for the reversal of deep rocuronium- or vecuronium-induced neuromuscular blockade under sevoflurane anesthesia," *Anesthesia & Analgesia*, vol. 110, no. 1, pp. 74–82, 2010.

[17] T. Suzuki, "A train-of-four ratio of 0.9 may not certify adequate recovery after sugammadex," *Acta Anaesthesiologica Scandinavica*, vol. 55, no. 3, pp. 368–369, 2011.

[18] Y. Morimoto, M. Mii, T. Hirata, H. Matayoshi, and T. Sakabe, "Target-controlled infusion of propofol for a patient with myotonic dystrophy," *Journal of Anesthesia*, vol. 19, no. 4, pp. 336–338, 2005.

12

Tracheal Intubation with Aura-i and aScope-2: How to Minimize Apnea Time in an Unpredicted Difficult Airway

Vittorio Pavoni,[1] Valentina Froio,[1] Alessandra Nella,[1] Martina Simonelli,[1] Lara Gianesello,[1] Andrew Horton,[2] Luca Malino,[3] and Massimo Micaglio[1]

[1]*Department of Anesthesia and Intensive Care, University-Hospital Careggi, Largo Brambilla 3, 50134 Firenze, Italy*
[2]*Faculty Practice Group, University of California, Los Angeles, CA 90095, USA*
[3]*Ambu Srl, Via Paracelso 18, Agrate Brianza, 20041 Milano, Italy*

Correspondence should be addressed to Vittorio Pavoni; pvv@unife.it

Academic Editor: Pavel Michalek

The supraglottic airway's usefulness as a dedicated airway is the subject of continuing development. We report the case of an obese patient with unpredicted difficult airway management in which a new "continuous ventilation technique" was used with the Aura-i laryngeal mask and the aScope-2 devices. The aScope-2/Aura-i system implemented airway devices for the management of predictable/unpredictable difficult airway. The original technique required the disconnection of the mount catheter from Aura-i, the introduction of the aScope-2 into the laryngeal mask used as a conduit for video assisted intubation and then towards the trachea, followed by a railroading of the tracheal tube over the aScope-2. This variation in the technique guarantees mechanical ventilation during the entire procedure and could prevent the risk of hypoventilation and/or hypoxia.

1. Introduction

Supraglottic airway devices (SADs) play a critical role in the management of difficult airway and their use in patients with difficult face-mask ventilation or failed tracheal intubation is widely recommended [1, 2]. Furthermore, SADs are well described as conduits to facilitate tracheal intubation [3], although most devices require fiber-optic bronchoscope (FOB) guidance to increase the rate of success [4–6]. With the aim of minimizing apnea time during the entire procedure, improving patient's safety, a continuous ventilation technique during the intubation procedure has been described, using a mount catheter with a fiber-optic cap attached to the tracheal tube (TT) [7].

We report a case of unpredicted difficult airway in which fiber-optic intubation was performed using a new "continuous ventilation technique" with combination of the Aura-i disposable laryngeal mask (Ambu A/S, Ballerup, Denmark) and the aScope-2 (Ambu A/S, Ballerup, Denmark).

The precurved disposable laryngeal mask Aura-i (Ambu A/S, Ballerup, Denmark) is a SAD designed to facilitate one-step tracheal intubation with FOB guidance [8], due to its anatomically correct curve and the presence of a navigation mark for guiding flexible scope. Its role has become still more interesting since the development of the aScope-2 (Ambu A/S, Ballerup, Denmark), a flexible intubation scope with its high-resolution specific monitor. Both devices are single use in order to reduce cross contamination and cleaning or repair costs [9].

2. Case Report

A 55-year-old female was scheduled to undergo elective cholecystectomy. Past medical history was significant for obesity (body mass index 31.2 Kg/m^2, obesity class I), tobacco smoking, and mild chronic obstructive pulmonary disease, treated with short-acting β_2-agonists. Preoperative arterial blood gas analysis showed PaO$_2$ 66 mmHg, PaCO$_2$

42 mmHg, HCO_3- 29 mEq/L, pH 7.39, and BE −3.0. On preoperative airway examination the Mallampati score oral opening view was evaluated to be class 2, with mouth opening of approximately 4 cm, a thyromental distance of 6.5 cm, and jaw protrusion was estimated as grade B and we noted also slightly limited neck extension. The patient exhibited slightly limited craniocervical extension. A borderline situation for possible difficult intubation was identified, but except for a light increase of BMI, no predictor of difficult mask ventilation was found. After routine monitoring, preoxygenation was performed and anesthesia was induced with propofol 170 mg and fentanyl 150 mcg i.v. After confirmation of the ability to ventilate the patient's lungs using a bag and mask, 80 mg of rocuronium was administered. Direct laryngoscopy was then performed, which revealed a grade III laryngeal view (Cormack and Lehane) due to a large floppy epiglottis. One attempt of gum elastic bougie-assisted tracheal intubation technique was unsuccessful. A size 4 Aura-i laryngeal mask was then easily inserted and the cuff inflated up to a pressure of 50–60 cmH$_2$O. Satisfactory ventilation was achieved in few seconds after connection to the ventilator (Drager Primus, Dragerwerk AG & Co.) using a volume controlled model (tidal volume 7 mL/kg, respiration rate 10 per min, PEEP 5 cmH$_2$O) and we considered the use of the SAD to facilitate tracheal intubation. With the aim of preventing hypoxia during the procedure, reducing the time of apnea, a variation in the intubation technique suggested from the manufacturer was introduced. Without discontinuing mechanical ventilation, the aScope-2 was guided inside the airway tube of Aura-i through a mount catheter with a fiber-optic cap (DAR-Covidien) and both its position and its anatomical relation with the glottis were checked. A partially obstructed view at the level of distal orifice of the Ambu-I LM was noted during the initial view; this was probably caused by malposition or downfolding of epiglottis. Following "up and down movements" of the LM, the view cleared up, with full view of the glottis displayed on the monitor, and the aScope-2 was withdrawn from the mask. The mount catheter was disconnected from the ventilatory circuit for few seconds to allow the distal end of a well lubricated 7.5 mm ID TT to be partially inserted into the airway tube of Aura-i. The TT cuff was inflated and the tube was connected to ventilator with unchanged ventilation mode. Then TT cuff was deflated and the TT was advanced over aScope-2 that was placed in the trachea and the TT connector hooked up to the anaesthesia circuit (Figure 1). Without discontinuing ventilation, the 630 mm insertion-cord of the aScope-2 was first guided inside the TT through the fiber-optic cap of the mount catheter and then into the airway tube of Aura-i to gain a full view of the glottic opening from the end of the SAD.

The cuff of the tracheal tube was deflated and the tube was then advanced over the aScope-2 used as a guide. Connector of the tracheal tube was attached to the anaesthesia circuit (Figure 1). Correct depth of the tracheal tube was checked and the aScope-2 was subsequently withdrawn. The TT cuff was inflated while the Aura-i cuff was deflated and kept in place, decreasing pressure on the pharyngeal mucosa. Anaesthesia and surgery proceeded uneventfully.

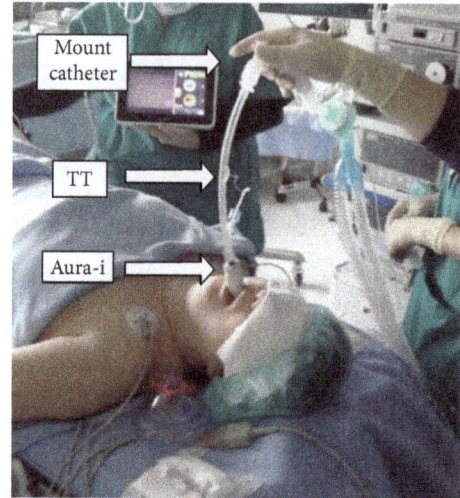

FIGURE 1: The patient is mechanically ventilated through a tracheal tube (TT) partially inserted in the airway tube of Aura-i and with the cuff inflated.

3. Discussion

Hypoxia may complicate difficult airway management representing a life-threatening event [10]. Obese patients have an elevated risk of hypoxia as compared to the nonobese population. The use of a SAD has been recently recommended in obese population instead of the face-mask ventilation in order to ease airway management and administer PEEP, thus preventing hypoxia [11].

Our patient did not show any feature that suggested difficulty in face-mask ventilation; therefore the early placement of SAD appeared not essential. On the other hand, our patient showed difficulty on direct laryngoscopy with tracheal intubation which was not predicted on the base of preoperative airway evaluation, if we exclude Mallampati class 2 and jaw protrusion grade B.

The usefulness of SADs both in unpredicted difficult airway and in predicted difficult intubation with conventional laryngoscopy was the subject of considerable interest [12, 13]. A number of studies have reported intubation through a SAD using a blind technique or assisted by light wands, optical stylets, and flexible fiber optic [14, 15]. Individual case reports have also described a variety of techniques.

The aScope-2/Aura-i system implements airway devices for the management of predictable/unpredictable difficult airway. The light weight of the "ergonomically designed" handle of the aScope-2 makes it easy to manipulate [16] (Figure 2). Furthermore the aScope-2 is less rigid than a fiberscope sparing the endotracheal tube to find resistance to progression through the laryngeal mask and the vocal cords. The portable monitor makes it easy to transport from one operating room to the other one and makes the system even more simple and friendly to use. Both the Aura-i laryngeal mask and the aScope-2 are disposable devices, so biological risks are minimized and they can be used in patients with infectious and transmissible diseases. They are always ready to use and there is no risk of damage during decontamination and storage.

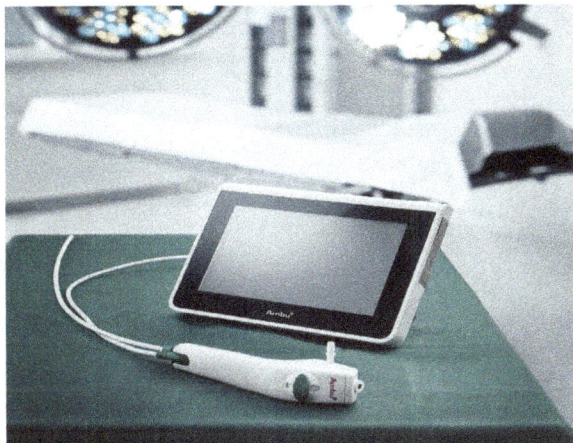

FIGURE 2: The aScope-2 with a transportable monitor.

The aScope-2 has a poor fiber-optic view comparing to a fiberscope and its tip is characterized by a lesser range of movement, with a limited angulation [9]. The aScope-2 has no suction port. Since outer diameter of the aScope-2 (5.3 mm) is larger than that of adult reusable fiber-optic scopes (3.5–4.2 mm), the Aintree Intubation Catheter, a device specifically designed to aid fibrescope guided tube placement through a laryngeal mask airway, cannot be used with it. When using a size 3 Aura-i laryngeal mask, a maximal ID size of the TT through this device is 6.5 mm. Positive pressure ventilation may be difficult through combination of the 6.5 mm ID TT and the aScope-2 [17]. The original technique needs the disconnection of the mount catheter from Aura-i, the introduction of the aScope-2 into the mask and then towards the trachea, followed by the introduction of the tracheal tube through the aScope-2. The variable time of apnea experienced during tracheal tube positioning could become critical in situations where the patient presents comorbidities that increase the risk related to hypoventilation and/or hypoxia. As previously described by Hammarskjöld et al. [18], conversion from laryngeal mask to endotracheal tube may be difficult. In their paper, where they intubated patients using a bougie guided technique through a laryngeal mask with a fiber-optic bronchoscope, the experienced time of apnoea was extremely variable: 17 patients were intubated within 2 minutes, 11 patients were intubated between 2 and 5 minutes, and one patient required 10 minutes. Variation of the intubation technique through the Aura-i laryngeal mask described in this case report guarantees adequate ventilation during the entire procedure and could prevent this risk.

4. Conclusion

Applying positive pressure ventilation during fiber-optic intubation through the SAD can reduce the potential risk of hypoxia and hypercapnia in case of unanticipated difficult airway.

References

[1] American Society of Anesthesiologists Task Force on Management of the Difficult Airway, "Practice guidelines for management of the difficult airway: an updated report by the American Society of Anesthesiologists Task Force on Management of the Difficult Airway," *Anaesthesiology*, vol. 118, pp. 251–270, 2013.

[2] F. Petrini, A. Accorsi, E. Adrario et al., "Recommendations for airway control and difficult airway management," *Minerva Anestesiologica*, vol. 71, no. 11, pp. 617–657, 2005.

[3] A. Timmermann, "Supraglottic airways in difficult airway management: successes, failures, use and misuse," *Anaesthesia*, vol. 66, no. 2, pp. 45–56, 2011.

[4] K. B. Greenland, H. Tan, and M. Edwards, "Intubation via a laryngeal mask airway with an Aintree catheter—not all laryngeal masks are the same," *Anaesthesia*, vol. 62, no. 9, pp. 966–967, 2007.

[5] M. Carron, U. Freo, and C. Ori, "Bronchoscope-guided intubation through a laryngeal mask airway supreme in a patient with a difficult-to-manage airway," *Journal of Anesthesia*, vol. 23, no. 4, pp. 613–615, 2009.

[6] P. Michalek, P. Hodgkinson, and W. Donaldson, "Fiberoptic intubation through an I-Gel supraglottic airway in two patients with predicted difficult airway and intellectual disability," *Anesthesia and Analgesia*, vol. 106, no. 5, pp. 1501–1504, 2008.

[7] M. Weiss, A. C. Gerber, and A. Schmitz, "Continuous ventilation technique for laryngeal mask airway (LMA) removal after fiberoptic intubation in children," *Paediatric Anaesthesia*, vol. 14, no. 11, pp. 936–940, 2004.

[8] F. McAleavey and P. Michalek, "Aura-i laryngeal mask as a conduit for elective fibreoptic intubation," *Anaesthesia*, vol. 65, no. 11, p. 1151, 2010.

[9] V. Krugel, I. Bathory, P. Frascarolo, and P. Schoettker, "Comparison of the single-use Ambu aScope 2 vs the conventional fibrescope for tracheal intubation in patients with cervical spine immobilisation by a semirigid collar," *Anaesthesia*, vol. 68, no. 1, pp. 21–26, 2013.

[10] T. M. Cook and S. R. Macdougall-Davis, "Complications and failure of airway management," *British Journal of Anaesthesia*, vol. 109, supplement 1, pp. i68–i85, 2012.

[11] A. Sinha, L. Jayaraman, D. Punhani, and B. Panigrahi, "ProSeal laryngeal mask airway improves oxygenation when used as a conduit prior to laryngoscope guided intubation in bariatric patients," *Indian Journal of Anaesthesia*, vol. 57, no. 1, pp. 25–30, 2013.

[12] D. G. Mathew, R. Ramachandran, V. Rewari, A. Trikha, and Chandralekha, "Endotracheal intubation with intubating laryngeal mask airway (ILMA), C- Trach , and Cobra PLA in simulated cervical spine injury patients: a comparative study," *Journal of Anesthesia*, vol. 28, no. 5, pp. 655–661, 2014.

[13] J. A. Law, N. Broemling, R. M. Cooper et al., "The difficult airway recommendations for management—part 2—the anticipated difficult airway," *Canadian Journal of Anesthesia*, vol. 60, no. 11, pp. 1119–1138, 2013.

[14] D. T. Wong, J. J. Yang, H. Y. Mak, and N. Jagannathan, "Use of intubation introducers through a supraglottic airway to facilitate tracheal intubation: a brief review," *Canadian Journal of Anesthesia*, vol. 59, no. 7, pp. 704–715, 2012.

[15] P. Michalek, W. Donaldson, C. Graham, and J. D. Hinds, "A comparison of the I-gel supraglottic airway as a conduit for tracheal intubation with the intubating laryngeal mask airway: a manikin study," *Resuscitation*, vol. 81, no. 1, pp. 74–77, 2010.

[16] T. Piepho, C. Werner, and R. R. Noppens, "Evaluation of the novel, single-use, flexible aScope for tracheal intubation in the simulated difficult airway and first clinical experiences," *Anaesthesia*, vol. 65, no. 8, pp. 820–825, 2010.

[17] K. Aoyama, E. Yasunaga, I. Takenaka, T. Kadoya, T. Sata, and A. Shigematsu, "Positive pressure ventilation during fibreoptic intubation: comparison of the laryngeal mask airway, intubating laryngeal mask and endoscopy mask techniques," *British Journal of Anaesthesia*, vol. 88, no. 2, pp. 246–254, 2002.

[18] F. Hammarskjöld, G. Lindskog, and P. Blomqvist, "An alternative method to intubate with laryngeal mask and see-through-bougie," *Acta Anaesthesiologica Scandinavica*, vol. 43, no. 6, pp. 634–636, 1999.

13

Venous Air Embolism Leading to Cardiac Arrest in an Infant with Cyanotic Congenital Heart Disease

Scott C. Watkins, Lewis McCarver, Alicia VanBebber, and David P. Bichell

Monroe Carell Jr. Children's Hospital at Vanderbilt, Vanderbilt University Medical Center, Nashville, N 37232, USA

Correspondence should be addressed to Scott C. Watkins, scott.watkins@vanderbilt.edu

Academic Editors: A. T. Han, C.-H. Hsing, P. Michalek, and D. A. Story

Gas emboli, including venous and arterial, are a rare but important complication of pediatric cardiac surgery. They have the potential to have devastating consequences and require prompt recognition and treatment. We present a case of gas embolism occurring in the immediate postoperative period in an infant with cyanotic congenital heart disease after palliative cardiac surgery resulting in cardiopulmonary arrest. The embolism was diagnosed by visualization of air within the vessel creating an airlock and occluding pulmonary blood flow.

1. Introduction

Venous and arterial gas emboli are a known and potentially devastating complication of surgical and nonsurgical procedures. Classically associated with neurosurgical procedures performed in the sitting position [1], advances in monitoring and improved awareness of gas embolism have broadened the scope of the problem to include many different surgical and nonsurgical procedures [2]. The number of novel etiologies for gas embolism is large and constantly expanding as technological advances improve recognition and increase the incidence of the problem. Gas emboli in pediatric cardiac surgery have been previously observed during central venous cannulation [3, 4], during sternotomy [5], while opening the heart chambers during cardiopulmonary bypass [6], and due to disconnects in the extracorporeal circuit [6]. We describe an unusual presentation of gas embolism occurring in the immediate postoperative period in an infant with cyanotic congenital heart disease after palliative cardiac surgery resulting in cardiopulmonary arrest.

2. Case Description

The patient was a 3-month-old male with cyanotic congenital heart disease consisting of double outlet right ventricle, near absent intraventricular septum, and aortic arch hypoplasia, who had previously undergone a Norwood stage I palliation with 3.5 mm modified Blalock-Taussig shunt (see Figure 1). He presented at 3 months of age for the next stage of palliation, a cavopulmonary anastomosis (bidirectional Glenn). His weight was 5.8 kg (31% percentile) and height was 58 cm (18% percentile). Pulse oximetry demonstrated O_2 saturations of 70 to 80%, which was appropriate for his lesion. Cardiac catheterization findings included a widely patent arch with estimated normal pulmonary artery (PA) pressures (mean of 12 mmHg in the RPA) by reverse pulmonary vein wedge, a BT shunt widely patent and arising from the innominate artery with flow to the branch pulmonary arteries. The preoperative CXR was unremarkable except for prior sternotomy. A preoperative echocardiogram demonstrated the above described anatomy, insignificant atrioventricular valve insufficiency, a patent modified Blalock-Taussig shunt, and patent proximal branch PA's.

Anesthesia was induced with fentanyl 50 mcg and pancuronium 1 mg, after premedication with intravenous midazolam 1 mg. After endotracheal intubation, anesthesia was maintained with a balanced anesthetic consisting of end tidal isoflurane concentrations of 0.4% and high-dose fentanyl (~100 mcg/kg) in air/oxygen mixture. A left subclavian central venous catheter was placed after induction. A right femoral arterial line was in place from earlier heart

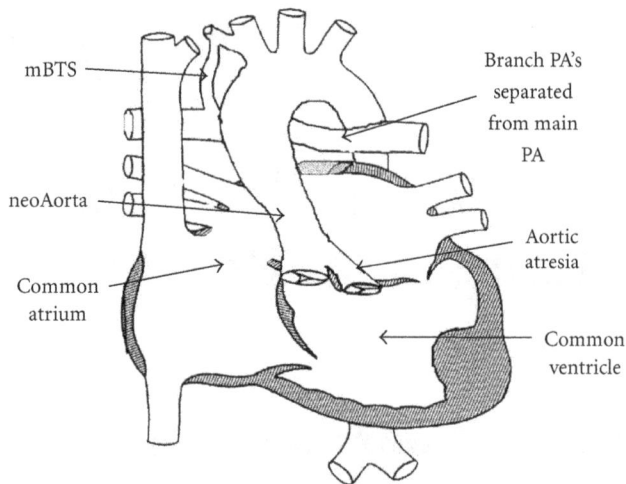

FIGURE 1: Preoperative anatomy (mBTS: modified Blalock-Taussig Shunt; PA: pulmonary artery).

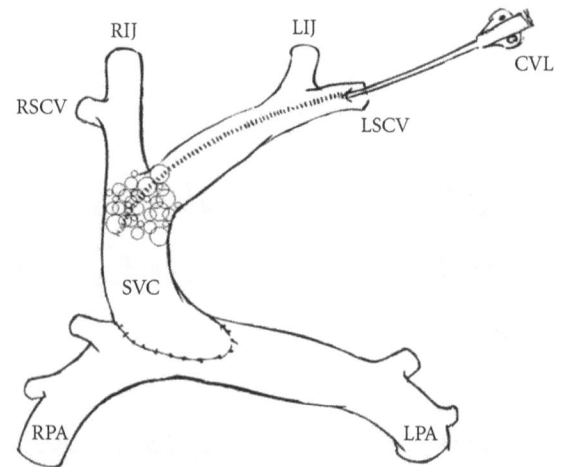

FIGURE 2: Depiction of surgical anastomosis with air bubbles at SVC-PA junction. (RSCV: right superior cava vein; LSCV: left superior cava vein; CVL: central venous line; RIJ: right internal jugular; LIJ: left internal jugular; SVC: superior vena cava; RPA: right pulmonary artery; LPA: left pulmonary artery).

catheterization. The patient tolerated anesthetic induction, placement of invasive lines and monitors and the pre-incision period with stable hemodynamics. In addition to standard ASA monitors, bilateral cerebral and somatic oximetry (Somanetics INVOS) was monitored throughout the case. Transesophageal echocardiography (TEE) was not used. It is not our practice to use TEE for cavopulmonary anastomosis procedures or procedures in which the cardiac chambers are not opened.

Cardiopulmonary bypass (CPB) commenced with bicaval venous cannulation at the inferior vena cava-right atrial (IVC-RA) junction and the innominate vein. The modified Blalock-Taussig shunt was ligated and divided at the initiation of cardiopulmonary bypass. The azygous vein was divided and the superior vena cava was separated from the right atrium. The bidirectional cavopulmonary anastomosis was constructed. The patient was weaned from CPB on dopamine (initially at 5 mcg/kg/min, range 0–5 mcg/kg/min) and milrinone (0.5 mcg/kg/min). Nitroprusside 0.5 mcg/kg/min, titrated to effect, was used briefly for a period of hypertension. Dexmedetomidine (0.7 mcg/kg/hr) was started during rewarming for post-op sedation. After successfully separating from cardiopulmonary bypass, O_2 saturations were near 100% and the transpulmonary gradient (CVP-LAP) was 8 to 9 mmHg. The left subclavian venous line tip was visible in the superior vena cava, near the innominate vein-superior vena cava (SVC) junction. Modified ultrafiltration was performed, protamine administered, and routine decannulation and sternotomy closure were performed. The cardiopulmonary bypass time was 36 minutes.

During the postbypass period the patient had stable vital signs with invasive blood pressures (IBPs) of ~90/40, heart rates (HRs) of ~150, oxygen saturations of 80–90% on 100% FiO_2, central venous pressures (CVPs) of 12, and transpulmonary gradient (CVP-LAP) of 7–9 mmHg. Cerebral and

somatic saturations were unchanged from baseline and the prebypass period.

Preparations were being made to transport the patient to the ICU when a sudden drop in SpO_2 to the 60's, a sudden rise in CVP to the mid 20's, ST segment elevation, and an acute change in the patient's color (head and face became profoundly plethoric) were noted. $EtCO_2$ was also markedly decreased although there was no change in ventilation. Bradycardia soon followed as oxygen saturations continued to decline. Cardiopulmonary resuscitation (CPR) was immediately started with chest compressions and administration of resuscitative drugs. Preparations for reopening the chest and initiating cardiopulmonary bypass (CPB) were made while CPR continued. Profound hypoxemia persisted despite good quality CPR, confirmed with an arterial pulse with compressions and adequate ventilation.

The chest was reopened during the administration of CPR with no evidence of tamponade. On examination of the superior vena cava, an abundant collection of air bubbles was visible through the wall of the vein, appearing to fill the entire superior vena cava from the pulmonary anastomosis to the innominate vein (see Figure 2). A needle was placed in the superior vena cava and a large amount of air escaped through the needle hole. Myocardial function had begun to decline despite some improvement in oxygenation, so the patient was placed emergently on cardiopulmonary bypass. Sixteen minutes had elapsed since hemodynamic collapse and initiation of full CPB. No air bubbles in the systemic circulation were observed at aortic cannulation, offering some assurance that the emboli were confined to the cavopulmonary circuit. Approximately 3 mL of air was aspirated from the SVC while the patient was on CPB. The patient was separated from cardiopulmonary bypass after 36 minutes, with hemodynamics nearly identical to those before arrest, the exception being slightly lower oxygen saturations, 80–85%. During the bypass period, efforts were made to determine the source of the emboli and prevent further expansion, but no definitive source was ever discovered. Unfortunately, echocardiography was not used during the initial procedure, so it was not available at the time of the arrest.

The patient remained stable after the second bypass period and tolerated chest closure. Systemic hypothermia was initiated Intra-op and continued for 24 hours post-op with a target temperature of 34-35°C. He was taken to the PICU in stable condition. The patient did well over the remainder of his hospital course with no discernible neurological or cardiovascular sequelae of the arrest and was discharged to home on POD 10.

3. Discussion

Gas emboli are relatively uncommon, but not rare occurrences in the setting of pediatric cardiac surgery and usually occur during central venous cannulation, during sternotomy, while opening the heart chambers during cardiopulmonary bypass, or due to disconnects in the extracorporeal circuit. This patient's complex anatomy and the timing of events, with the arrest occurring after surgical closure, make this case unusual. Patients with cavopulmonary connections have passive pulmonary circulation and are dependent on venous return from the superior vena cava for all pulmonary blood flow. In this patient, the venous air embolism caused complete obstruction to pulmonary blood flow resulting in cardiopulmonary arrest. In patients with cavopulmonary anastomosis, venous return from the upper extremities and the head drain via the SVC to the pulmonary circuit, while blood return from the lower extremity and viscera drain via the IVC to the heart. This separation of venous return from the upper and lower body allowed us to narrow the source of air embolism to the upper compartment. Possible sources include the left subclavian central line or upper extremity intravenous line, accumulation of air from multiple medication injections throughout the case, residual air in the SVC from the anastomosis, or air trapped in the pulmonary arterial tree during the CPB period. Due to the acuteness of the arrest, we believe that it was a sudden bolus or entrainment of air from an intravascular line rather than an accumulation or residual air, although we are not aware of such a bolus of air occurring. We meticulously inspected all intravenous tubing following the arrest for loose connections, cracks, or disconnects that might have allowed air to be entrained but found none. We think residual air from the surgical procedure or air that might have been introduced during CPB, would have long since passed and is an unlikely source.

The event occurred as the child was being prepared for transport from the OR to the ICU, which is a time when the anesthesia provider is distracted by the act of transferring multiple lines, monitors, and critical medical equipment. During this period of time, vigilance may be diminished, and the anesthesia provider may be distracted by the multitasking required to prepare the patient for transport. Yet, this remains one of the more critical times during the case, as the patient's anesthetic requirements and hemodynamic parameters may be fluctuating requiring titration of

anesthetic levels and hemodynamic infusions. The anesthesia providers caring for this patient were experienced in caring for children with congenital heart disease and are cognizant of the need to de-air tubing and the need to aspirate for air prior to injecting, but it is possible that due to distraction or diminished vigilance air may have been injected or infused unnoticed.

A potential source that was explored was the pressure bag attached to the transducer for the CVP line. It has been our practice to leave the drip chamber half full to allow visualization of fluid dripping when the transducer is flushed. We also use the CVP transducer port as a medication push port and flush medications by using the pig tail on the transducer. If the pressure bag is inverted, as might occur as a patient is being transported, this can allow the air in the drip chamber to be flushed into the patient.

In summary, gas emboli are a rare but important complication of pediatric cardiac surgery, as they may have devastating consequences. This is an unusual case of gas embolism involving a patient with single ventricle physiology after cavopulmonary connection leading to complete obstruction to pulmonary blood flow and cardiopulmonary arrest. Venous air embolism has not previously been reported as a cause of hypoxia following cavopulmonary connection. The exact etiology and source of the emboli in our patient remains unknown although presumably it was introduced into the circulation via an intravascular catheter. Prevention of gas emboli requires vigilance on the part of the entire perioperative team. Successful outcomes depend on prompt recognition and aggressive treatment, with the goal of treatment being to reduce the size of the embolus and minimize end-organ damage. In this case, resuscitation and outcome was successful due to the immediate recognition, good quality CPR and immediate access to hypothermic CPB.

References

[1] S. C. Palmon, L. E. Moore, J. Lundberg, and T. Toung, "Venous air embolism: a review," *Journal of Clinical Anesthesia*, vol. 9, no. 3, pp. 251–257, 1997.

[2] M. A. Mirski, A. V. Lele, L. Fitzsimmons, and T. J. K. Toung, "Diagnosis and treatment of vascular air embolism," *Anesthesiology*, vol. 106, no. 1, pp. 164–177, 2007.

[3] C. H. Leicht and J. Waldman, "Pulmonary air embolism in the pediatric patient undergoing central catheter placement: a report of two cases," *Anesthesiology*, vol. 64, no. 4, pp. 519–521, 1986.

[4] S. M. Bhananker, D. W. Liau, P. K. Kooner, K. L. Posner, R. A. Caplan, and K. B. Domino, "Liability related to peripheral venous and arterial catheterization: a closed claims analysis," *Anesthesia and Analgesia*, vol. 109, no. 1, pp. 124–129, 2009.

[5] I. Keidan, Y. Mardor, S. Preisman, and D. Mishaly, "Venous embolization during sternotomy in children undergoing corrective heart surgery," *Journal of Thoracic and Cardiovascular Surgery*, vol. 128, no. 4, pp. 636–638, 2004.

[6] P. K. Neema, S. Pathak, P. K. Varma et al., "Case 2-2007 systemic air embolization after termination of cardiopulmonary bypass," *Journal of Cardiothoracic and Vascular Anesthesia*, vol. 21, no. 2, pp. 288–297, 2007.

14

Prothrombin Complex Concentrate for Rapid Reversal of Warfarin Anticoagulation to Allow Neuraxial Blockade

Conor Skerritt and Stephen Mannion

Department of Anaesthesia, South Infirmary, Victoria University Hospital, Old Blackrock Road, Cork, Ireland

Correspondence should be addressed to Conor Skerritt; skerritc@tcd.ie

Academic Editors: R. S. Gomez, L. Hebbar, D. Lee, and J.-j. Yang

The development of Prothrombin Complex Concentrates (PCCs) has led to better outcomes in patients receiving emergency reversal of warfarin. However, most published data describes the use of PCCs in the setting of major bleeding or emergent major surgery, with little information on neuraxial blockade. We describe a case of rapid warfarin reversal using PCC and subsequent surgery under spinal anaesthesia in an 87-year-old lady, for whom general anaesthesia was deemed high risk. Her international normalised ratio (INR) on the morning of surgery was 1.8, precluding neuraxial blockade; however, it was felt that given, the need for imminent surgery, immediate reversal of the warfarin was indicated. We administered a single dose of 23 units/kg PCC and 5 mg vitamin K. Her INR 1 hour following PCC was 1.2, and spinal anesthetic was administered. The patient then underwent excision of melanoma deposits from her leg and groin dissection. There were no complications, the patient recovered satisfactorily, and there were no thrombotic or hemorrhagic events at 30 days postoperatively. This case study demonstrates a novel use of PCCs; in certain patients, PCCs may be safely used for immediate reversal of warfarin to allow for neuraxial blockade, safer anaesthesia, and better outcomes.

1. Introduction

The development of Prothrombin Complex Concentrates (PCCs) has led to better outcomes in patients receiving emergency reversal of warfarin anticoagulation [1–4]. However, most of the published data describes the use of PCCs in the setting of major bleeding or emergent major abdominal surgery, with a dearth of information on neuraxial blockade. We describe a case of rapid warfarin reversal using PCC and subsequent surgery under spinal anaesthesia, with a good surgical outcome and no thrombotic or haemorrhagic events at 30 days.

2. Case/Methods

An 87-year-old lady was scheduled for urgent palliative removal of malignant melanoma and satellite lesions from her lower leg and ipsilateral groin dissection for metastatic disease. Her background history included atrial fibrillation which was rate controlled (digoxin) and required anticoagulation (warfarin). Her background also included mitral regurgitation, hypertension, and hypothyroidism. As her mobility was severely limited by osteoarthritis of the hip, it was difficult to clinically establish her exercise tolerance, and it was decided that she would be more suitable for neuraxial blockade than general anaesthesia. She was instructed to discontinue warfarin for 4 days prior to her planned surgery, which she did. However, on the day of her planned procedure, her international normalised ratio (INR) was 1.8. A decision was made to rapidly reverse her anticoagulation and proceed with the surgery under spinal anaesthesia. Postponing her surgery would have caused a delay of a number of days, due to the specifics of scheduling her case, and it was felt that, given the existing tumour burden, a delay of this magnitude was not acceptable.

A decision was made that rapid reversal of anticoagulation was needed and that, based on current evidence in medical literature, a combination of intravenous vitamin K and

PCC would be most effective [5]. 5 mg intravenous vitamin K was given as a slow bolus, and using the hospital's protocol regarding the administration of blood products, 1500 units of Octaplex (PCC containing factors II, VII, IX, X, and proteins C and S) were given over 35 minutes. The total volume of this solution was 60 mL. The patient's INR was rechecked 1 hour following completion of the PCC infusion and was found to be 1.2, within the acceptable recommended range (i.e., <1.5) [6]. A single shot spinal anaesthesia was performed by an experienced anesthesiologist, with the patient in the sitting position. Using an $L_{4/5}$ paramedian approach and a 22 G spinal needle, 1.5 mL 0.5% heavy bupivacaine and 25 μg of fentanyl were injected intrathecally in an atraumatic fashion (first pass, CSF identified, and no blood seen).

3. Results

The block was then clinically evaluated, and, finding good blockade (loss of temperature sensation at T_{10}), surgery was commenced. The patient did not receive any hypnotic or sedative medication in the perioperative period.

The surgery carried out was a right sided groin dissection, excision of melanoma deposits from right lower leg, split skin graft, and diathermy ablation of melanoma satellite lesions. The surgery was uncomplicated, intraoperative blood loss was minimal (<250 mL), and the sensory blockade was adequate. The duration of surgery was approximately 100 minutes.

Examination of the patient at 60 minutes postoperatively (160 minutes after spinal) revealed return of gross motor function to both lower limbs and sensation at T_{10}. Further examination at 250 minutes postoperatively (310 minutes after spinal) revealed full return of motor function and full sensation in both lower limbs, with a pain score of 3/10 on oral analgesics. The patient received her usual dose of warfarin that evening.

At 30-day followup, there were no thrombotic or haemorrhagic events, the surgical wounds were satisfactory, and the skin graft was intact.

4. Discussion

Prothrombin Complex Concentrates (PCCs) are pooled plasma products which contain a mixture of vitamin K dependent clotting factors. Originally designed for the treatment of haemophilias, they are now used for reversal of coagulopathies of the vitamin K dependent pathways, both congenital and acquired or iatrogenic. PCC has been used to rapidly correct various abnormalities of coagulation in patients with haemorrhage or the need for immediate surgical or invasive medical intervention [1–4]. It has been found to be superior to vitamin K alone in the reversal of the effects of warfarin [7]. However, there is little published evidence regarding the use of PCC for reversal of warfarin prior to spinal anaesthesia or other forms of neuraxial anaesthesia. Single shot spinal anaesthesia in the presence of coagulopathy has been classified as "very high risk" by the American Society of Regional Anaesthesia (ASRA), the European Society of Regional Anaesthesia (ESRA), and the Association of Anaesthetists of Great Britain and Ireland (AAGBI) and, as such, should not be attempted with an INR >1.4.

The optimal dose of PCC for the rapid reversal of warfarin has been extensively investigated, and numerous data on the subject have been published [7–9]. Mean doses in these articles of research have ranged from 12 units/kg to 28.5 units/kg. The recommendations of the manufacturer are as follows [10]: in a patient whose INR is 2–2.5, normalisation of INR (i.e., INR ≤1.2) within 1 hour may be achieved with a single dose of 0.9–1.3 mL/kg, which equates to 22.5–32.5 units/kg. However, our patient's initial INR was 1.8, and the manufacturer's published data did not refer to INRs of <2.0. Therefore, the manufacturer's recommendations were used as guidelines and interpreted alongside other published data. Our patient received a single dose of 23 units/kg. This not only reflects the data we extrapolated from the manufacturer's guidelines, but also reflects the more recently published articles on the matter.

The usefulness of contemporaneous vitamin K with PCC to achieve more timely reversal of anticoagulation has also been described [5], and it is for this reason that we included it as part of our treatment.

The rapid reversal of anticoagulation will, of course, predispose the patient to thrombotic events (stroke, coronary ischemia, peripheral ischemia, and disseminated intravascular coagulation), but the likelihood of these depends also on the initial indication for anticoagulation, as well as the dose of PCC given. Other potential adverse effects include hypersensitivity, headache, transmitted viral illnesses, and transient hepatic transaminitis. Our patient was anticoagulated because she had atrial fibrillation, and although her relative risk of a thrombotic event was high if she was not anticoagulated [11], a brief window of normal INR was estimated to be low risk, and, indeed, at 30 days after intervention, there were no thrombotic events in our case study.

5. Conclusion

In conclusion, our case study demonstrates that Prothrombin Complex Concentrate (PCC), as a single dose of 23 units/kg, can be used to acutely reverse the anticoagulant effect of warfarin, such that effective spinal anaesthesia may be safely administered. The novel usage of this well-established product means that neuraxial blockade may be administered in cases where the risk of bleeding complications would previously have precluded its use, thus allowing for safer anaesthesia and better outcomes for our patients.

Authors' Contribution

Conor Skerritt attests that this paper is his own creation; he gathered the necessary information, obtained consent from the patient, followed up the patient, created the first drafts, researched the reference material, and submitted it for publication; he was also involved in the clinical decision making at the time of the procedure. Stephen Mannion attests that he oversaw creation of this paper, edited the drafts, performed the procedure in question, and was involved in the clinical decision making at the time of the procedure.

References

[1] J. Huhtakangas, S. Tetri, S. Juvela et al., "Improved survival of patients with warfarin-associated intracerebral hemorrhage: a retrospective longitudinal population-based study," *International Journal of Stroke*, 2012.

[2] J. A. Quick, A. N. Bartels, J. P. Coughenour, and S. L. Barnes, "Experience with prothrombin complex for the emergent reversal of anticoagulation in rural geriatric trauma patients," *Surgery*, vol. 152, no. 4, pp. 722–726, 2012.

[3] S. Jalini, A. Y. Jin, and S. W. Taylor, "Reversal of warfarin anticoagulation with prothrombin complex concentrate before thrombolysis for acute stroke," *Cerebrovascular Diseases*, vol. 33, no. 6, article 597, 2012.

[4] Y. Wong, "Use of prothrombin complex concentrate for vitamin K antagonist reversal before surgical treatment of intracranial hemorrhage," *Clinical Medicine Insights*, vol. 4, pp. 1–6, 2011.

[5] M. Yasaka, T. Sakata, H. Naritomi, and K. Minematsu, "Optimal dose of prothrombin complex concentrate for acute reversal of oral anticoagulation," *Thrombosis Research*, vol. 115, no. 6, pp. 455–459, 2005.

[6] Regional Anaesthesia in Patients with Abnormalities in Coagulation http://www.aagbi.org/sites/default/files/RAPAC%20for%20consultation.pdf.

[7] S. A. Chapman, E. D. Irwin, A. L. Beal, N. M. Kulinski, K. E. Hutson, and M. A. Thorson, "Prothrombin complex concentrate versus standard therapies for INR reversal in trauma patients receiving warfarin," *Annals of Pharmacotherapy*, vol. 45, no. 7-8, pp. 869–875, 2011.

[8] P. Toth, J. J. Van Veen, K. Robinson et al., "Real world usage of PCC to "rapidly" correct warfarin induced coagulopathy," *Blood Transfusion*, vol. 11, no. 4, pp. 500–505, 2012.

[9] M. Wozniak, A. Kruit, R. Padmore, A. Giulivi, and J. Bormanis, "Prothrombin complex concentrate for the urgent reversal of warfarin. Assessment of a standard dosing protocol," *Transfusion and Apheresis Science*, vol. 46, no. 3, pp. 309–314, 2012.

[10] Summary of Product Characteristics and dosing suggestions for OCTAPLEX http://www.octapharma.ca/fileadmin/user_upload/octapharma.ca/20120613_PM_Octaplex_approved.pdf.

[11] "Cerebral Embolism Task Force. Cardiogenic brain embolism," *Archives of Neurology*, vol. 43, no. 1, pp. 71–84, 1986.

15

Sympathetic Blocks Provided Sustained Pain Relief in a Patient with Refractory Painful Diabetic Neuropathy

Jianguo Cheng,[1] Anuj Daftari,[2] and Lan Zhou[3]

[1] Department of Pain Management, Cleveland Clinic, 9500 Euclid Avenue, Cleveland, OH 44195, USA
[2] Department of Physical Medicine and Rehabilitation, Metrohealth Medical Center, 2500 Metrohealth Drive, Cleveland, OH 44109, USA
[3] Department of Neurology, Cleveland Clinic, 9500 Euclid Avenue, Cleveland, OH 44195, USA

Correspondence should be addressed to Jianguo Cheng, chengj@ccf.org

Academic Editor: A. Apan

The sympathetic nervous system has been implicated in pain associated with painful diabetic neuropathy. However, therapeutic intervention targeted at the sympathetic nervous system has not been established. We thus tested the hypothesis that sympathetic nerve blocks significantly reduce pain in a patient with painful diabetic neuropathy who has failed multiple pharmacological treatments. The diagnosis of small fiber sensory neuropathy was based on clinical presentations and confirmed by skin biopsies. A series of 9 lumbar sympathetic blocks over a 26-month period provided sustained pain relief in his legs. Additional thoracic paravertebral blocks further provided control of the pain in the trunk which can occasionally be seen in severe diabetic neuropathy cases, consequent to extensive involvement of the intercostal nerves. These blocks provided sustained and significant pain relief and improvement of quality of life over a period of more than two years. We thus provided the first clinical evidence supporting the notion that sympathetic nervous system plays a critical role in painful diabetic neuropathy and sympathetic blocks can be an effective management modality of painful diabetic neuropathy. We concluded that the sympathetic nervous system is a valuable therapeutic target of pharmacological and interventional modalities of treatments in painful diabetic neuropathy patients.

1. Introduction

Diabetic polyneuropathy is one of the most common forms of peripheral neuropathy. It afflicts patients of both type 1 and type 2 diabetes with an increased prevalence as the disease progresses [1–3]. Up to 50% of all diabetics with long-duration diabetes have polyneuropathy which is a major cause of morbidity and is associated with increased mortality. Up to 26% of diabetics develop painful diabetic neuropathy (PDN) with debilitating effects on quality of life [4–6]. Management of PDN remains an enormous challenge to both the patients and the clinicians as we have recently reviewed [7]. The current strategy includes mandatory glycemic control and pain control by pharmacological treatment with local anesthetic patches, anticonvulsants, tricyclic antidepressants, selective serotonin and noradrenalin reuptake inhibitors, and/or opioids. Spinal cord stimulation has been tested in a few studies involving a small number of highly selected patients who failed to respond to conservative treatments, with some degree of positive effects [8, 9]. However, the pain control of diabetic neuropathy remains a daunting challenge and the overall outcomes of the current management of diabetic neuropathy are not satisfactory.

Although diabetic polyneuropathy is clinically known for over a century, the pathophysiological mechanisms were only recently better understood. It is recognized that the microvascular dysfunction, secondary to chronic hyperglycemia and dyslipidemia, is a common pathophysiological basis of polyneuropathy and other microvascular complications with diabetes. There is also evidence that the sympathetic nervous system may play an important role in painful diabetic neuropathy. Circulating norepinephrine is higher in painful than painless diabetic neuropathy, and its concentration is correlated with the severity of neuropathic pain [10]. Thus, painful diabetic neuropathy is suggested to be associated with a relatively higher number of functioning

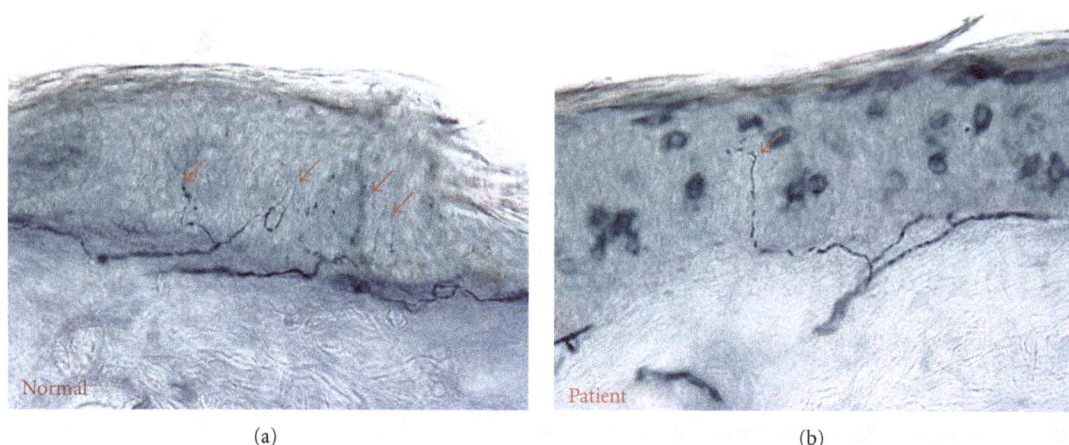

FIGURE 1: PGP9.5 immunostaining of skin biopsies at the distal leg. The patient with painful diabetic neuropathy (b) showed reduced intraepidermal nerve fibers (red arrow), in comparison to a normal subject (a) who showed many intraepidermal nerve fibers (red arrows).

sympathetic fibers that may contribute to pain. Damaged peripheral nerves became hyperexcitable through abnormal electrical connections that may have resulted in ephaptic transmission or "crosstalking" between sensory and sympathetic nerve fibers [11, 12]. Indeed, norepinephrine excited the ongoing ephaptic activity in damaged peripheral nerves through activation of alpha receptors [11]. Furthermore, patients with PDN had impaired sympathetically mediated vasoconstriction, contributing to inappropriate local blood flow regulation in these patients [13].

Based on these observations, we hypothesized that sympathetic nerve blocks may reduce pain associated with diabetic neuropathy by reducing sympathetic outflow and improving circulation. We tested this hypothesis in a patient with severe PDN refractory to multiple pain medications by treating him with lumbar and thoracic sympathetic blocks. The diagnosis of small fiber sensory neuropathy was based on clinical presentations and confirmed by skin biopsies. A series of 9 lumbar sympathetic blocks over a 26-month period provided sustained pain relief in his legs. Additional thoracic paravertebral blocks further provided control of his pain in the trunk from dermatomes T6 to L1, consequent to extensive involvement of PDN. These blocks significantly improved his quality of life over a period of more than two years.

2. Case Report

The patient is a 37-year-old right-handed Caucasian man who was in his usual state of health until December 2006 when he started to notice that his feet were cold, numb, and had a tingling sensation (described as pins and needles) from the ankles down. In a few weeks, the tingling sensation progressed up to the knees which remained stable for the next three months. In April 2007, he also noted the tingling sensation in the arms.

At time of his presentation to our pain clinic and neurology clinic in October 2007, he reported diffuse constant tingling sensation, mostly involving his arms, legs, and face,

which was accompanied by sharp pains, mostly in the feet and distal legs. The pain was rated on average as an 8 on a numerical rating scale (NRS) (0 is no pain and 10 is most severe pain imaginable). He also reported episodic lower extremity allodynia to light touch and burning dysesthesia in his trunk and hands. These symptoms kept him up at night and disturbed his sleep. He began to experience symptoms of depression secondary to the relentless pain condition. He denies weakness. Physical examination at the time of presentation was significant for decreased light touch sensation and hyperalgesia to pinprick in a stocking-glove distribution. Motor strength, proprioception, and tendon reflexes were well preserved.

A nerve conduction study and electromyography was normal showing no evidence of a large fiber peripheral neuropathy or radiculopathy. We further conducted skin biopsies at the distal leg (DL), distal thigh (DT), and proximal thigh (PT) in the Cleveland Clinic Cutaneous Nerve Laboratory and carried out intraepidermal nerve fiber density (IENFD) analysis as previously described [14, 15]. Intraepidermal nerve fiber density was significantly reduced at the distal leg as compared to normal control (Figure 1), which indicates a distal small fiber sensory neuropathy. The neuropathy etiology evaluation was significant for diabetes mellitus as revealed by oral glucose tolerance test with a 2-hour glucose level being 220 mg/dL. ESR, ANA, ENA, rheumatoid factor, ACE level, ANCAs, TSH, free T4, serum and urine immunofixation, folic acid, vitamin B12, RPR, Lyme serology, and heavy metal screen were all unremarkable.

He was diagnosed with painful diabetic small fiber sensory neuropathy and started on Glucophage. In terms of his neuropathic pain control, however, he had failed to respond to multiple pain medications, including Topiramate, Oxcarbazepine, Duloxetine, Amitriptyline, Darvocet, Tramadol, and Lidocaine transdermal patches. Gabapentin only offered minimal pain relief. Given the unsatisfactory outcomes of conservative treatment, we decided to try a lumbar sympathetic block for his pain and allodynia in the low extremities. We used the classic approach for

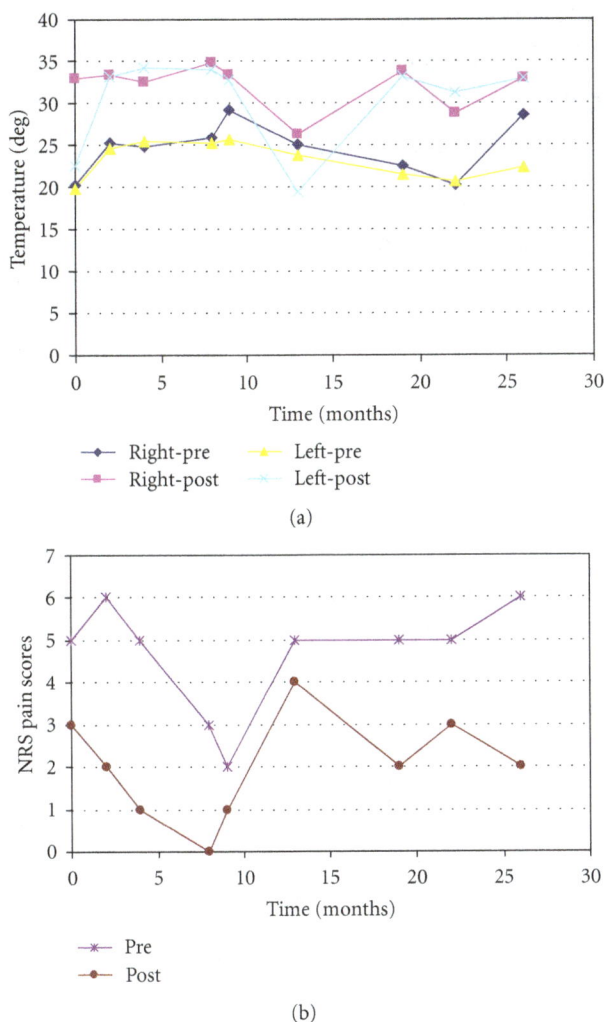

FIGURE 2: Sympathetic block-induced changes in temperature and NRS pain scores. (a) The peak temperatures, monitored at the plantar surface of the toes with an electronics device, increased significantly in both sides after bilateral lumbar sympathetic blocks (post) compared to the baseline values taken before the blocks (pre). (b) The NRS pain scores, evaluated in the preprocedure room before the blocks (pre) and in the recovery room after the block (post), decreased significantly after each lumbar sympathetic block.

bilateral lumbar sympathetic block at the level of L3 under fluoroscopic guidance and injected a mixture of 12 mL of 1% Lidocaine and 20 mg Triamcinolone on each side. The temperatures, monitored in the plantar surface of the big toes (LS 14000 Temperature Monitor and Skin Temperature Probe, NovaMed, NY, USA), increased significantly, and NRS pain scores decreased substantially after the procedure as shown in Table 1 (initial block) and Figure 2.

At his 2-month followup, the patient reported "excellent" relief of his foot pain bilaterally for over 6 weeks, but became more cognizant of his thoracic and hand pain. A decision was made to proceed with a repeat lumbar sympathetic block to further enhance the pain relief. Subsequent temperature and pain score changes were again noted as shown in Table 1 (2 months) and Figure 2. Management of his thoracic pain was

further considered at the following office visit. At a follow-up visit 4 weeks later, the patient again reported "significant, sustained" relief of his bilateral foot pain. He felt "dramatic" improvement of the "coldness and tingling pain" with the first injection with sustained relief that was further enhanced with the second procedure.

At this point, his chief complaint became the "hypersensitive, pins and needles, burning" thoracic and abdominal pain that was described as occupying a discrete antero-/posteroarea of his thorax, roughly covering the T6 to the L1 dermatomes. Physical examination, as previously described, was significant only for bilateral lower extremity stocking-distribution decrease in sensation to light touch and pinprick. He returned 2 weeks later for a T8 bilateral paravertebral sympathetic nerve block, which was performed in the classic fashion, under fluoroscopic guidance. A solution of 1% Lidocaine 10 mL and 20 mg Triamcinolone was injected on each side. The patient was maintained on the same doses of Gabapentin and Tramadol. Upon his return to the clinic 4 weeks later, he reported "70%" relief of his thoracic pain following his T8 paravertebral block. By this point, his bilateral foot pain was 5 on the NRS three months following his second lumbar sympathetic block; therefore, a third bilateral lumbar sympathetic block was performed (Table 1, 4 months). Pain medications remained the same, and the patient was followed up in three months.

Over the next two years, the patient continued to have lower extremity neuropathic pain as described above with good, sustained pain relief after each of subsequent lumbar sympathetic blocks. The intervals of each block are shown in Table 1 (Figure 2) with the corresponding temperature changes and the NRS pre- and postblock pain scores. He additionally underwent two thoracic paravertebral blocks at the T6 level in April and May of 2010 with good relief following each procedure. The remainder of his clinical course was uneventful.

3. Discussion

We observed that lumbar and thoracic sympathetic nerve blocks significantly improved the circulations and reduced neuropathic pain in this patient with diabetic small fiber sensory neuropathy. The analgesic effects are reproducible upon repeated blocks and are long-lasting (sustained 2–4 months after each block). These observations support the notion that the sympathetic nervous system plays a critical role in the pathophysiological mechanisms of painful diabetic polyneuropathy. This case report thus provides the first clinical evidence supporting the notion that the pain in diabetic neuropathy may be sympathetically mediated to a significant extent that has not been recognized previously. Given the sustained pain relief after each sympathetic block, the sympathetic nervous system may prove to be an important therapeutic target of pharmacological and interventional treatments for painful diabetic neuropathy.

Painful diabetic neuropathy is a relatively common medical condition, which can predominantly affect small sensory nerve fibers [16]. Glucose dysmetabolism, including diabetes and prediabetes, is present in about 1/3 of patients with

TABLE 1: Sympathetic block-induced changes in temperature and NRS pain score.

| Number of blocks (months after initial block) | Temperature | | | | NRS | |
| | Right toe | | Left toe | | | |
	Pre	Post	Pre	Post	Pre	Post
1 Initial	20.2	33.0	19.7	22.6	5	3
2 (2)	25.3	33.4	24.5	33.2	6	2
3 (4)	24.8	32.6	25.4	34.2	5	1
4 (8)	25.9	34.8	25.2	33.9	3	0
5 (9)	29.2	33.4	25.7	32.7	2	1
6 (13)	24.9	26.3	23.7	19.4	5	4
7 (19)	22.5	33.7	21.5	33.2	5	2
8 (22)	20.2	28.7	20.6	31.3	5	3
9 (26)	28.5	33.0	22.2	33.0	6	2
Average	24.6	32.1	23.2	30.4	4.7	2

painful sensory neuropathy and nearly 50% of otherwise idiopathic small fiber neuropathy [17–20]. Neuropathic pain can be the presenting symptom of diabetes, as seen in this patient. It is one of the most distressing symptoms of diabetic polyneuropathy and the main reason for seeking medical attention. Typical of painful diabetic neuropathy sufferers, this patient experienced a progressive buildup of unpleasant sensory symptoms that include tingling or "pins and needles" (paresthesia), and/or pain characteristic of burning, shooting (like "electric shock" down the legs), lancinating (stabbing or knifelike), and deep aching quality. The patient also developed allodynia and hyperalgesia. Furthermore, the patient experienced pain extended from the lower limbs to the upper limbs and trunk and face, as sometimes seen in advanced cases. Consequently, the patient suffered disturbed sleep and depressive mood after multiple failures to pharmacological treatments.

The patient's neuropathy is consistent with small fiber sensory neuropathy based on his clinical features and skin biopsy findings. Additionally, the patient presented with thoracic and abdominal pain in a dermatomal distribution from T6 to L1 bilaterally. This form of pain can be seen in diabetic peripheral neuropathy although it is not very common [21, 22]. Because the pain in his feet and trunk was most debilitating, we targeted these areas by performing lumbar and thoracic sympathetic blocks. While lumbar sympathetic blocks have been widely used in treating patients with chronic pain conditions in the lower limbs such as complex regional pain syndromes [23–25], paravertebral blocks have predominantly been used for surgical and acute pain management [26]. We utilized the combination of the two blocks and successfully maintained control of the pain in both his legs and trunk for more than 2 years. The novel application of both techniques may thus represent a valuable addition to the armamentarium of interventional pain management.

Although the mechanism of how a mixture of a local anesthetic and a steroid medication can produce long-lasting pain relief is not completely understood as in the case of epidural steroid injections for radicular pain [27], it has been shown that steroids can block nociceptive input.

Corticosteroids suppress discharges in chronic neuromas and prevent ectopic discharge in experimental neuromas, likely through a direct action on cell membrane [28]. The application of methylprednisolone has been shown to block C-fibers but not $A\beta$ fibers [29]. Damaged nerve fibers often have high accumulation of expressed sodium channels that are particularly sensitive to local anesthetics such as Lidocaine [30]. Therefore, the sympathetic blocks with local anesthetics and steroids may provide pain relief through similar pharmacological actions on nociceptive fibers. Alternatively, the blocks may reduce sympathetic outflow and circulating norepinephrine, thereby diminishing alpha receptor stimulation of injured peripheral nerve fibers [11]. A third explanation for the pain relief may be due to a sympathectomy-induced improvement in microvascular circulation as indicated by the dramatic increase in temperature of the toes after the blocks (Figure 2), relieving ischemia of nociceptors. It has been recognized that, in addition to a direct toxic effect of glucose on nerve cells, the damage of the nerve structures is accompanied by a microvascular dysfunction, which damages the vasa nervorum. The latter is secondary to the oxidative stress caused by hyperglycemia and other metabolic/homeostatic disorders. This is consistent with the fact that neuropathy and neuropathic pain occur more often in patients whose diabetes is chronically poorly controlled and who also have other cardiovascular risk factors such as hypertension and hyperlipidemia.

While recognizing the limitations of a case study, the findings are evidently intriguing and justify further large-scale studies. Given the inefficiency of current treatment options [7, 31], search for new therapeutic modalities is particularly needed. Interventions targeting at the sympathetic nervous system and its receptors are likely to represent a novel direction of effective therapy.

Disclosure

This work has not been presented in any meetings or published in any forms.

References

[1] M. J. Young, A. J. M. Boulton, A. F. Macleod, D. R. R. Williams, and P. H. Sonksen, "A multicentre study of the prevalence of diabetic peripheral neuropathy in the United Kingdom hospital clinic population," *Diabetologia*, vol. 36, no. 2, pp. 150–154, 1993.

[2] J. Pirart, "Diabetes mellitus and its degenerative complications: a prospective study of 4,400 patients observed between 1947 and 1973," *Diabetes Care*, vol. 1, no. 3, pp. 168–188, 1979.

[3] S. Tesfaye, L. K. Stevens, J. M. Stephenson et al., "Prevalence of diabetic peripheral neuropathy and its relation to glycaemic control and potential risk factors: the EURODIAB IDDM Complications Study," *Diabetologia*, vol. 39, no. 11, pp. 1377–1384, 1996.

[4] M. Davies, S. Brophy, R. Williams, and A. Taylor, "The prevalence, severity, and impact of painful diabetic peripheral neuropathy in type 2 diabetes," *Diabetes Care*, vol. 29, no. 7, pp. 1518–1522, 2006.

[5] S. J. Benbow, M. E. Wallymahmed, and I. A. Macfarlane, "Diabetic peripheral neuropathy and quality of life," *QJM*, vol. 91, no. 11, pp. 733–737, 1998.

[6] S. Tesfaye and D. Selvarajah, "Recent advances in the pharmacological management of painful diabetic neuropathy," *The British Journal of Diabetes and Vascular Disease*, vol. 9, no. 6, pp. 283–287, 2009.

[7] W. Pluijms, F. Huygen, M. van Kleef et al., "Evidence-based interventional pain medicine according to clinical diagnoses 19: diabetic polyneuropathy," *Pain Practice*, vol. 11, no. 2, pp. 191–198, 2011.

[8] N. A. Mekhail, J. Cheng, S. Narouze, L. Kapural, M. N. Mekhail, and T. Deer, "Clinical applications of neurostimulation: forty years later," *Pain Practice*, vol. 10, no. 2, pp. 103–112, 2010.

[9] N. A. Mekhail, M. Mathews, F. Nageeb, M. Guirguis, M. N. Mekhail, and J. Cheng, "Retrospective review of 707 cases of spinal cord stimulation: indications and complications," *Pain Practice*, vol. 11, no. 2, pp. 148–153, 2011.

[10] C. Tsigos, P. Reed, C. Weinkove, A. White, and R. J. Young, "Plasma norepinephrine in sensory diabetic polyneuropathy," *Diabetes Care*, vol. 16, no. 5, pp. 722–727, 1993.

[11] P. D. Wall and M. Gutnick, "Ongoing activity in peripheral nerves: the physiology and pharmacology of impulses originating from a neuroma," *Experimental Neurology*, vol. 43, no. 3, pp. 580–593, 1974.

[12] Z. Seltzer and M. Devor, "Ephaptic transmission in chronically damaged peripheral nerves," *Neurology*, vol. 29, no. 7, pp. 1061–1064, 1979.

[13] C. Quattrini, N. D. Harris, R. A. Malik, and S. Tesfaye, "Impaired skin microvascular reactivity in painful diabetic neuropathy," *Diabetes Care*, vol. 30, no. 3, pp. 655–659, 2007.

[14] N. R. Holland, T. O. Crawford, P. Hauer, D. R. Cornblath, J. W. Griffin, and J. C. McArthur, "Small-fiber sensory neuropathies: cinical course and neuropathology of idiopathic cases," *Annals of Neurology*, vol. 44, no. 1, pp. 47–59, 1998.

[15] B. G. McCarthy, S. T. Hsieh, A. Stocks et al., "Cutaneous innervation in sensory neuropathies: evaluation by skin biopsy," *Neurology*, vol. 45, no. 10, pp. 1848–1855, 1995.

[16] J. Tavee and L. Zhou, "Small fiber neuropathy: a burning problem," *Cleveland Clinic Journal of Medicine*, vol. 76, no. 5, pp. 297–305, 2009.

[17] J. R. Singleton, A. G. Smith, and M. B. Bromberg, "Increased prevalence of impaired glucose tolerance in patients with painful sensory neuropathy," *Diabetes Care*, vol. 24, no. 8, pp. 1448–1453, 2001.

[18] S. P. Novella, S. E. Inzucchi, and J. M. Goldstein, "The frequency of undiagnosed diabetes and impaired glucose tolerance in patients with idiopathic sensory neuropathy," *Muscle and Nerve*, vol. 24, no. 9, pp. 1229–1231, 2001.

[19] A. G. Smith and J. R. Singleton, "The diagnostic yield of a standardized approach to idiopathic sensory-predominant neuropathy," *Archives of Internal Medicine*, vol. 164, no. 9, pp. 1021–1025, 2004.

[20] C. J. Sumner, S. Sheth, J. W. Griffin, D. R. Cornblath, and M. Polydefkis, "The spectrum of neuropathy in diabetes and impaired glucose tolerance," *Neurology*, vol. 60, no. 1, pp. 108–111, 2003.

[21] G. F. Longstreth, "Diabetic thoracic polyradiculopathy," *Best Practice and Research: Clinical Gastroenterology*, vol. 19, no. 2, pp. 275–281, 2005.

[22] V. Bansal, J. Kalita, and U. K. Misra, "Diabetic neuropathy," *Postgraduate Medical Journal*, vol. 82, no. 964, pp. 95–100, 2006.

[23] I. Carroll, J. D. Clark, and S. Mackey, "Sympathetic block with botulinum toxin to treat complex regional pain syndrome," *Annals of Neurology*, vol. 65, no. 3, pp. 348–351, 2009.

[24] F. van Eijs, M. Stanton-Hicks, J. Van Zundert et al., "Complex regional pain syndrome," *Pain Practice*, vol. 11, no. 1, pp. 70–87, 2011.

[25] K. M. Tran, S. M. Frank, S. N. Raja, H. K. El-Rahmany, L. J. Kim, and B. Vu, "Lumbar sympathetic block for sympathetically maintained pain: changes in cutaneous temperatures and pain perception," *Anesthesia and Analgesia*, vol. 90, no. 6, pp. 1396–1401, 2000.

[26] M. K. Karmakar, "Thoracic paravertebral block," *Anesthesiology*, vol. 95, no. 3, pp. 771–780, 2001.

[27] K. Van Boxem, J. Cheng, J. Patijn et al., "Evidence-based Interventional Pain Medicine according to clinical diagnoses 11: lumbar radicular pain," *Pain Practice*, vol. 10, pp. 339–358, 2010.

[28] M. Devor, R. Govrin-Lippmann, and P. Raber, "Corticosteroids suppress ectopic neural discharge originating in experimental neuromas," *Pain*, vol. 22, no. 2, pp. 127–137, 1985.

[29] A. Johansson and G. J. Bennett, "Effect of local methylprednisolone on pain in a nerve injury model a pilot study," *Regional Anesthesia*, vol. 22, no. 1, pp. 59–65, 1997.

[30] M. J. Craner, J. P. Klein, M. Renganathan, J. A. Black, and S. G. Waxman, "Changes of sodium channel expression in experimental painful diabetic neuropathy," *Annals of Neurology*, vol. 52, no. 6, pp. 786–792, 2002.

[31] A. Veves, M. Backonja, and R. A. Malik, "Painful diabetic neuropathy: epidemiology, natural history, early diagnosis, and treatment options," *Pain Medicine*, vol. 9, no. 6, pp. 660–674, 2008.

16

Negative Pressure Pulmonary Edema after Reversing Rocuronium-Induced Neuromuscular Blockade by Sugammadex

Manzo Suzuki,[1] **Toshiichiro Inagi,**[1] **Takehiko Kikutani,**[2] **Takuya Mishima,**[3] **and Hiroyasu Bito**[1]

[1] Department of Anesthesiology, Musashikosugi Hospital, Nippon Medical School, 1-396 Kosugi-cho, Nakahara-ku, Kanagawa 211-8533, Japan

[2] Department of Anesthesiology, Higashitotuka Memorial Hospital, 548-7 Shinano-cho, Totsuka-ku, Yokohama-shi, Kanagawa 244-0801, Japan

[3] Department of Surgery, Higashitotuka Memorial Hospital, 548-7 Shinano-cho, Totuka-ku, Yokohama-shi, Kanagawa 244-0801, Japan

Correspondence should be addressed to Manzo Suzuki; manzo@nms.ac.jp

Academic Editors: A. Han and T. Suzuki

Negative pressure pulmonary edema (NPPE) is a rare complication that accompanies general anesthesia, especially after extubation. We experienced a case of negative pressure pulmonary edema after tracheal extubation following reversal of rocuronium-induced neuromuscular blockade by sugammadex. In this case, the contribution of residual muscular block on the upper airway muscle as well as large inspiratory forces created by the respiratory muscle which has a low response to muscle relaxants, is suspected as the cause.

1. Introduction

Upper airway closure after tracheal extubation is a crucial event during general anesthesia. Postoperative negative pressure pulmonary edema is an uncommon but well-described complication of upper airway obstruction [1]. Most cases of NPPE develop under the presence of laryngospasm which occurs at the time of extubation due to incomplete recovery from anesthesia, secretion, or blood irritating the vocal cord [2].

Sugammadex, a modified gamma-cyclodextrin, is a novel selective agent that can reverse rocuronium-induced neuromuscular blockade [3]. It achieves reversal of muscle relaxation by complex formation with free muscle relaxant molecules. The manufacturer recommends administration of 2 mg/kg of sugammadex after the second twitch of train of four stimulation (TOF) is obtained and extubation after the presence of TOF ratio of over 0.9 [3]. We report a case of postoperative negative pressure pulmonary edema after reversal of muscle relaxation by sugammadex due to dissociated recovery from the neuromuscular agent between the

upper airway smooth muscle and respiratory muscles such as the diaphragm.

2. Case Report

A 41-year-old man with a weight of 70 kg and height of 163 cm underwent laparoscopic appendectomy for the diagnosis of acute appendicitis. He was generally healthy but had a history of asthma as a child. In the operating room, neuromuscular function was monitored using mechanomyography by train of four (TOF) built in the anesthesia monitor (S5 TM, GE Healthcare TM, Milwaukee, WI, USA). Calibration was performed at the right adductor pollicis. General anesthesia was induced by intravenous administration of propofol 120 mg and a bolus of remifentanil 0.05 mg followed by continuous infusion of remifentanil 0.2 µg/kg/min; rocuronium 60 mg facilitated tracheal intubation. Bilateral transversus abdominis plane (TAP) block using 0.375% ropivacaine (20 mL, each) was performed using the ultrasound technique. General anesthesia was maintained by sevoflurane 1–1.5% and continuous infusion of remifentanil 0.1-0.2 µg/kg/min, and an additional 10 mg bolus of rocuronium was given at the appearance

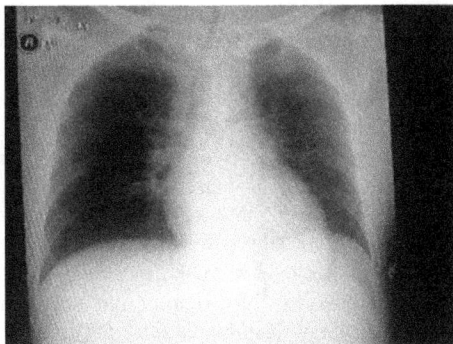

FIGURE 1: Chest roentgenogram obtained just before extubation in our patient.

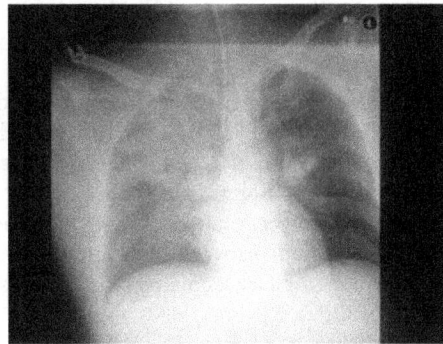

FIGURE 2: Chest roentgenogram after reintubation is shown. Marked shadow of the butterfly is seen.

of the second twitch of TOF. The duration of surgery was 51 minutes, and the surgery was finished uneventfully. At the time of skin closure, continuous administration of fentanyl 30 μg/hr was started for postoperative pain using a patient-controlled analgesia pump (Sylinjector PCA TM, Daiken TM, Tokyo, Japan). Forty-five minutes after the final administration of rocuronium, the fourth twitch of TOF was confirmed. Sugammadex, 140 mg (2 mg/kg), was given, and infusion of remifentanil as well as propofol was discontinued. The total dose of rocuronium administered during surgery was 70 mg. The patient began spontaneous ventilation, regained consciousness, and responded to commands. The value of the T4/T1 ratio in TOF was over 90%. Chest X-ray was obtained as a routine procedure in the hospital and showed no abnormal signs (Figure 1). The tidal volume was over 400 mL and respiratory rate was over 15 breaths/min. After suctioning the sputum in the trachea and oropharynx, the trachea was extubated. Just after the extubation, the patient began to choke and developed marked respiratory depression. The airway was secured by jaw tilting, spontaneous respiration resumed with stridor, and the anesthesiologist began manual bag ventilation. Even though manual bag ventilation was possible, oxygen saturation remained at around 90%. Arterial blood gas analysis revealed marked hypercapnia and hypoxia (pH, 7.14; P_{CO_2}, 61.8 mmHg; P_{O_2}, 145.8 mmHg; Base Excess, -9.4, $FiO_2 = 1.0$). Bilateral auscultation revealed abnormal breath sounds. During mask ventilation, frothy pink sputum was noted to be coming from the patient's mouth. A bolus of propofol 40 mg and the residual bolus of rocuronium 30 mg, which remained in the syringe, were given to reintubate.

The trachea was reintubated. High airway pressure was required to obtain adequate tidal volume. Chest X-ray obtained after reintubation revealed marked bilateral pulmonary edema (NPPE) (Figure 2). Arterial blood gas analysis showed remarkable hypercapnia and hypoxia (pH, 7.18; P_{CO_2}, 60.0 mmHg; P_{O_2}, 240 mmHg; and Base Excess, -7.0, $FiO_2 = 1.0$). The patient was admitted to the ICU and received continuous positive airway pressure ventilation and administration of furosemide for two days after the surgery. The trachea was extubated two days after surgery and no clinical problems remained.

3. Discussion

We experienced a case of NPPE after administration of sugammadex in a healthy patient. Acute upper airway obstruction had developed after extubation. The pathophysiology of negative pressure pulmonary edema is well described as follows: a large inspiratory force in the presence of upper airway obstruction induces extremely negative intrathoracic pressure, increases blood flow into the pulmonary vasculature, and increases hydrostatic pressure and pulmonary vessel distension [4]. Among adult cases, NPPE was due to laryngospasm in more than 50% of the patients [2]. In the present case, although we suspected laryngospasm or glottic closure reflex, since we were able to secure the airway without a neuromuscular blocking agent or hypnotics, laryngospasm was more likely. Laryngospasm is defined as occlusion of the glottis secondary to contraction of laryngeal constrictors (interarytenoid, lateral cricoarytenoids, and internal and external thyroarytenoids) and is a protective reflex against mechanical or chemical internal stimuli or painful external stimuli. It involves all of the muscles of the larynx. The larynx is composed of special visceral structures that permit both voluntary and involuntary actions and is very sensitive to neuromuscular blocking agents [5]. In the present case, laryngospasm followed by NPPE developed after extubation under TOF ratio >0.9. Eikermann et al. [6] demonstrated that recovery of TOF ratio >0.9 is highly likely in the absence of neuromuscular blocking agent-induced upper airway obstruction without reversal by sugammadex. However, in the same study [6], 2 out of 70 patients presented impairment of swallowing, suggesting partial neuromuscular blockade. Herbstreit et al. demonstrated that residual neuromuscular block increases upper airway collapsibility even if the TOF ratio recovers to more than 0.8, and it does not reach the preadministration level even after TOF = 1.0 is obtained [7]. The important thing to keep in mind is that upper airway collapse is induced by the relationship between negative pharyngeal pressure by inspiratory force and upper airway patency [7]. There is a different degree of sensitivity to muscle relaxant between the upper airway muscle and diaphragm [8]. In an in vivo study in rats, after administration of sugammadex at the time of T4/T1 = 0.5, the time for recovery in respiratory function such as tidal volume was shorter than that for the time T4/T1 became 1.0 [9]. Thus, in the present patient who presented TOF >0.9, there is still a possibility that upper airway obstruction was induced by increased upper airway collapsibility and large inspiratory forces by the diaphragm that had fully recovered from muscle relaxation by sugammadex. Thus far, the difference in recovery profile between the diaphragm and upper airway muscle by sugammadex has not been elucidated in humans. There is a possibility that rapid recovery of respiratory forces in the presence of upper airway collapsibility results in the development of NPPE.

In the present case, it is controversial whether we should have given an additional bolus of sugammadex. In critical situations such as the presence of laryngospasm, reestablishment of muscle relaxation to release the closure of vocal cord or for reintubation is required. Before reintubation, muscle relaxation was reestablished after administration of low-dose rocuronium (30 mg). Again, after anesthesia, patients who present TOF >0.9 or =1.0 after muscle relaxation do not recover from upper airway collapsibility up to the preanesthetic level [7]. An additional dose of sugammadex may have led to missing an opportunity to reestablish muscle relaxation for reintubation [10, 11].

Patients who receive sugammadex and present TOF >0.9 may develop upper airway obstruction and NPPE. We experienced a case of NPPE after reversal of rocuronium-induced muscle relaxation by sugammadex.

References

[1] Y.-C. Chuang, C.-H. Wang, and Y.-S. Lin, "Negative pressure pulmonary edema: report of three cases and review of the literature," *European Archives of Oto-Rhino-Laryngology*, vol. 264, no. 9, pp. 1113–1116, 2007.

[2] J. D. Goldenberg, L. G. Portugal, B. L. Wenig, and R. T. Weingarten, "Negative-pressure pulmonary edema in the otolaryngology patient," *Otolaryngology—Head Neck Surgery*, vol. 117, no. 1, pp. 62–66, 1997.

[3] I. F. Sorgenfrei, K. Norrild, P. B. Larsen et al., "Reversal of rocuronium-induced neuromuscular block by the selective relaxant binding agent sugammadex: a dose-finding and safety study," *Anesthesiology*, vol. 104, no. 4, pp. 667–674, 2006.

[4] D. J. Krodel, E. A. Bittner, R. Abdulnour, R. Brown, and M. Eikermann, "Case scenario: acute postoperative negative pressure pulmonary edema," *Anesthesiology*, vol. 113, no. 1, pp. 200–207, 2010.

[5] K. Deepika, C. A. Kenaan, A. M. Barrocas, J. J. Fonseca, and G. B. Bikazi, "Negative pressure pulmonary edema after acute upper airway obstruction," *Journal of Clinical Anesthesia*, vol. 9, no. 5, pp. 403–408, 1997.

[6] M. Eikermann, M. Blobner, H. Groeben et al., "Postoperative upper airway obstruction after recovery of the train of four ratio of the adductor pollicis muscle from neuromuscular blockade," *Anesthesia and Analgesia*, vol. 102, no. 3, pp. 937–942, 2006.

[7] F. Herbstreit, J. Peters, and M. Eikermann, "Impaired upper airway integrity by residual neuromuscular blockade: increased airway collapsibility and blunted genioglossus muscle activity in response to negative pharyngeal pressure," *Anesthesiology*, vol. 110, no. 6, pp. 1253–1260, 2009.

[8] T. Osawa, "Different recovery of the train-of-four ratio from rocuronium-induced neuromuscular blockade in the diaphragm and the tibialis anterior muscle in rat," *Journal of Anesthesia*, vol. 22, no. 3, pp. 236–241, 2008.

[9] M. Eikermann, S. Zaremba, A. Malhotra, A. S. Jordan, C. Rosow, and N. L. Chamberlin, "Neostigmine but not sugammadex impairs upper airway dilator muscle activity and breathing," *British Journal of Anaesthesia*, vol. 101, no. 3, pp. 344–349, 2008.

[10] H. D. de Boer, J. J. Driessen, J. van Egmond, and L. H. Booij, "Non-steroidal neuromuscular blocking agents to re-establish paralysis after reversal of rocuronium-induced neuromuscular block with sugammadex," *Canadian Journal of Anesthesia*, vol. 55, no. 2, pp. 124–125, 2008.

[11] J. Fabregat-López, G. Veiga-Ruiz, N. Dominguez-Serrano, and M. R. García-Martinez, "Re-establishment of neuromuscular block by rocuronium after sugammadex administration," *Canadian Journal of Anesthesia*, vol. 58, no. 7, pp. 658–659, 2011.

17

Anesthetic Management of a Child with Mitochondrial Neurogastrointestinal Encephalopathy

Vianey Q. Casarez, Acsa M. Zavala, Pascal Owusu-Agyemang, and Katherine Hagan

Department of Anesthesiology & Perioperative Medicine, The University of Texas MD Anderson Cancer Center,
1515 Holcombe Boulevard, Unit 409, Houston, TX 77030, USA

Correspondence should be addressed to Vianey Q. Casarez; vcasarez@mdanderson.org

Academic Editor: Renato Santiago Gomez

Mitochondrial neurogastrointestinal encephalomyopathy (MNGIE) is an autosomal recessive disorder associated with deficiency of thymidine phosphorylase (TP). Associated manifestations include visual and hearing impairments, peripheral neuropathies, leukoencephalopathy, and malnutrition from concomitant gastrointestinal dysmotility and pseudoobstruction. Given the altered metabolic state in these patients, specific consideration of medication selection is advised. This case report will describe the anesthetic management used in a 10-year-old girl with MNGIE. She had multiple anesthetics while undergoing allogeneic hematopoietic stem cell transplantation. This case report will discuss the successful repeated use of the same anesthetic in this pediatric patient, with the avoidance of volatile anesthetic agents, propofol, and muscle relaxant.

1. Introduction

MNGIE is a rare autosomal recessive genetic disorder directly associated with a deficiency of thymidine phosphorylase (TP) [1–4]. MNGIE results from a mutation in the TYMP gene (ECGF 1 gene) that encodes for thymidine phosphorylase (TP). This mutation results in a reduction or elimination of TP activity. TP breaks down thymidine and regulates the levels of thymidine and deoxyuridine in the body via negative feedback loop, so shortage of TP allows thymidine to build up [2–4]. Mitochondria use thymidine to build new molecules of mitochondrial DNA (mtDNA), so the excess of thymidine can result in mutations that damage the replication, maintenance, and repair of mtDNA. Patients with MNGIE have low levels of TP; therefore, toxic levels of thymidine and deoxyuridine are responsible for causing irreversible mitochondrial mutations in these patients [4]. These mutations can result in a decrease in ATP production via oxidative phosphorylation in the respiratory chain found in mitochondria, affecting tissues that have high energy demands including cardiac, nervous, and skeletal muscle tissue. Mutated mitochondrial protein production can also

affect the tissues where the protein is found, resulting in GI and hepatic disease.

Clinically, this disorder is difficult to diagnose given the array of symptoms that present concurrently with one another. These patients typically present with visual and hearing impairments, peripheral neuropathy, and leukoencephalopathy. Other prominent symptoms include malnutrition from concomitant gastrointestinal dysmotility and pseudoobstruction [3–5]. Given the concerning gastrointestinal symptoms that ensue in these patients, MNGIE patients commonly require anesthetic services for exploratory laparotomies and diagnostic endoscopies throughout the progression of their disease.

MNGIE patients are now being offered an option to undergo allogeneic hematopoietic stem cell transplantation (HSCT) [2–4]. Although this innovation is new and has only been used successfully in nine MNGIE patients, this treatment is yielding promising results as it aims to normalize thymidine phosphorylase (TP) levels [2, 6]. Studies have shown that early HSCT treatment in these patients helps deter disease progression by reversing the toxic nucleoside levels of thymidine and deoxyuridine found in patients with this disorder [2–4]. While stem cell transplantation has not been found to reverse mitochondrial mutations or help with neurological symptoms, improved gastrointestinal relief has been noted with this treatment. For this reason, HSCT treatments have been found to decrease the morbidity and mortality that are attributed to the diminished gastrointestinal health found in MNGIE patients [2].

Given the altered metabolic state, medications administered to these patients should be carefully selected [7]. There is no preferred anesthetic for these patients. Although the medical literature describes many anesthetic approaches, individuals with MNGIE respond atypically to common anesthetic agents [8, 9]. With written permission from this patient's father and local IRB approval, this case report presents our approach in the care of a 10-year-old girl with MNGIE undergoing stem cell transplantation.

2. Case Presentation

A 10-year-old girl previously diagnosed with MNGIE disease presented to the anesthesia assessment center for preoperative evaluation the day before her scheduled surgery. The patient was scheduled to undergo anesthesia for placement of a central venous catheter for her upcoming stem cell transplantation. The patient presented with hearing deficits, visual abnormalities, cognitive delays, small stature, chronic malnutrition, and unsteady gait. Given her complicated disease process, the decision was made to admit the patient to the hospital that evening in anticipation for surgery the following morning. In an effort to maintain adequate hydration and oxygenation during the preoperative fast, an intravenous saline solution with 5% dextrose was administered as a continuous infusion overnight.

The patient weighed 17 kg and was 109 cm tall. Her previous surgical history included a right cochlear implant four years priorly and no anesthetic complications at that time. Preoperatively, the patient was awake, cachectic, and frail. She was accompanied by her father, sitting up in bed, and spontaneously breathing room air. Her vital signs included tachycardia of 124 beats per minute, her airway exam was normal, and her laboratory examination showed slight hypoalbuminemia of 3 g/dL and low total protein of 5.4 g/dL. The anesthesia plan was to intubate the patient as the patient had GI dysmotility and abdominal pain.

Upon arrival to the operating room suite, monitors were placed, preoxygenation was provided, and general anesthesia was induced. The induction agents of choice included 0.15 mg/kg of midazolam, 3 mcg/kg of fentanyl, and 1 mg/kg of ketamine. Continuous infusions of 0.7 mcg/kg/min of dexmedetomidine and 15 mcg/kg/min of ketamine were also initiated at the start of induction and maintained throughout the case. After adequate depth of anesthesia was established, the patient was easily intubated with a 5.0 mm cuffed endotracheal tube following topical laryngotracheal anesthesia with an LTA using 1 cc of 4% lidocaine. The use of volatile anesthetic agents, muscle relaxants, and propofol was omitted in the care of this patient. The patient remained hemodynamically stable throughout the procedure. Once a left subclavian

triple lumen catheter was placed, the dexmedetomidine and ketamine infusions were both discontinued. Spontaneous ventilation was established; the patient was extubated shortly thereafter and transported to the postoperative recovery unit.

Throughout this patient's hospital stay, our anesthetic team had the privilege of caring for this patient on two other occasions and the same anesthetic plan was utilized. The other two procedures included a repeated central line venous insertion and a liver biopsy. The liver biopsy was performed after she developed abnormal liver function tests (increased AST, ALT, alkaline phosphate, and bilirubin) following her stem cell transplant from a matched unrelated donor. Due to the patient's young age and the anticipated discomfort of the procedure, the decision was made to anesthetize the patient for the liver biopsy. After each of these anesthetics, the patient was closely monitored and no apparent postoperative complications were reported.

3. Discussion

Patients with mitochondrial abnormalities create evident challenges for anesthetic providers for a multitude of reasons. Not only do mitochondrial syndromes involve multisystem organ impairments, but also the lack of well-defined guidelines in the care of these patients makes it even more cumbersome. There is minimal published information on the anesthetic management of patients with MNGIE; thus, anesthesia personnel are limited not only to making clinical decisions and medication selections based upon the patient's past medical history but also to limited published reports on anesthetic effects on mitochondria [8].

During the preoperative period, the patient was provided with continuous intravenous solution to prevent dehydration. A retrospective case review published in the British Journal of Anaesthesia found that preoperative fasting can be detrimental to patients with mitochondrial disease when not adequately hydrated during the fasting period. Recommendations in that study support the use of lactate-free intravenous fluids with dextrose to prevent lactic acidosis in all patients with mitochondrial disorders. The article further notes that excessive glucose oxidation can increase levels of lactate in the blood when normal glucose levels are not maintained [7, 10]. The normal glucose levels would be 70–110 fasting and less than 140 mg/dL two hours after eating a meal.

When comparing the most commonly used induction agents in anesthesia, propofol has been discovered to affect mitochondrial function the most when compared to ketamine, etomidate, and barbiturates [8, 11, 12]. While the latter three agents have been found to only inhibit one mechanism of mitochondrial function, propofol has been found to depress mitochondrial function via four different pathways [8]. Although some case reports have successfully reported the use of propofol in patients with mitochondrial disease, other studies have found an increased sensitivity of propofol infusion syndrome and delayed sequela from the use of propofol in mitochondrial patients

[8, 11–13]. For this reason, we decided to avoid the use of propofol.

Volatile anesthetic gases have also been found to inhibit mitochondria [13]. Although anesthetic gases are minimally metabolized, avoiding the use of volatile anesthetics is ideal in patients of mitochondrial disease given the mitochondrial mutations found with these syndromes. Metabolic derangements alter the utilization of full oxygen capacity and ATP production and ultimately increase the sensitivity that these patients have to volatile anesthetics [8, 14]. The use of sevoflurane has been suggested as the maintenance anesthetic of choice for mitochondrial patients; however, sevoflurane sensitivity has also been linked to some patients with mitochondrial disease [13].

To date, there is no data suggesting that muscle relaxants or narcotics contribute to the inhibition of mitochondrial pathways [8]. Although neuromuscular blocking agents were not used in this patient, the decision was solely based on the type of procedures conducted and the proposed lengths of surgery. We were able to successfully secure an endotracheal tube with the combination of laryngotracheal anesthesia, midazolam, fentanyl, and ketamine in this patient. By utilizing current literature to develop the anesthetic plan, this case report effectively demonstrates the specific considerations that were taken to avoid further deterioration of this patient's ongoing metabolic derangements.

Adequate hydration, oxygenation, and limited stress are important in the preoperative, intraoperative, and postoperative care of these patients [7]. Choosing the safest combination of anesthetic agents for patients with MNGIE is challenging given that all general anesthetic medications have been found to inhibit mitochondrial function to varying degrees [8, 11, 12, 15]. Until more studies are conducted regarding the anesthetic management of patients with specific mitochondrial disorders, anesthetic providers are expected to devise an individualized anesthetic care plan that is safest for the patient based on current recommendations, current medical history, and their best clinical judgment.

Authors' Contribution

All authors contributed in paper preparation.

References

[1] M. Hirano, G. Silvestri, D. M. Blake et al., "Mitochondrial neurogastrointestinal encephalomyopathy (MNGIE): clinical, biochemical, and genetic features of an autosomal recessive mitochondrial disorder," *Neurology*, vol. 44, no. 4, pp. 721–727, 1994.

[2] M. Filosto, M. Scarpelli, P. Tonin et al., "Course and management of allogeneic stem cell transplantation in patients with mitochondrial neurogastrointestinal encephalomyopathy," *Journal of Neurology*, vol. 259, no. 12, pp. 2699–2706, 2012.

[3] M. Hirano, R. Martí, C. Casali et al., "Allogeneic stem cell transplantation corrects biochemical derangements in MNGIE," *Neurology*, vol. 67, no. 8, pp. 1458–1460, 2006.

[4] E. Hussein, "Non-myeloablative bone marrow transplant and platelet infusion can transiently improve the clinical outcome of mitochondrial neurogastrointestinal encephalopathy: a case report," *Transfusion and Apheresis Science*, vol. 49, no. 2, pp. 208–211, 2013.

[5] J. E. Teitelbaum, C. B. Berde, S. Nurko, C. Buonomo, A. R. Perez-Atayde, and V. L. Fox, "Diagnosis and management of MNGIE syndrome in children: case report and review of the literature," *Journal of Pediatric Gastroenterology and Nutrition*, vol. 35, no. 3, pp. 377–383, 2002.

[6] J. Halter, W. M. M. Schüpbach, C. Casali et al., "Allogeneic hematopoietic SCT as treatment option for patients with mitochondrial neurogastrointestinal encephalomyopathy (MNGIE): a consensus conference proposal for a standardized approach," *Bone Marrow Transplantation*, vol. 46, no. 3, pp. 330–337, 2011.

[7] J. L. Edmonds Jr., "Surgical and anesthetic management of patients with mitochondrial dysfunction," *Mitochondrion*, vol. 4, no. 5-6, pp. 543–548, 2004.

[8] J. Niezgoda and P. G. Morgan, "Anesthetic considerations in patients with mitochondrial defects," *Paediatric Anaesthesia*, vol. 23, no. 9, pp. 785–793, 2013.

[9] H. Ellinas and E. A. M. Frost, "Mitochondrial disorders: a review of anesthetic considerations," *Middle East Journal of Anesthesiology*, vol. 21, no. 2, pp. 235–244, 2011.

[10] E. J. Footitt, M. D. Sinha, J. A. J. Raiman, A. Dhawan, S. Moganasundram, and M. P. Champion, "Mitochondrial disorders and general anaesthesia: a case series and review," *British Journal of Anaesthesia*, vol. 100, no. 4, pp. 436–441, 2008.

[11] J. J. Wallace, H. Perndt, and M. Skinner, "Anaesthesia and mitochondrial disease," *Paediatric Anaesthesia*, vol. 8, no. 3, pp. 249–254, 1998.

[12] E. A. Shipton and D. O. Prosser, "Mitochondrial myopathies and anaesthesia," *European Journal of Anaesthesiology*, vol. 21, no. 3, pp. 173–178, 2004.

[13] P. G. Morgan, C. L. Hoppel, and M. M. Sedensky, "Mitochondrial defects and anesthetic sensitivity," *Anesthesiology*, vol. 96, no. 5, pp. 1268–1270, 2002.

[14] E.-B. Kayser, P. G. Morgan, and M. M. Sedensky, "GAS-1: a mitochondrial protein controls sensitivity to volatile anesthetics in the nematode caenorhabditis elegans," *Anesthesiology*, vol. 90, no. 2, pp. 545–554, 1999.

[15] Ò. Miró, A. Barrientos, J. R. Alonso et al., "Effects of general anaesthetic procedures on mitochondrial function of human skeletal muscle," *European Journal of Clinical Pharmacology*, vol. 55, no. 1, pp. 35–41, 1999.

18

Pycnodysostosis: An Anaesthetic Approach to This Rare Genetic Disorder

Rajeev Puri,[1] Arpita Saxena,[1] Awak Mittal,[2] Zia Arshad,[1] Yogita Dwivedi,[1] Trilok Chand,[1] Apurva Mittal,[1] Archna Agrawal,[1] Jay Prakash,[1] and Sathiyanarayanan Pilendran[1]

[1] Department of Anaesthesia and Critical Care, S. N. Medical College, Agra, India
[2] Department of Orthopaedics, S. N. Medical College, Agra, India

Correspondence should be addressed to Rajeev Puri; drrajp00747@gmail.com

Academic Editors: A. Apan, E. Farag, A. Han, C.-H. Hsing, E. W. Nielsen, and D. A. Story

Pycnodysostosis (the Toulouse-Lautrec syndrome) is a rare autosomal-recessive disorder of osteoclast dysfunction. This disorder was first described by Maroteaux and Lamy in 1962. We describe anaesthetic management of a 35-year-old female having pyknodysostosis with fracture shaft left femur with anticipated difficult intubation. Therefore, spinal anesthesia was planned for her fracture fixation. The intra- and postoperative period remains uneventful.

1. Introduction

Pycodysostosis is a rare autosomal-recessive disorder of osteoclast dysfunction due to mutation of cathepsin K gene [1] causing osteosclerosis. The disease shows equal sex distribution with high parental consanguinity, having an incidence of 1.7 per 1 million births [2, 3]. This disorder is characterized by short stature, increased bone density, short and stubby fingers, fragile bones that may fracture easily, and craniofacial abnormalities caused by delayed suture closure. Patients usually present with frequent fractures even after minor trauma.

2. Case Report

A 34-year-old, 45 kg patient having Pycodysostosis was planned for elective femur plating under spinal anesthesia. The patient had past history of spontaneous fractures which were managed conservatively. Her mental and sexual developments were normal. Patient had large protruding tongue (Figure 1) and Mallampati grade IV with a history of snoring. Patient had characteristic short stature, particularly limbs, short broad hands, frontal and occipital bossing, and chest deformities. Radiograph demonstrates increased bone density with hypoplastic clavicle, narrow intervertebral spaces, and bowing long bones (Figure 2). The patient height was 130 cm, upper limb to lower limb ratio was 60/76, and arm span was 128 cm. Patient had no known history of allergy to any drug. Laboratory investigations including serum electrolytes, ECG, and X-ray of chest were within normal limits.

Inside the operation theatre intravenous access was secured with an 18-gauge cannula, and preloading was done with 500 mL of Ringer's lactate. Urinary catheterization was done. Monitoring of electrocardiograph, heart rate, SpO2, and NIBP was done. Patient preoperative vitals were within normal limits. Ceftriaxone 1 gm was administered. Under strict aseptic conditions, spinal anesthesia was given at lumber space L2-3 with 26-gauge spinal needle in sitting position. Drug used was 2.5 mL of bupivacaine heavy (0.5%). The patient then positioned supine, and a sensory level up to T12 was achieved. 1 mL of midazolam was given to the patient to allay operative anxiety. Total duration of surgery was 80 minutes. Intraoperative and postoperative period was uneventful.

3. Discussion

Pycodysostosis is a rare autosomal-recessive disorder of osteoclast dysfunction [4], and the understanding of early

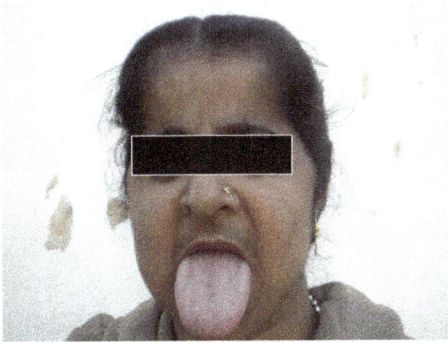

FIGURE 1: Patient with large protruding tongue.

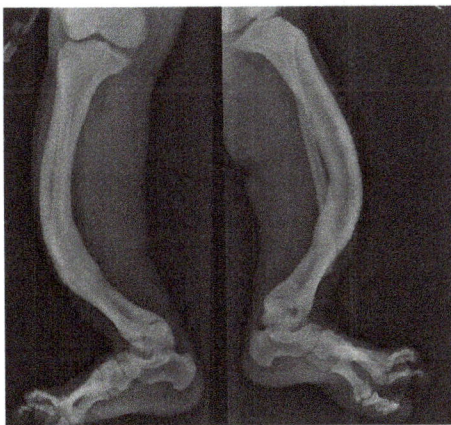

FIGURE 3: X-ray showing sclerosis of terminal phalanges.

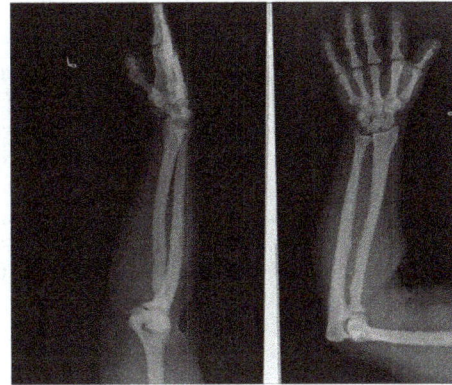

FIGURE 2: X-ray showing bowing of long bones.

and delayed radio-clinical manifestations of pycnodysostosis is very important since it resembles cleidocranial dysostosis and osteopetrosis [5]. The features which differentiates it are short stature, brachycephaly, generalized diffuse osteosclerosis, sclerosis of the terminal phalanges (Figure 3), hypoplastic clavicles, and history of multiple fractures of long bones [6]. The jaw and collar bone (clavicles) are also particularly prone to fractures.

Craniofacial features include a large head with front parietal bossing, open soft cranial sutures and fontanelles, depressed nasal bridge, a high arched grooved palate, maxillary hypoplasia, mandibular fractures, osteomyelitis, malpositioned teeth, elongated soft palate precipitating mouth breathing, and heavy snoring in addition to periapical cementoma-like lesions in the mandible [7, 8]. Many of these findings were present in our case which differentiates her from osteopetrosis and cleidocranial dysostosis. In osteopetrosis, there is no delayed closure of cranial sutures, no phalangeal, or clavicle hypoplasia. Cleidocranial dysostosis is transmitted by autosomal dominant inheritance, open fontanels and cranial sutures are also observed at an advanced age, and there is no phalangeal or clavicle hypoplasia.

Pycodysostosis has been described all over the world with minimal difference affecting all races regardless of sex and age; the youngest patient reported was a nine-month-old baby and the oldest was 45 years in age [2]. PKD in children is commoner in males than in females, occurring at a ratio of 2 : 1 [9]. The sclerosing activity of Pycodysostosis is due to a genetic defect located on chromosome 1q21. This anomaly consists of mutations that produce changes in a lysosomal cystine protease, cathepsin K [4], the expression of which is reduced in the osteoclasts of these patients [10]. Patient's one elder brother also had similar features.

Various reports have been published regarding Pycodysostosis which presents clinical and radiological features which differentiates it from others, but little or none have been talked about giving anaesthesia in these patients. We were dealing with a very rare case with anticipated difficult intubation due to high arched palate, mandibular hypoplasia, and large protruding tongue, which made it Mallampati grade IV. Also sniffing position and airway manipulations during endotracheal intubation may predispose patient to trauma and fracture. So general anaesthesia was avoided, and spinal anaesthesia was chosen for femoral plating. History of obstructive sleep apnea may have a risk of airway obstruction in postoperative period; hence, it should be carefully addressed.

The diagnosis of Pycodysostosis is primarily based on clinical features and radiographs. In lack of any specific treatment of Pycodysostosis, which is mainly supportive, our main aim is to prevent minor trauma, which may cause iatrogenic fracture in the patient. Such precautions include careful handling of an affected patient, with minimal manipulations that are safe and do not require too much impact.

In conclusion, undoubtedly these patients pose challenge to anaesthesiologists, but proper preoperative patient assessment, planning, and multidisciplinary approach are the keys to successful outcome in these patients.

Acknowledgments

The authors would like to acknowledge Dr. Nitika Mittal, Department of Anaesthesia and Critical Care, S. N. Medical College, Agra, and Dr. Vivek Mittal, Department of Orthpaedics, S. N. Medical College, Agra.

References

[1] S. M. Krane and A. L. Schiller, "Hyperostosis, fibrous dysplasia, and other dysplasias of bone and cartilage," in *Harrison's Principles of Internal Medicine*, A. S. Fauci, E. Braunwald, K. J. Isselbacher et al., Eds., pp. 2269–2275, McGraw-Hill, New York, NY, USA, 1998.

[2] K. W. Fleming, G. Barest, and O. Sakai, "Dental and facial bone abnormalities in pyknodysostosis: CT findings," *American Journal of Neuroradiology*, vol. 28, no. 1, pp. 132–134, 2007.

[3] Q. Mujawar, R. Naganoor, H. Patil, A. N. Thobbi, S. Ukkali, and N. Malagi, "Pycnodysostosis with unusual findings: a case report," *Cases Journal*, vol. 2, no. 7, p. 6544, 2009.

[4] S. Kiran, M. Goel, P. Singhal, M. K. Goel, and R. Gupta, "Pyknodysostosis: anaesthetic considerations-a case report," *The Internet Journal of Anesthesiology*, vol. 21, no. 2, p. 13, 2009.

[5] P. Beighton, F. Horan, and H. Hamersma, "A review of the osteopetroses," *Postgraduate Medical Journal*, vol. 53, no. 622, pp. 507–516, 1977.

[6] Z. S. Kundu, K. M. Marya, S. Magu, S. Rohilla, and V. Yadav, "Radiological quiz-musculoskeletal: pyknodysostosis," *Indian Journal of Radiology and Imaging*, vol. 12, no. 3, pp. 435–436, 2002.

[7] R. J. Bathi and V. N. Masur, "Pyknodysostosis-a report of two cases with a brief review of the literature," *International Journal of Oral and Maxillofacial Surgery*, vol. 29, no. 6, pp. 439–442, 2000.

[8] C. M. Jones, J. S. Rennie, and A. S. Blinkhorn, "Pycnodysostosis. A review of reported dental abnormalities and a report of the dental findings in two cases.," *British dental journal*, vol. 164, no. 7, pp. 218–220, 1988.

[9] D. Wolfgang, *Radiology Review Manual*, Wolters Kluwer Health, New Delhi, India, 6th edition, 2007.

[10] G. Motyckova and D. E. Fisher, "Pycnodysostosis: role and regulation of cathepsin K in osteoclast function and human disease," *Current Molecular Medicine*, vol. 2, no. 5, pp. 407–421, 2002.

19

Diagnosis and Rescue of a Kinked Pulmonary Artery Catheter

Nicolas J. Mouawad,[1] Erica J. Stein,[2] Kenneth R. Moran,[2]
Michael R. Go,[1] and Thomas J. Papadimos[2]

[1]Department of Surgery, The Ohio State University Wexner Medical Center, 410 West 10th Avenue, Columbus, OH 43210, USA
[2]Department of Anesthesiology, The Ohio State University Wexner Medical Center, 410 West 10th Avenue, Columbus, OH 43210, USA

Correspondence should be addressed to Thomas J. Papadimos; papadimos.1@osu.edu

Academic Editor: Pavel Michalek

Invasive hemodynamic monitoring with a pulmonary catheter has been relatively routine in cardiovascular and complex surgical operations as well as in the management of critical illnesses. However, due to multiple potential complications and its invasive nature, its use has decreased over the years and less invasive methods such as transesophageal echocardiography and hemodynamic sensors have gained widespread favor. Unlike these less invasive forms of hemodynamic monitoring, pulmonary artery catheters require an advanced understanding of cardiopulmonary physiology, anatomy, and the potential for complications in order to properly place, manage, and interpret the device. We describe a case wherein significant resistance was encountered during multiple unsuccessful attempts at removing a patient's catheter secondary to kinking and twisting of the catheter tip. These attempts to remove the catheter serve to demonstrate potential rescue options for such a situation. Ultimately, successful removal of the catheter was accomplished by simultaneous catheter retraction and sheath advancement while gently pulling both objects from the cannulation site. In addition to being skilled in catheter placement, it is imperative that providers comprehend the risks and complications of this invasive monitoring tool.

1. Introduction

The flow-directed balloon-tipped pulmonary artery catheter (PAC), also known as the Swan-Ganz catheter, has been in widespread clinical use for over 40 years. In fact, for patients in the United States, as many as 1 million PACs and 5 million central venous catheters are placed annually [1]. Invasive hemodynamic monitoring with the PAC has been relatively routine in cardiovascular and complex surgical operations as well as in the management of critical illness. Although the American College of Cardiology published a consensus statement in 1998 regarding the use of the PAC in cardiac disease, there are no validated indications for its general use.

The advent of more noninvasive methods to determine cardiovascular status has led way to a decrease in the use of the PAC, however, and more junior physicians are less experienced in the management of PACs and their potential complications. A recent study by Koo et al. evaluating over 15,000 patients over a 5-year period noted that 12.8% had a PAC placed; over the same study period, the adjusted rate of

use of the PAC decreased from 16.4% to 6.5% [2]. The determinants of PAC use did not change over time, but the largest nonpatient related factor for PAC use was the attending physician's base specialty and intensive care unit status.

With such widespread use, it is imperative on the part of the provider to be well versed in the technique, possible complications, and rescue maneuvers should they be necessary. Perforation of the access vessels leading to hemothorax or perforation of the pleura with subsequent pneumothorax is a known complication. Perforation of the aorta with ensuing cardiac tamponade can occur if the cannula-site perforation is within the pericardial sac; this is usually associated with a mortality of 90% [3]. Arrhythmias constitute the most common complication in relation to PAC insertion. These are usually premature ventricular contractions or nonsustained ventricular tachycardia that usually resolve by retracting the catheter back into the right atrium from the right ventricle or advancing it in the pulmonary artery. Right bundle branch block is another complication and, in patients with existing left bundle branch block, care must be taken to avoid precipitating complete heart block. Necessary adjunctive medications and a temporary pacemaker should be kept nearby in such situations. Cardiac damage and valvular and structural heart injury as well as pulmonary artery vessel injury with resultant hemoptysis are also devastating potential complications.

Here, we describe the case of a patient with a PAC in which significant resistance was encountered during removal attempts due to kinking and twisting of the catheter tip and present rescue options for such a situation.

2. Case Description

A 57-year-old African American woman with a longstanding history of dilated cardiomyopathy secondary to mitral insufficiency was evaluated for a mitral valve repair and MAZE procedure at an outside hospital (OSH). Preoperative hemodynamic monitoring was instituted with a single stick left transinternal jugular PAC placed in the standard fashion as well as a left radial arterial line. The PAC was easily advanced using pressure curves and secured for periodic evaluation of pulmonary capillary wedge pressure. On induction of anesthesia at the OSH she had severe hypotension with pulseless electrical activity for 15 minutes. She was resuscitated with multiple boluses of epinephrine and subsequent infusions of norepinephrine, milrinone, and amiodarone. Median sternotomy was performed emergently; however the procedure was aborted and an intra-aortic balloon pump (IABP) was placed for supportive care and resuscitation. The sternotomy was then closed without placing the patient on cardiopulmonary bypass and she was transferred to our tertiary level care center for critical care management and a mitral valve repair.

On arrival, the norepinephrine was discontinued and she was placed on a dobutamine infusion; milrinone and amiodarone were continued. Preoperatively her transesophageal echocardiogram demonstrated severe systolic dysfunction with an ejection fraction of <20%, a normal sized right ventricle with moderately reduced systolic function, an enlarged left atrium, and severe mitral regurgitation with a thickened mitral valve. Six days after admission she successfully underwent a redo sternotomy with repair of the mitral valve using a 26 mm Edwards annuloplasty band. She arrived in the intensive care unit with infusions of dobutamine, milrinone, and amiodarone and the IABP still in place.

Two days after surgery the drips were discontinued and the IABP was removed. That same afternoon the decision was made to remove the PAC from her left internal jugular vein. After appropriate positioning, sterile technique, and assurance that the catheter balloon was deflated, the catheter sleeve was disconnected from the introducer sheath. A slow, smooth, and steady motion was employed to pull back the catheter and met with significant resistance. Two subsequent attempts at pulling and advancing the catheter were attempted to no avail, suggesting a problem. Chest radiography at the bedside was performed which demonstrated kinked PAC at the confluence of the left internal jugular vein and left subclavian vein (Figure 1). The chest roentgenogram from that same morning demonstrated that the pulmonary

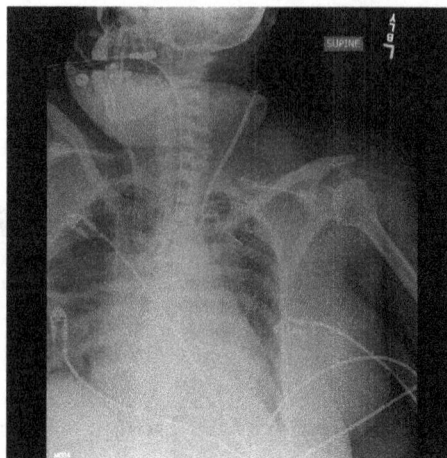

Figure 1: Chest radiography of kinked PAC at the confluence of the left internal jugular vein and left subclavian vein.

artery catheter was in proper position without any kinks. Vascular surgery was consulted for recommendations regarding its removal.

After review of the chest X-ray, gentle initial traction was applied in an attempt to remove the catheter; significant resistance was again noted. A hybrid operating room was prepared in order to pass a semistiff or stiff guide wire to help straighten out the catheter. While awaiting transfer to the operating room the decision was made to attempt to deepen the sheath over the catheter to help straighten it out. Ultimately, with a combination of steady backward traction and forward advancement of the sheath, the catheter was retracted into the sheath allowing for a successful and safe recovery. Once the sheath was removed, the coil pattern, or kinking, of the catheter was evident and reproducible (Figure 2).

Hemostasis was achieved with a manual compression. The patient tolerated the procedure well and ultimately was discharged from the hospital to a skilled nursing facility for convalescence.

3. Discussion

Although the use of the PAC has decreased over time and given way to more noninvasive methods such as transesophageal echocardiography and infrared sensors that evaluate stroke volume variation and cardiac output, it still remains a well-established tool in the management of critically ill patients [2, 4]. The use of PACs allows invasive monitoring capabilities for practitioners to manage a variety of critical and cardiac conditions. It is imperative that the provider be very skilled in catheter placement as well as comprehending the risks and complications of this invasive monitoring tool.

Complications of the PAC are divided into initial vascular access, insertion technique of the PAC, and maintenance of the PAC in a branch of the pulmonary artery (right or left). Clearly, the incidence of complications relates to operator skill and technique as well as patient status and selection.

With regard to initial vascular access, strong consideration is necessary for route selection. Arterial puncture can

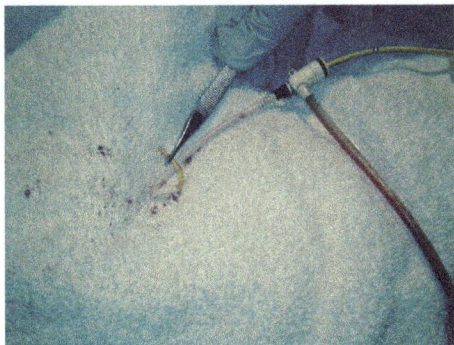

FIGURE 2: Ex vivo photograph of the PAC maintaining its kinked position.

occur with an incidence of 2–16% [5]. This complication can result in a hemothorax if the subclavian route is attempted, whereas a carotid artery hematoma may manifest itself if inadvertent carotid injury occurs during internal jugular cannulation. A carotid artery to internal jugular vein arteriovenous fistula has been reported also when inadvertent cannulation of the carotid artery has occurred [5]. Most of these concerns can be mitigated by using ultrasound guidance during vascular access. In fact, a Cochrane Database Review by Brass and colleagues conducted an extensive search ranging from 1966 until 2013 and identified over 730 studies that fit the search criteria; their analysis noted that use of two-dimensional ultrasound rather than classic anatomic landmarks decreased the total complication rate of vascular access by 71% and of inadvertent arterial access by 72% [6]. In addition, success on the first attempt increased by 57% using ultrasound guidance [6].

Arrhythmias constitute the most common complication in relation to PAC insertion. These are usually premature ventricular contractions or nonsustained ventricular tachycardia. Furthermore, catheter resistance, endocarditis, endocardial damage, pseudoaneurysms, and cardiac valve injury are all possible complications of PAC insertion. Rupture of the pulmonary artery is the most devastating complication of PAC maintenance, with a mortality rate reaching approximately 50% [5].

Avoiding serious complications, in the use of a PAC, requires a proactive awareness of potential catheter complications, in particular when unexpected resistance is felt during catheter withdrawal attempts [7, 8]. Patients with dilated cardiac chambers, as in this case, are more prone to catheter kinking and knotting [8]. The larger chamber dimensions allow the catheter considerable opportunities for locomotion thereby enabling coiling, knotting, or kinking. Interestingly, these catheters function fine and it is only during withdrawal attempts or catheter repositioning that the kinking or coiling is suspected, as noted in our case as well [9–11]. Coiling or knotting of the catheter is usually confirmed by radiography. Management techniques for dealing with a kinked catheter can be nonsurgical or surgical.

List of Nonsurgical and Interventional/Surgical Options for Bail Out of Kinked and Knotted PAC

Nonsurgical

(i) Steady and smooth traction.

(ii) Extraction using a larger sheath.

(iii) Extraction using a semistiff or stiff guide wire to straighten the catheter.

Interventional and/or Surgical

(i) Cut-down over insertion site.

(ii) Snare technique and use of the basket under fluoroscopy.

(iii) Contrast venography with balloon venoplasty to correct stenoses.

(iv) Sternotomy and open surgical extraction.

(v) In cases of fixed catheters from cardiac surgical suture line, cardiotomy is necessary.

It is important that appropriate consultations are employed, in particular vascular surgeons and interventional radiologists. The use of advanced interventional techniques are usually very helpful in correcting intravascular foreign body issues, and, in fact, endovascular methods are the preferred modality if amenable [12–14]. Appropriate fluoroscopy capabilities including percutaneous access from the femoral vein (unilateral or bilateral approach) may be necessary. The use of snaring techniques or endovascular basket catheters as well as balloon venoplasty may be helpful in dilating stenoses, grasping the foreign body and unwinding. It is imperative that a clear understanding of the technique, pitfalls, complications, and rescue solutions is necessary on the part of the practitioner as the continued use of these catheters is employed.

References

[1] H. S. Mueller, K. Chatterjee, K. B. Davis et al., "ACC expert consensus document. Present use of bedside right heart catheterization in patients with cardiac disease. American College of Cardiology," *Journal of the American College of Cardiology*, vol. 32, no. 3, pp. 840–864, 1998.

[2] K. K. Y. Koo, J. C. J. Sun, Q. Zhou et al., "Pulmonary artery catheters: evolving rates and reasons for use," *Critical Care Medicine*, vol. 39, no. 7, pp. 1613–1618, 2011.

[3] P. Fangio, E. Mourgeon, A. Romelaer, J.-P. Goarin, P. Coriat, and J.-J. Rouby, "Aortic injury and cardiac tamponade as a complication of subclavian venous catheterization," *Anesthesiology*, vol. 96, no. 6, pp. 1520–1522, 2002.

[4] M. A. Hamilton, M. Cecconi, and A. Rhodes, "A systematic review and meta-analysis on the use of preemptive hemodynamic intervention to improve postoperative outcomes in moderate and high-risk surgical patients," *Anesthesia & Analgesia*, vol. 112, no. 6, pp. 1392–1402, 2011.

[5] T. A. Bowdle, "Complications of invasive monitoring," *Anesthesiology Clinics of North America*, vol. 20, no. 3, pp. 333–350, 2002.

[6] P. Brass, U. Boerner, M. Hellmich et al., "Traditional landmark versus ultrasound guidance for central vein catheterization," *Cochrane Database of Systematic Reviews*, no. 1, Article ID CD006962, 2008.

[7] L. Eshkevari and B. M. Baker, "Occurrence and removal of a knotted pulmonary artery catheter: a case report," *AANA Journal*, vol. 75, no. 6, pp. 423–428, 2007.

[8] T. Asteri, I. Tsagaropoulou, K. Vasiliadis, I. Fessatidis, E. Papavasiliou, and P. Spyrou, "Beware Swan-Ganz complications. Perioperative management," *Journal of Cardiovascular Surgery*, vol. 43, no. 4, pp. 467–470, 2002.

[9] B. W. Bottiger, H. Schmidt, H. Bohrer, and E. Martin, "Nonsurgical removal of a knotted pulmonary artery catheter," *Anaesthesist*, vol. 40, no. 12, pp. 682–686, 1991.

[10] Y. Lubliner, H. I. Miller, V. Yakirevich, and B. Vidne, "Knotting of a Swan-Ganz catheter in the right ventricle," *Heart and Lung*, vol. 13, no. 4, pp. 419–420, 1984.

[11] M. C. Lopes, R. d. Cleva, B. Zilberstein, and J. J. Gama-Rodrigues, "Pulmonary artery catheter complications: report on a case of a knot accident and literature review," *Revista do Hospital das Clínicas*, vol. 59, no. 2, pp. 77–85, 2004.

[12] Q. Wang, B. Xiong, C. Zheng, G. Feng, M. Liang, and H. Liang, "Percutaneous retrieval of PICC fractures via the femoral vein in six cancer patients," *The Journal of Vascular Access*, vol. 16, no. 1, pp. 47–51, 2015.

[13] H.-S. Han, Y.-T. Jeon, H.-S. Na, J.-Y. Hwang, E.-J. Choi, and M.-H. Kim, "Successful removal of kinked J-guide wire under fluoroscopic guidance during central venous catheterization—a case report-," *Korean Journal of Anesthesiology*, vol. 60, no. 5, pp. 362–364, 2011.

[14] G. K. Jalwal, V. Rajagopalan, A. Bindra et al., "Percutaneous retrieval of malpositioned, kinked and unraveled guide wire under fluoroscopic guidance during central venous cannulation," *Journal of Anaesthesiology Clinical Pharmacology*, vol. 30, no. 2, pp. 267–269, 2014.

20

Unexpected High Sensory Blockade during Continuous Spinal Anesthesiology (CSA) in an Elderly Patient

R. Ketelaars and A. P. Wolff

Department of Anaesthesia, Radboud University Nijmegen Medical Centre, P.O. Box 9101,
6500 HB Nijmegen, The Netherlands

Correspondence should be addressed to R. Ketelaars, r.ketelaars@anes.umcn.nl

Academic Editors: A. Apan, M. Dauri, and R. Riley

A 98-year-old woman presented for a hemiarthroplasty of the left hip. Because of her age and cardiac and pulmonary co-existing diseases we decided to provide adequate regional anesthesia by continuous spinal anesthesia. Fragmented doses of isobaric bupivacaine 0.5% were administered through a system consisting of a spinal catheter connected to an antimicrobial filter. After an uneventful surgical procedure, prior to removal of the catheter, this system was flushed with 10 mL of normal saline in order to try to prevent post-dural-puncture headache. After arrival at the postanesthesia care unit and fifteen minutes after removal of the catheter the patient suffered an unexpected high thoracic sensory blockade and hypotension requiring treatment. The continuous spinal anesthesia technique can be used in selected cases to be able to administer local anesthetic agents in a slow and controlled manner to reach the desired effect. The risk of post-dural-puncture headache using this technique in elderly patients is very low and therefore precludes the need to try to prevent it. We have described a potentially dangerous complication of flushing a bupivacaine-filled system into the spinal canal of an elderly patient resulting in an undesirable high sensory blockade.

1. Introduction

Continuous spinal anesthesia (CSA) is an accepted technique of achieving regional anesthesia for surgery below the waist in elderly patients [1, 2]. Its advantages are the superior control by the physician on the type and dosage of drugs administered intrathecally. Consequently the level of sensory blockade can be controlled very precisely leading to minimal respiratory, hemodynamic and mental implications [3].

The height of a sensory block achieved with a single-shot spinal anesthesia (SSA) depends on various patient factors including age [4]. Advanced age also influences cardiovascular instability following spinal anesthesia, CSA may therefore be preferred over SSA for elderly patients [5]. Moreover the extent and intensity of the intrathecal blockade induced with local anesthetic agents influences cardiovascular instability. Concomitant conditions like cardiomyopathy or aortic valve stenosis may increase this risk of hemodynamic instability and cardiovascular complications further, strengthening the indication for CSA.

The downside of CSA over SSA is its higher rate of complications such as infection, epidural hematomas, post-dural-puncture headache (PDPH), and cauda equina syndrome [6–9].

This report is, as far as we know, the first one describing unintentional and unexpected high sensory blockade following CSA. We do not believe this to be an uncommon or even unrecognized complication but it nevertheless appears to be an underreported one.

2. Case Presentation

A 98-year-old woman suffered a left-sided femoral neck fracture caused by a fall and presented for a hip hemiarthroplasty. Her medical record shows paroxysmal atrial fibrillation, hypertension, recurrent complaints attributed to cardiac decompensation, a cardiac murmur and hypoxemic chronic obstructive pulmonary disease (COPD), global initiative for chronic obstructive lung disease (GOLD) classification stage II (moderate severity), for which she received supplemental oxygen therapy at home. Her symptoms of dyspnea have remained constant over the last few weeks. She had contracted pulmonary tuberculosis in the past and had recently been treated with an antibiotic and prednisolone because of recurrent pneumonia and COPD exacerbation. Over the last few years the number of falls she sustained had increased.

Additional medication consisted of a loop diuretic, calcium channel inhibitor, nebulized combination of a β2-agonist and an anticholinergic agent, and acetaminophen. She took no antiplatelet drugs or vitamin-K antagonists.

On physical examination she had a respiratory frequency of 17 per minute, peripheral oxygen saturation (SpO_2) 92% with nasal administration of O_2 at two liters per minute. Blood pressure was 144/72 mmHg and heart rate 81 beats per minute (bpm). A cardiac murmur was heard over the chest. Electrocardiography showed a normal sinus rhythm.

The transthoracic echocardiogram revealed a moderate aortic valve stenosis and a hypertrophied left ventricle with a good systolic function.

Because of the patients advanced age, aortic valve stenosis and the kind of surgery required, we formulated a plan to pursue a hemodynamic situation within normal limits for this patient with minimal impact on pulmonary and cerebral function. We decided to provide adequate regional anesthesia by CSA.

We undertook this procedure starting an hour before surgery at the postanesthesia care unit (PACU) with monitoring of pulse, ECG, and blood pressure. In a complete sterile manner with the patient in a sitting position we introduced an 18-gauge Tuohy needle (Perican; B. Braun Melsungen AG, Melsungen, Germany) in the midline at the level of the spinous process of the third and fourth lumbar vertebrae. After we punctured the duramater and observed a free flow of spinous fluid, we introduced a 20 gauge, 104 cm catheter (Perifix Softtip; B.Braun), and five centimeters intrathecally. This catheter was connected to an antimicrobial filter (Perifix; B.Braun), flushed with normal saline (NaCl 0.9%), and fixed to the patients back with adhesive film and tape. This procedure using these materials describes the standard operating procedure to introduce an intrathecal catheter for CSA in our institution.

Approximately 45 minutes before surgery we administered 0.5 mL of a 0.5% isobaric bupivacaine solution (2.5 mg; AstraZeneca, London, United Kingdom). Fifteen minutes later we administered another 0.25 mL (1.25 mg) of this solution. To assess the extent of sensory blockade a refrigerated metal "hammer" was used. The patient was able to adequately report cold sensation while touching the skin of the thorax, abdomen, and upper legs on both sides of the body, moving in a craniocaudal direction. Five minutes after having administered the second dose of the local anesthetic agent we tested sensory blockade and determined it to be symmetrically at the level of the eleventh thoracic dermatome and below. After this we introduced a urinary catheter and placed the patient in the right dependent position and surgery commenced.

An hour after the second dose of bupivacaine we administered a third dose of 0.5 mL (2.5 mg) and another hour later a fourth dose of 0.5 mL. Upon completion of the

surgery and 50 minutes after the last dose of bupivacaine, we removed the spinal catheter. Immediately prior to removing the catheter we injected 10 mL of normal saline to reduce the risk of developing PDPH and the patient was transported to the PACU.

During surgery all monitored physiological variables stayed within normal values. We administered 500 mL of a colloidal solution and 250 mL of normal saline. The course of surgery was as planned. Blood loss was 500 milliliters.

Fifteen minutes after removal of the catheter her blood pressure decreased to a minimum of 75/35 mmHg with a heart rate of 80 bpm. After administration of up to a total of 350 μg of phenylephrine, her pulse slowed to 60 bpm and blood pressure improved. Examination revealed an unexpected symmetric sensory blockade at the third thoracic dermatome and below. She reported no pain and was unable to move her legs and feet.

Besides frequent hemodynamic monitoring, sensory blockade was monitored every 15 minutes. We considered requesting a magnetic resonance imaging scan to rule out an epidural hematoma being a deleterious side effect of introducing or removing neuraxial catheters. Fortunately 130 minutes after the first occurrence of high sensory blockade and hypotension, sensory blockade finally regressed to a level below the sixth thoracic dermatome. Thereafter motor and sensory blockade regressed swiftly.

Pain after regression of the blockade was successfully treated with fragmented doses of intravenous morphine.

The patient was discharged on the fifth day after surgery after an otherwise uneventful hospital stay. She never complained about headaches.

3. Discussion

The CSA technique can be used to titrate local anesthetic agents to accomplish an adequate height of sensory blockade for patients having surgery. The wide spread of local anesthetic agents when using a CSA technique can in many cases occur after start of titration of the doses, if they are administered too fast or in higher doses than necessary. This adverse effect is thought to be known by most anesthesiologists. While there are reports of intrathecal catheters resulting in abnormal spread or inadequate sensory blocks, to date there are no reports in medical literature of the potentially dangerous complication we have described [10].

We hypothesized that the 10 mL flush of normal saline prior to the removal of the intrathecal catheter caused the late and high level of the unintended intrathecal anesthesia. The system we used consisted of a 104 cm catheter connected with a connector to an antimicrobial filter, closed with a cap. This system contains a total volume of 0.8 mL. In the worst case scenario this system would contain undiluted bupivacaine 0.5% and thus a dose of 4 mg. By flushing the system with normal saline we diluted and flushed most of the bupivacaine into the cerebrospinal fluid (CSF). We hypothesized that the resulting effect resembled a technique called barbotage in which during the performance of a SSA a local anesthetic agent is injected while intermittently CSF is aspirated and reinjected to dilute the local anesthetic and to induce a certain current in the CSF. The rationale of the barbotage technique is to increase sensory block height using a relatively low dose of local anesthetic drugs, however evidence is lacking [4, 11].

Elderly patients may have a lower lumbosacral cerebrospinal fluid (CSF) volume with lower CSF pressures [12]. The combination of 4 mg bupivacaine and its dilution with 10 mL normal saline into a relatively small volume of CSF might also have contributed to the unexpected large extent of intrathecal anesthesia up to the 3rd thoracic dermatome.

When using the CSA technique, the risk of PDPH is slightly higher, but probably still very low. By injecting normal saline, we intended to reduce the risk of PDPH, despite the incidence of this occurring after an SSA decreases with age [13]. In addition there appears to be little evidence, if any, for a single intrathecal injection of normal saline before removing a catheter to prevent the occurrence of post-dural-puncture headache [9, 14, 15].

In conclusion we recommend that regional anesthesia by CSA be the technique of choice in the elderly high-risk patient requiring hip surgery. In this case the procedure went well until we flushed the intrathecal catheter with 10 mL saline before catheter removal. This probably caused an unintended and undesirable high sensory blockade because the intrathecal system contained enough bupivacaine to block the spinal afferent and efferent nerves up to a high thoracic level in an elderly patient.

This case demonstrates that the injection of normal saline through the intrathecal catheter before removal in order to reduce the chance on PDPH in elderly patients is debatable and not without risk. Anesthesiologists may be aware of this potential event, but as far as we know an incident like this has not been reported in literature previously.

References

[1] P. A. Sutter, Z. Gamulin, and A. Forster, "Comparison of continuous spinal and continuous epidural anaesthesia for lower limb surgery in elderly patients. A retrospective study," *Anaesthesia*, vol. 44, no. 1, pp. 47–50, 1989.

[2] J. F. Favarel-Garrigues, F. Sztark, M. E. Petitjean, M. Thicoïpé, P. Lassié, and P. Dabadie, "Hemodynamic effects of spinal anesthesia in the elderly: single dose versus titration through a catheter," *Anesthesia and Analgesia*, vol. 82, no. 2, pp. 312–316, 1996.

[3] T. Okutomi, M. Saito, M. Koura, and S. Hoka, "Spinal anesthesia using a continuous spinal catheter for cesarean section in a parturient with prior surgical correction of scoliosis," *Journal of Anesthesia*, vol. 20, no. 3, pp. 223–226, 2006.

[4] G. Hocking and J. A. W. Wildsmith, "Intrathecal drug spread," *British Journal of Anaesthesia*, vol. 93, no. 4, pp. 568–578, 2004.

[5] M. Goyal, S. Taxak, K. K. Kshetrapal, and M. K. Goel, "Continuous spinal anesthesia in a high risk elderly patient using epidural set," *Journal of Anaesthesiology Clinical Pharmacology*, vol. 27, no. 1, pp. 139–141, 2011.

[6] T. Volk, A. Wolf, H. Van Aken, H. Bürkle, A. Wiebalck, and T. Steinfeldt, "Incidence of spinal haematoma after epidural puncture: analysis from the German network for safety in regional anaesthesia," *European Journal of Anaesthesiology*, vol. 29, no. 4, pp. 170–176, 2012.

[7] M. L. Rigler, K. Drasner, T. C. Krejcie et al., "Cauda equina syndrome after continuous spinal anesthesia," *Anesthesia and Analgesia*, vol. 72, no. 3, pp. 275–281, 1991.

[8] B. S. Rasmussen, L. Blom, P. Hansen, and S. S. Mikkelsen, "Postspinal headache in young and elderly patients. Two randomised, double-blind studies that compare 20- and 25-gauge needles," *Anaesthesia*, vol. 44, no. 7, pp. 571–573, 1989.

[9] S. Abdulla, W. Abdulla, and R. Eckhardt, "Caudal normal saline injections for the treatment of post-dural puncture headache," *Pain Physician*, vol. 14, no. 3, pp. 271–279, 2011.

[10] L. M. M. Morrison, J. H. McClure, and J. A. W. Wildsmith, "Clinical evaluation of a spinal catheter technique in femoro-popliteal graft surgery," *Anaesthesia*, vol. 46, no. 7, pp. 576–578, 1991.

[11] P. J. Nightingale, "Barbotage and spinal anaesthesia. The effect of barbotage on the spread of analgesia during isobaric spinal anaesthesia," *Anaesthesia*, vol. 38, no. 1, pp. 7–9, 1983.

[12] W. W. Tourtellotte, W. G. Henderson, R. P. Tucker, O. Gilland, J. E. Walker, and E. Kokman, "A randomized, double-blind clinical trial comparing the 22 versus 26 gauge needle in the production of the post-lumbar puncture syndrome in normal individuals," *Headache*, vol. 12, no. 2, pp. 73–78, 1972.

[13] D. Bezov, R. B. Lipton, and S. Ashina, "Post-dural puncture headache: part i diagnosis, epidemiology, etiology, and pathophysiology," *Headache*, vol. 50, no. 7, pp. 1144–1152, 2010.

[14] M. M. Charsley and S. E. Abram, "The injection of intrathecal normal saline reduces the severity of postdural puncture headache," *Regional Anesthesia and Pain Medicine*, vol. 26, no. 4, pp. 301–305, 2001.

[15] C. C. Apfel, A. Saxena, O. S. Cakmakkaya, R. Gaiser, E. George, and O. Radke, "Prevention of postdural puncture headache after accidental dural puncture: a quantitative systematic review," *British Journal of Anaesthesia*, vol. 105, no. 3, pp. 255–263, 2010.

21

Sugammadex and Reversal of Neuromuscular Block in Adult Patient with Duchenne Muscular Dystrophy

Ahmed Abdelgawwad Wefki Abdelgawwad Shousha, Maria Sanfilippo, Antonio Sabba, and Paolo Pinchera

Department of Anesthesiology and Intensive Care, Sapienza University, Viale del policlinico 155, 00161 Rome, Italy

Correspondence should be addressed to Ahmed Abdelgawwad Wefki Abdelgawwad Shousha; dott.ahmed@gmail.com

Academic Editors: A. Han, J. G. Jakobsson, T. Suzuki, and E. A. Vandermeersch

Duchenne's muscular dystrophy (DMD) is the most common and severe form of myopathy. Patients with DMD are more sensitive to sedative, anesthetic, and neuromuscular blocking agents which may result in intraoperative and early postoperative cardiovascular and respiratory complications, as well as prolonged recovery from anesthesia. In this case report, we describe a 25-year-old male patient admitted for cholecystectomy under general anesthesia. We induced our anesthesia by oxygen, propofol, fentanyl, and rocuronium bromide. Maintenance was done by fentanyl, rocuronium bromide, sevoflurane, and O_2. We report in this case the safety use of sugammadex to antagonize the neuromuscular block and rapid recovery in such category of patients.

1. Introduction

Duchenne muscular dystrophy (DMD) is a rare genetic X-linked recessive disorder but it is one of the most frequent genetic conditions affecting approximately 1 in 3,500 male births worldwide. It is usually recognized between three and six years of age. DMD is characterized by weakness and wasting (atrophy) of the muscles of the pelvic area followed by the involvement of the shoulder muscles. As the disease progresses, muscle weakness and atrophy spread to affect the trunk and forearms and gradually progress to involve additional muscles of the body [1, 2].

The anesthetic management of these patients is complicated not only by muscle weakness but also by cardiac and pulmonary manifestations.

However there is no definite recommendation for either general or regional anaesthesia.

Succinylcholine and volatile anaesthetics have been best avoided because there is a risk of hyperkalemic cardiac arrest or severe rhabdomyolysis [3].

Some authors have suggested intubation and anesthesia without resorting to muscle relaxants, in order to avoid postoperative respiratory failure related to the usage of muscle relaxants and the other complications induced by acetylcholinesterase inhibitors. However, anesthesia without muscle relaxants might not always be suitable for some surgical procedures like such as in our patient [4].

Case reports in patients with myasthenia gravis document the successful use of sugammadex (six case reports). For other rare muscular diseases like Duchenne muscular dystrophy recent reports document the successful reversal of rocuronium with sugammadex in pediatric patients [5–9].

And in this case report we document the sugammadex safety in an adult Duchenne disease patient.

2. Case Presentation

A 25-year-old male with DMD with a modified Barthel index of 23 (Barthel index is an ordinal scale used to measure performance in activities of daily living) [10] (BMI 25,6, ASA III) was scheduled for open cholecystectomy under general anesthesia. The surgery duration was about 240 minutes and this prolongation was due to further undiagnosed stenosis of the biliary tract. His medical history revealed DMD disability, moderate restrictive pulmonary dysfunction, mild hypokalemia, and hypertension.

TABLE 1: Hemogasanalysis at the middle of the surgery.

Temperature (37.0°C)	
pH	7.37
pCO$_2$	34 mmHg
pO$_2$	322 mmHg
Na$^+$	141 mmol/L
K$^{+\prime}$	2.8 mmol/L
Ca^{++}	1.48 mmol/L
Glu	95 mg/dL
Lac	0.5 mmol/L
Oximeter	
tHb	12.4 g/dL
°2 Hb	96.3%
COHb	1.8%
MetHb	1.6%
HHb	0.3%
5°2	99.7%
Derivatives	
TCO$_2$	20.7 mmol/L
BEecf	−5.6 mmol/L
BE (B)	−4.8 mmol/L
Ca^{++} (7.4)	1.46 mmol/L
SO$_2$ (C)	99.9%
HCO$_3$-(c)	19.7 mmol/L
HCO$_{3\,standard}$	21.2 mmol/L
Hct (c)	37%

TABLE 2: Hemogasanalysis 1 hour after the end of surgery.

Temperature (37.0°C)	
pH	7.24
pCO$_2$	45 mmHg
pO$_2$	137 mmHg
Na$^+$	142 mmol/L
K$^{+\prime}$	4.9 mmol/L
Ca^{++}	1.39 mmol/L
Glu	109 mg/dL
Lac	0.7 mmol/L
Oximeter	
tHb	13.9 g/dL
°2 Hb	96.4%
COHb	2.1%
MetHb	1.2%
HHb	0.3%
5°2	99.7%
Derivatives	
TCO$_2$	20.7 mmol/L
BEecf	−8.1 mmol/L
BE (B)	−8.0 mmol/L
Ca^{++} (7.4)	1.30 mmol/L
SO$_2$ (C)	98.6%
HCO$_3$-(c)	19.3 mmol/L
HCO$_{3\,standard}$	19.3 mmol/L
Hct (c)	42%

His preoperative laboratory tests were hemoglobin 13.9 g^{-1}, hematocrit 43.5%, platelets 202,000 mm^{-3}, sodium 141 mmom·L^{-1}, potassium 3 mmol·L^{-1}, magnesium 0.58 mg·dL^{-1}, creatinine 0.06 mg·dL^{-1}, total calcium 8.72 mg·dL^{-1}, lactic dehydrogenase (LDH) 230 U·L^{-1}, direct bilirubin 230 U·L^{-1}, and alkaline phosphatase 130 U·L^{-1}.

For the common difficulty to obtain a peripheral venous access in such patients, a central venous access was established by ultrasound guided cannulation of the internal right jugular vein.

In the preoperative room we prepared our patient by antibiotics prophylaxis: ciprofloxacin 2 gm; metronidazole 500 mg; and an antiemetic agent ondansetron 4 mg.

Our patient was monitored by pulse oximetry, expiratory capnography, invasive and noninvasive blood pressure, electrocardiogram, neuromuscular transmission by train-of-four repeated every 12 seconds at the adductor pollicis muscle (TOF Guard Organon Teknika B.V, Boxtel, The Netherlands), and diuresis.

We induced our anesthesia by oxygen, propofol 150 mg, fentanyl 200 mcg, and rocuronium bromide 10 mg, and then we proceeded to a rapid sequence endotracheal intubation (tube diameter was 7.5 mm).

The maintenance of the anesthesia was achieved by fentanyl in a total dose of 400 mcg (200-100-100), rocuronium bromide 5 mg repeated every 45 minutes at T4/T1 recovery of 25%, sevoflurane 2%, and O$_2$ 40% in air. The fluid replacement was calculated depending on his diuresis, plasma fluid, and intraoperative blood loss and he had received a total fluids amount of Ringer Lactate 1500 mL and Nacl 0.9% 1000 mL. He was mechanically ventilated with these parameters: IPPV with respiratory frequency 12 incursions per minute, tidal volume of 550 mL, PEEP 5 cm H$_2$O, and inspiratory/expiratory time ratio 1 : 2.

Blood gas analysis was performed twice (at the middle of the surgery and one hour after the end of surgery) by obtaining blood samples through the arterial catheter used for invasive blood pressure monitoring. For hypokalemia we administered KCl 40 mEq (Tables 1 and 2).

At the end of surgery and immediately before the emergence phase we registered that TOF ratio was 25%; we administrated Sugammadex at a single dose of 150 mg; in 5 minutes we obtained a TOF ratio of 75% increasing; for another 5 minutes TOF ratio reached 90%; the patient was extubated with careful monitoring for his cardiovascular and respiratory functions.

After 15 minutes we got the complete recovery of our patient; he was awake with excellent and stabile both hemodynamic and respiratory functions.

3. Conclusion

However there are few studies which can confirm the safety use of Sugammadex in patients with muscular dystrophic diseases and however mainly these few studies were implicated on pediatric population and especially in patients with myasthenia gravis. In our case we had the fortune to confirm the effectiveness and the safety of the drug in an adult patient with Duchenne dystrophy as we registered the rapid emergence without any postoperative residual curarization.

Also we recommend whenever it is necessary the use of rocuronium in such category of patient; the Sugammadex can provide a rapid and safe reversal moderate neuromuscular block after administration of rocuronium in dose of $2\,mg\cdot kg^{-1}$.

References

[1] "Duchenne muscular dystrophy: MedlinePlus Medical Encyclopedia," 2013, http://www.nlm.nih.gov/ .

[2] A. Woodhead, *Molecular Biology of Aging*, Plenum Press, 1985.

[3] "Lange anesthesiology: chapter 37," Anesthesia for Patients with Neuromuscular Disease.

[4] N. Abe, T. Kunisawa, T. Sasakawa, O. Takahata, and H. Iwasaki, "Anesthetic management using remifentanil target controlled infusion without muscle relaxants in two patients with myasthenia gravis," *Masui*, vol. 59, no. 6, pp. 727–730, 2010.

[5] C. Unterbuchner, H. Fink, and M. Blobner, "The use of sugammadex in a patient with myasthenia gravis," *Anaesthesia*, vol. 65, no. 3, pp. 302–305, 2010.

[6] A. M. Petrun, D. Mekiš, and M. Kamenik, "Successful use of rocuronium and sugammadex in a patient with myasthenia," *European Journal of Anaesthesiology*, vol. 27, no. 10, pp. 917–918, 2010.

[7] H. D. de Boer, J. van Egmond, J. J. Driessen, and L. H. J. D. Booij, "Sugammadex in patients with myasthenia gravis," *Anaesthesia*, vol. 65, no. 6, p. 653, 2010.

[8] A. Rudzka-Nowak and M. Piechota, "Anaesthetic management of a patient with myasthenia gravis for abdominal surgery using sugammadex," *Archives of Medical Science*, vol. 7, no. 2, pp. 361–364, 2011.

[9] V. Garcia, P. Diemunsch, and S. Boet, "Use of rocuronium and sugammadex for caesarean delivery in a patient with myasthenia gravis," *International Journal of Obstetric Anesthesia*, vol. 21, no. 3, pp. 286–287, 2012.

[10] C. Collin, D. T. Wade, S. Davies, and V. Horne, "The Barthel ADL index: a reliability study," *International Disability Studies*, vol. 10, no. 2, pp. 61–63, 1988.

22

Intralipid Therapy for Inadvertent Peripheral Nervous System Blockade Resulting from Local Anesthetic Overdose

Ihab Kamel, Gaurav Trehan, and Rodger Barnette

Temple University School of Medicine, 3401 N. Broad Street, 3rd Floor Outpatient Building, Zone B, Philadelphia, PA 19140, USA

Correspondence should be addressed to Ihab Kamel; ihab.kamel@tuhs.temple.edu

Academic Editor: Renato Santiago Gomez

Although local anesthetics have an acceptable safety profile, significant morbidity and mortality have been associated with their use. Inadvertent intravascular injection of local anesthetics and/or the use of excessive doses have been the most frequent causes of local anesthetic systemic toxicity (LAST). Furthermore, excessive doses of local anesthetics injected locally into the tissues may lead to inadvertent peripheral nerve infiltration and blockade. Successful treatment of LAST with intralipid has been reported. We describe a case of local anesthetic overdose that resulted in LAST and in unintentional blockade of peripheral nerves of the lower extremity; both effects completely resolved with administration of intralipid.

1. Introduction

Local anesthetics are well established in the practice of anesthesia. Although local anesthetics have an acceptable safety profile, significant morbidity and mortality have been associated with their use. Inadvertent intravascular injection of local anesthetics and/or the use of excessive doses have been the most frequent causes of local anesthetic systemic toxicity (LAST). Excessive doses of local anesthetics injected at the surgical site may lead to inadvertent peripheral nerve infiltration and blockade. We describe a case of local anesthetic overdose that resulted in early manifestations of LAST and unintentional sensory and motor blockade of peripheral nerves of the lower extremity. The concurrent sensory and motor blockade of the lower extremity completely resolved with intralipid that was administered to treat early symptoms of LAST.

2. Case Report

A 51-year-old, 163 cm, 74 kg, ASA-2 female was scheduled for posterior colpoperineorrhaphy and transobturator sling insertion. Her past medical history was significant for asthma, urinary incontinence, and multiple uneventful cesarean deliveries. The patient received general endotracheal anesthesia using propofol, vecuronium, sevoflurane, and fentanyl.

Surgery was performed with the patient in the lithotomy position. Shortly prior to the conclusion of the procedure 80 mL of 0.5% bupivacaine with epinephrine was injected by the surgeon into the surgical incision site for postoperative analgesia. The surgical procedure lasted for 90 minutes.

In the postanesthesia care unit (PACU) the patient experienced dizziness, agitation, posturing, and oculogyric symptoms and stated that she "felt funny." The patient further stated that she could not feel or move her left lower extremity and that it felt "numb." On examination the left lower extremity revealed nonflaccid loss of motor power (1/5) in the hip flexors and adductors and inability to articulate the left knee joint. She had decreased touch sensation over the anterior and medial aspect of the left thigh and the left leg (L2–L5 dermatomes). The neurology service was immediately consulted to evaluate the patient for the possibility of stroke. Approximately 20 minutes after arriving at PACU, the patient was treated with 100 mL of intralipid 20% I.V. fat emulsion (Baxter Healthcare Corporation, Deerfield, IL) over one minute, followed by 400 mL of intralipid 20% over 20 minutes. Immediately upon completion of the initial intralipid loading dose, the patient's overall condition improved; the intermittent oculogyric symptoms resolved and she became less agitated and stated that she "felt better." During the subsequent intralipid infusion the patient stated that she could now feel her left lower extremity and slight knee movement was noted. On examination, the patient regained sensation over the medial and anterior left thigh and the left leg. Motor evaluation revealed return of motor power to left hip flexors and adductors and the ability to articulate the left knee joint. Following completion of the infusion the patient had restoration of motor function and sensation to the left lower extremity. The neurology service arrived approximately 30 minutes after the patient's arrival at PACU and concluded that her left lower extremity symptoms were likely due to the excessive dose of local anesthetic injected during the procedure, rather than a cerebrovascular accident. They also noted that the patient's left lower extremity weakness and sensory loss were significantly improving with intralipid injection. The patient maintained awareness and spontaneous ventilation with a SpO$_2$ of 98% or higher throughout the event. EKG showed sinus rhythm without evidence of ectopy or arrhythmia. A 12-lead EKG revealed no change in comparison to the preoperative EKG. Prior to administration of intralipid, she experienced one episode of hypotension that was successfully treated with 100 mcg of phenylephrine. The patient continued to complain of left lower extremity parasthesias; however these had resolved completely by the next morning. The patient was discharged home on the first postoperative day without sequelae.

3. Discussion

Successful intralipid treatment of cardiovascular and central nervous system (CNS) local anesthetic toxicity has been reported [1–5]. This patient received approximately twice the maximum recommended dose of bupivacaine and appeared to experience early manifestations of central nervous system local anesthetic toxicity. The patient inadvertently received 80 mL of 0.5% bupivacaine (400 mg) instead of 0.25% (200 mg). This occurred because the operating room technician did not dilute the 0.5% bupivacaine solution as instructed. The onset of symptoms occurred gradually as the bupivacaine injected at the surgical site was absorbed into the blood stream. Because of the gradual and partial absorption of bupivacaine and epinephrine into the blood stream the patient did not experience acute full-blown manifestations of LAST and tachycardia. These findings prompted rapid treatment and all signs and symptoms of LAST resolved with administration of intralipid. The use of intralipid upon identifying early premonitory symptoms and signs can prevent further clinical manifestations of CNS toxicity and progression to cardiovascular toxicity [2, 6–8]. Atypical presentation has been reported in approximately 40% of patients experiencing LAST [7], and cases in which patients had minimal premonitory signs of CNS toxicity, such as oculogyric movement and agitation, have progressed to cardiac arrest [9]. Airway management and circulatory support have been reported to be crucial to successful treatment of LAST. However, in this case, the patient maintained adequate respiratory and cardiovascular functions.

In this patient, local anesthetic overdose was associated with a new onset unilateral lower extremity peripheral nerve block. While gradual systemic absorption of the excessive bupivacaine dose is responsible for LAST, diffusion of the excessive bupivacaine and local infiltration of surrounding tissues could explain the concomitant peripheral nerve blockade of the left femoral and obturator nerves. Postoperative unilateral lower extremity peripheral nerve blockade due to local anesthesia injection during transobturator sling placement has been reported [10].

The rapid temporally associated resolution of both sensory and motor symptoms in the left lower extremity during the administration of intralipid in the absence of any other interventions raises the possibility of a cause-effect relationship. This observation deserves further investigation in regard to the effect of intralipid on peripheral nerve local anesthetic blockade. Despite the plethora of reports and studies on intralipid use to treat LAST, our review of the current literature did not reveal any reports on the effect of intralipid on peripheral nerve local anesthetic blockade. The ability to reverse peripheral nerve blockade could allow early neurological examination and potentially prevent delays in diagnosis, thus reducing the risk of permanent neurological damage.

The mechanism of action of intralipid is incompletely understood. It is believed that intralipid provides an intravascular compartment for lipid soluble drugs [11]. Intralipid may affect metabolism, distribution, and displacement of local anesthetics from receptors into lipids within the tissues [4, 11] and counteract the inhibitory effect of bupivacaine on fatty acid transport at the inner mitochondrial membrane [11]. Although the safety profile of acute lipid emulsion infusion is not completely understood, there are no published reports of adverse outcomes [5].

4. Conclusion

We report a case in which administration of intralipid to treat LAST resulted in complete and rapid resolution of concomitant peripheral nerve blockade symptoms caused by local infiltration of bupivacaine overdose. Intralipid could be used to reverse prolonged or inadvertent peripheral nerve blocks allowing for earlier neurological evaluation.

Ethical Approval

The responsible institutional review board gave permission to publish this report.

Disclosure

This report was previously presented, in part, at the Medically Challenging Case poster presentation at the ASA Annual Meeting 2013.

References

[1] A. G. Spence, "Lipid reversal of central nervous system symptoms of bupivacaine toxicity," *Anesthesiology*, vol. 107, no. 3, pp. 516–517, 2007.

[2] R. J. Litz, T. Roessel, A. R. Heller, and S. N. Stehr, "Reversal of central nervous system and cardiac toxicity after local anesthetic intoxication by lipid emulsion injection," *Anesthesia and Analgesia*, vol. 106, no. 5, pp. 1575–1577, 2008.

[3] S. L. Corman and S. J. Skledar, "Use of lipid emulsion to reverse local anesthetic-induced toxicity," *Annals of Pharmacotherapy*, vol. 41, no. 11, pp. 1873–1877, 2007.

[4] J. C. Rowlingson, "Lipid rescue: a step forward in patient safety? Likely so!," *Anesthesia and Analgesia*, vol. 106, no. 5, pp. 1333–1336, 2008.

[5] G. L. Weinberg, "Treatment of local anesthetic systemic toxicity (LAST)," *Regional Anesthesia and Pain Medicine*, vol. 35, no. 2, pp. 188–193, 2010.

[6] S. J. Brull, "Lipid emulsion for the treatment of local anesthetic toxicity: patient safety implications," *Anesthesia and Analgesia*, vol. 106, no. 5, pp. 1337–1339, 2008.

[7] J. M. Neal, C. M. Bernards, J. F. Butterworth IV et al., "ASRA practice advisory on local anesthetic systemic toxicity," *Regional Anesthesia and Pain Medicine*, vol. 35, no. 2, pp. 152–161, 2010.

[8] J. M. Neal, M. F. Mulroy, and G. L. Weinberg, "American society of regional anesthesia and pain medicine checklist for managing local anesthetic systemic toxicity: 2012 version," *Regional Anesthesia and Pain Medicine*, vol. 37, no. 1, pp. 16–18, 2012.

[9] P. Chazalon, J. P. Tourtier, T. Villevielle et al., "Ropivacaine-induced cardiac arrest after peripheral nerve block: successful resuscitation," *Anesthesiology*, vol. 99, no. 6, pp. 1449–1451, 2003.

[10] A. J. Park, J. L. Fisch, and M. D. Walters, "Transient obturator neuropathy due to local anesthesia during transobturator sling placement," *International Urogynecology Journal and Pelvic Floor Dysfunction*, vol. 20, no. 2, pp. 247–249, 2009.

[11] G. L. Weinberg, "Lipid infusion therapy: translation to clinical practice," *Anesthesia and Analgesia*, vol. 106, no. 5, pp. 1340–1342, 2008.

23

Paraplegia after Gastrectomy in a Patient with Cervical Disc Herniation

Qingfu Zhang, Wei Jiang, Quanhong Zhou, Guangyan Wang, and Linlin Zhao

Department of Anesthesiology, Shanghai Jiao Tong University Affiliated Shanghai Sixth People's Hospital, 600 Yishan Road, Shanghai 200233, China

Correspondence should be addressed to Wei Jiang; jiangw@sjtu.edu.cn

Academic Editors: C.-H. Hsing and D. Lee

Paraplegia is a rare postoperative complication. We present a case of acute paraplegia after elective gastrectomy surgery because of cervical disc herniation. The 73-year-old man has the medical history of cervical spondylitis with only symptom of temporary pain in neck and shoulder. Although the patient's neck was cautiously preserved by using the Discopo, an acute paraplegia emerged at about 10 hours after the operation. Severe compression of the spinal cord by herniation of the C4-C5 cervical disc was diagnosed and emergency surgical decompression was performed immediately. Unfortunately the patient showed limited improvement in neurologic deficits even after 11 months.

1. Introduction

Paraplegia is a rare postoperative complication, and the pathology is various. We present a case of acute paraplegia after elective gastrectomy surgery because of cervical disc herniation. The IRB of Shanghai Sixth People's Hospital reviewed the case report and gave permission for us to publish the report.

2. Case Description

A 73-year-old man with peptic ulcer and bleeding was checked into the Department of Gastroenterology due to brown vomit and drain black stool once. The patient has a past medical history of duodenal ulcer for 18 years and complained from abdominal discomfort for 4 days. He received medical treatment with omepazole for 10 days and then was referred to the Department of General Surgery for selective gastrectomy. He denied any other medical history or other medication during preoperative visit by anesthetist.

General anesthesia was induced by intravenous administration of 15 μg/kg fentanyl, 2 mg/kg propofol, and 0.1 mg/kg rocuronium. As the patient had loosened teeth, Discopo was taken for orotracheal intubation. During the whole process, the patient's neck was placed in a neutral position.

The patient was mechanically ventilated with the settings of FiO_2 1.0, tidal volume 8 mL/kg, respiratory rate 10/min, and inspiration/expiration 1/2 and one minimum alveolar concentration of sevoflurane was administered during the surgery. In the meantime, propofol (2 mg/kg/h) and fentanyl (3 μg/kg/h) were also infused.

Subtotal gastrectomy was performed, and gastrointestinal tract was reconstructed with the method of Billroth II. The operation, which lasted about 2 hours, was uneventful with a total blood loss of 250 mL. There was no hemodynamic instability during surgery. The patient was sent to the postoperative care unit (PACU) and extubated 30 minutes later. The recovery process was smooth, and the patient was transferred to surgery intensive care unit (SICU). Ten hours after the arrival at SICU, the patient was found to be flaccid in both his legs. Neurological examinations revealed complete paralysis of the bilateral lower extremities, bilateral weakness of upper extremities, and absence of deep and superficial sensation below T4 level. CT scan was negative for intracranial lesions. Further, when asked about previous medical history, he said he had cervical spondylosis before, with the only symptom of intermittent pain in neck and shoulder. A preoperative MRI showed a protruded intervertebral disc between C3 and C4, C4 and C5, C5 and C6, and corresponding spinal canal stenosis (Figure 1). Repeated MRI of the neck at 20 hours

TABLE 1: Reported cases of nontraumatic acute myelopathy due to cervical disc herniation.

Authors	Year	Country	Age/sex	After general anesthesia	level	Spinal stenosis	Operation	Recovery of motor function
Lourie et al. [1]	1973	USA	37/M	–	C6-C7	–	ASF	+
Kawaguchi et al. [18]	1991	USA	61/M	+	C6-C7	–	ASD	+
Ueyama et al. [3]	1999	Japan	61/F	–	C6-C7	+	ASF	+
Suzuki et al. [4]	2003	Japan	29/M	–	C6-C7	+	ASF	–
Chen et al. [5]	2005	Taiwan	54/M	+	C6-C7	–	ASF	–
Hirose and Akhrass [6]	2005	USA	65/M	+	C7-T1	–	ASF	–
Tsai et al. [7]	2006	Taiwan	32/F	–	C3-c4	–	ASF	+
Hwang et al. [8]	2008	Singapore	63/M	+	C5-C6, C6-C7	+	No operation	+
Liu et al. [9]	2010	China	75/M	–	C4-C5	+	ASF	–
Gorur et al. [19]	2010	Turkey	62/M	+	C5-C6	–	ASF	+
Kato et al. [10]	2010	Japan	48/M	–	C6-C7	–	ASF	+
Ikeda et al. [11]	2012	Japan	21/F	–	C3-C4	+	ASF	+
Ahmed et al. [12]	2013	Egypt	48/F	–	C5-C6	+	ASF	+
Present case	2013	China	73/M	+	C4-C5	+	ASF	–

M: male; F: female; ASF: anterior spine fusion; ASD: anterior spine decompression.

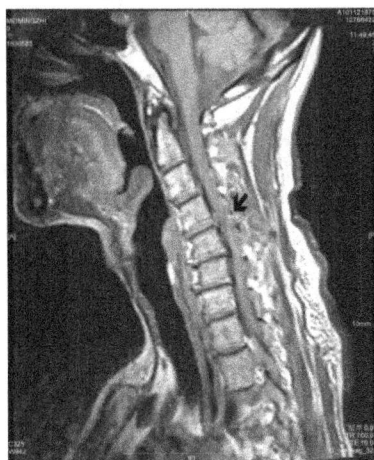

FIGURE 1: T2-weighted MRI demonstrates disc protrusion at C3-C4, C4-C5, and C5-C6 and corresponding spinal canal stenosis (preoperative MRI). Arrow shows the lesion at the C4-5 level before the operation.

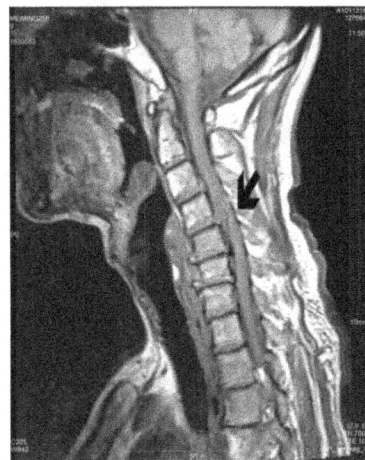

FIGURE 2: T2-weighted MRI demonstrates disc protrusion at C3-C4, C4-C5, and C5-C6, with spinal cord degeneration at 20 hours after gastrectomy. Arrow shows the lesion at the C4-5 level after the operation.

after gastrectomy demonstrated a posterior disc herniation at C4-5, and spinal canal stenosis from C3 to C6, with spinal cord degeneration (Figure 2). After consultation with neurosurgeons, an emergency anterior approach to the C3–C5 vertebral disectomy was performed immediately, followed by C4 vertebral resection and interbody fusion with iliac crest bone graft. After the surgery, the patient's upper extremities improved, however, lower extremities remained paralyzed without significant improvement at 11 months of follow up.

3. Discussion

Nontraumatic paraplegia caused by cervical disc herniation is rare. Since it was first reported in 1973 [1], more cases have

been described in detail [2–12], especially in the last decade (Table 1). We present postoperative paraplegia due to acute compression of spinal cord secondary to the protrusion of cervical disc.

Nontraumatic paraplegia is an emergent condition. It is difficult to make an accurate diagnosis if there was no obvious injury. Paraplegia caused by cervical disc herniation after general anesthesia was even more rare. The possible etiology of cervical herniation during operation was not clear. Various etiologies should be kept in mind, such as intracranial lesions, spinal infarction, disorders of muscle, or neuromuscular junctions [9]. For this case, CT scan of the brain was negative. The patient denied any disorders of muscle or neuromuscular junctions.

Among our review of the literature, there are 5 cases that had apparent cause for the onset of paraplegia. Two developed following bending forward to do something [9, 12], 1 following being fixed to the headrest of the MRI instrument [10], 1 following rolling in bed on the left side [4], and 1 is in association with labor [7]. These events may have led to the posterior movement of the disk, which in turn caused herniation, increasing the compression on the dural sac and leading to severe mechanical compression and ischemia of the spinal cord [10]. It is likely that extension of the cervical spine loosened the tension of the posterior longitudinal ligament and caused posterior listhesis of the vertebra.

Excessive neck extension in intubation and changing the position of neck during general anesthesia and loss of muscle support may aggravate spinal cord injury [5]. Coexisting cervical spine disorders, such as spondylosis, bulging disc, and spinal canal stenosis, are not uncommon in the elderly patients, which raises the possibility of spinal cord injury during general anesthesia. In our case, the medical history of cervical spondylosis and previous MRI test led us to suspect a lesion within the cervical cord.

The incidence rate in Asians is higher than others. This could be explained by the narrower spinal canal anatomy among Asians [9, 13, 14]. In the present case, the patient had spinal canal stenosis which made him more vulnerable to compressive disturbances [15, 16]. To make things worse, the patient did not mention his previous cervical spondylosis history. His previous MRI was overlooked by all medical staff before the gastrectomy. Although careful history taking was performed, details not shared with medical staff might cause serious consequences as in this case.

There are many techniques of intubation commonly used for patients with cervical spondylosis such as awake endotracheal intubation, flexible fiberoptic bronchoscope, and Discopo [17]. Unfortunately, complications still happened. Deem et al. [2] reported quadriplegia after thoracolumbar surgery in a patient with severe cervical spondylosis, despite the fact that awake oral tracheal intubation under direct visual laryngoscopy was performed without difficulty. Hwang et al. [8] described quadriparesis after CABG in a patient with a history of cervical spondylosis although all precautions to prevent hyperextension of the neck during intubation and patient positioning were considered. In the present case, although Discopo was used to minimize the movement of the neck and to keep the head in neutral position, for endotracheal intubation, the cervical herniation still happened. The lesson from the case is to keep the neck support for cervical spondylosis during noncervical surgery. We also suggest that, in patients with significant cervical diseases undergoing elective noncervical spine surgery, cervical decompression should be considered as the initial treatment.

In conclusion, paraplegia after noncervical spine surgery under general anesthesia is a devastating complication, which often results in permanent disability or neurological deficit in patients with preexisting cervical spine diseases. Anesthesiologists and surgeons should pay much attention to this complication and share details of history with each other in order to exclude the coexisting cervical spine disorders. Excessive neck movement is believed to be trigging factor and skillful intubation and neck supporting are recommended to reduce spinal cord injury.

References

[1] H. Lourie, M. C. Shende, and D. H. Stewart Jr., "The syndrome of central cervical soft disk herniation," *Journal of the American Medical Association*, vol. 226, no. 3, pp. 302–305, 1973.

[2] S. Deem, H. M. Shapiro, and L. F. Marshall, "Quadraplegia in a patient with cervical spondylosis after thoracolumbar surgery in the prone position," *Anesthesiology*, vol. 75, no. 3, pp. 527–528, 1991.

[3] T. Ueyama, N. Tamaki, T. Kondoh, H. Miyamoto, H. Akiyama, and T. Nagashima, "Non-traumatic acute paraplegia associated with cervical disc herniation: a case report," *Surgical Neurology*, vol. 52, no. 2, pp. 204–207, 1999.

[4] T. Suzuki, E. Abe, H. Murai, and T. Kobayashi, "Nontraumatic acute complete paraplegia resulting from cervical disc herniation: a case report," *Spine*, vol. 28, no. 6, pp. E125–E128, 2003.

[5] S. H. Chen, Y. L. Hui, C. M. Yu, C. C. Niu, and P. W. Lui, "Paraplegia by acute cervical disc protrusion after lumbar spine surgery," *Chang Gung Medical Journal*, vol. 28, no. 4, pp. 254–257, 2005.

[6] H. Hirose and R. Akhrass, "Tetraplegia after coronary artery bypass, a rare complication," *Annals of Thoracic and Cardiovascular Surgery*, vol. 11, no. 4, pp. 270–272, 2005.

[7] H. H. Tsai, T. Y. Li, and S. T. Chang, "Nontraumatic acute myelopathy associated with cervical disc herniation during labor," *Journal of Back and Musculoskeletal Rehabilitation*, vol. 19, no. 2-3, pp. 97–100, 2006.

[8] N. C. Hwang, P. Singh, and Y. L. Chua, "Quadriparesis after cardiac surgery," *Journal of Cardiothoracic and Vascular Anesthesia*, vol. 22, no. 4, pp. 587–589, 2008.

[9] C. Liu, Y. Huang, H. X. Cai, and S. W. Fan, "Nontraumatic acute paraplegia associated with cervical disk herniation," *Journal of Spinal Cord Medicine*, vol. 33, no. 4, pp. 420–424, 2010.

[10] Y. Kato, N. Nishida, and T. Taguchi, "Paraplegia caused by posture during MRI in a patient with cervical disk herniation," *Orthopedics*, vol. 33, no. 6, pp. 448–450, 2010.

[11] H. Ikeda, J. Hanakita, T. Takahashi, K. Kurasishi, and M. Watanabe, "Nontraumatic cervical disc herniation in a 21-year-old patient with no other underlying disease," *Neurologia Medico-Chirurgica*, vol. 52, no. 9, pp. 652–656, 2012.

[12] E. S. Ahmed, M. Gouda, W. Stephan, and B. Heinrich, "Acute nontraumatic cervical disk herniation with incomplete tetraplegia. A case report and review of literature," *European Orthopaedics and Traumatology*, vol. 4, no. 4, pp. 267–272, 2013.

[13] T. E. Geyer, M. J. Naik, and R. Pillai, "Anterior spinal artery syndrome after elective coronary artery bypass grafting," *Annals of Thoracic Surgery*, vol. 73, no. 6, pp. 1971–1973, 2002.

[14] S. Fujioka, Y. Niimi, K. Hirata, I. Nakamura, and S. Morita, "Tetraplegia after coronary artery bypass grafting," *Anesthesia and Analgesia*, vol. 97, no. 4, pp. 979–980, 2003.

[15] Z. Naja, A. Zeidan, H. Maaliki et al., "Tetraplegia after coronary artery bypass grafting in a patient with undiagnosed cervical

stenosis," *Anesthesia and Analgesia*, vol. 101, no. 6, pp. 1883–1884, 2005.

[16] K. J. Song and K. B. Lee, "Non-traumatic acute myelopathy due to cervical disc herniation in contiguous two-level disc spaces: a case report," *European Spine Journal*, vol. 14, no. 7, pp. 694–697, 2005.

[17] Q. J. Chu, A. M. Yang, Z. Jia, G. L. Xie, and W. Zhang, "A new visual stylet (Discopo): early clinical experience in patients with difficult intubation," *Anaesthesia and Intensive Care*, vol. 39, no. 3, pp. 512–513, 2011.

[18] Y. Kawaguchi, A. Miyasaka, and K. Sugatani, "Acute paraplegia due to cervical disk herniation: a case report," *Rinsho Seikei Geka*, vol. 26, pp. 1395–1398, 1991.

[19] A. Gorur, N. Ali Aydemir, N. Yurtseven, and M. S. Bilal, "Tetraplegia after coronary artery bypass surgery in a patient With cervical herniation," *Innovations*, vol. 5, no. 2, pp. 134–135, 2010.

24

Anaesthetic Management of Two Patients with Pompe Disease for Caesarean Section

I. J. J. Dons-Sinke, M. Dirckx, and G. P. Scoones

Department of Anesthesiology, Erasmus MC-Sophia, Postbus 2060, 3000 CB Rotterdam, The Netherlands

Correspondence should be addressed to I. J. J. Dons-Sinke; i.dons@erasmusmc.nl

Academic Editors: M. Dauri, Y. Demiraran, and C. Seefelder

The introduction of enzyme replacement therapy and the resultant stabilisation or improvement in mobility and respiratory muscle function afforded to patients with late-onset Pompe may lead to an increased number of Pompe patients prepared to accept the challenges of parenthood. In this case report, we describe our anaesthetic management of two patients with Pompe disease for a caesarean section.

1. Introduction

Pompe disease (PD), also referred to as acid maltase deficiency (AMD) or glycogen storage disease type II (GSDII), is an autosomal recessive disorder caused by a deficiency of the lysosomal enzyme acid-α-glucosidase (GAA) [1]. In PD, lysosomal glycogen accumulates in many tissues with skeletal, cardiac, and smooth muscle most prominently involved. Severity varies according to the age of onset; the degree and severity of skeletal, cardiac, and respiratory muscle involvement; and rate of disease progression. The combined incidence of all forms of PD is estimated to be 1 : 40.000 [2]. In general, disease severity is inversely related to residual acid-α-glucosidase activity.

Although PD is often classified into two separate phenotypes—infantile and late onset—based on age of onset of symptoms, PD is a clinical disease spectrum. Patients with infantile PD, present in the first few months of life with a hypertrophic cardiomyopathy, generalized muscle weakness and hypotonia. Without enzyme treatment death due to cardiorespiratory failure occurs within the first year of life. Late-onset PD can present at any age and is characterized by the absence of cardiac involvement and a less dismal short-term prognosis. Symptoms are related to progressive skeletal muscle dysfunction. Proximal lower limb and paraspinal trunk muscles are usually affected first, followed by involvement of the diaphragm and accessory muscles of respiration.

As the muscle weakness worsens, patients often become wheelchair dependent and may require assisted ventilation. Respiratory failure is the usual cause of increasing morbidity and mortality.

Alglucosidase alfa (recombinant GAA (rhGAA), Myozyme/Lumizyme) has been shown to be effective in the treatment of patients with early- and late-onset PD [3]. Individual response to enzyme replacement therapy (ERT) is however variable and determined by many factors: age of presentation, the rate of disease progression, muscle fibre type, defective autophagy, underlying genotype, and the development of rhGAA specific antibodies.

In this case report we describe the anaesthetic management of two patients with PD for a caesarean section.

2. Case Description

2.1. Patient 1. A 41-year-old nulliparous female (1.73 m/67 kg) with PD had been treated with enzyme therapy for 18 months at time of presentation. Before starting enzyme therapy there was a marked deterioration in muscle function, which manifested as a limb girdle weakness and a decrease in respiratory function, for which she needed nocturnal mechanical ventilation. After starting enzyme replacement therapy, there was a significant improvement in muscle strength.

As her pregnancy progressed, she noticed a marked deterioration in her effort tolerance. She needed more sleep, her walking distance decreased, and she felt short of breath. At 20 weeks pregnancy, her lung function tests showed a functional vital capacity of 1.61 (40% of normal predicted value) sitting and FVC of 1.11 (26%) supine. These results were similar to her lung function results prior to her pregnancy and were therefore related to the increased metabolic and respiratory demands of pregnancy rather than deterioration in her muscle function.

Following a multidisciplinary discussion, it was decided to do a caesarean section at 38 weeks of gestation, under combined spinal-epidural anaesthesia (CSE). In the normal healthy population, there is an increased risk of pelvic floor problems (including faecal and urinary incontinence) with a vaginal delivery. The recently reported incidence of previously unrecognised and underreported gastrointestinal symptoms including malabsorption and diarrhoea in patients with PD was a reason to avoid a vaginal delivery [4, 5]. Furthermore, there may be glycogen storage in the uterus as well, with unknown consequences during vaginal delivery.

The patient received our routine antacid prophylaxis, for example, oral ranitidine, sodium citrate, and metoclopramide. Monitoring was done by pulse oximeter, ECG, and automatic noninvasive blood pressure, set to record every 2.5 minutes. Combined spinal-epidural anaesthesia (CSE) at the L3-4 interspace was performed with the patient being in the sitting position. 1.6 mL bupi 0.5%/sufentanil (6.4 mg hyperbaric bupivacaine and 1.6 mcg sufentanyl) was injected intrathecally. Voluven coload of 500 mL and a phenylephrine infusion at 0.1 mcg/kg/min were commenced. The patient was placed supine in left lateral tilt position. She put on her own CPAP mask to assist her own ventilation. Throughout the operation her oxygen saturation remained above 95%. An adequate sensory block was reached 13 minutes after spinal injection. The phenylephrine infusion was increased to 0.24 mcg/kg/min to maintain baseline mean BP (80 mmHg). A live male infant was delivered 10 minutes after incision. Oxytocin 5 IU was titrated slowly intravenously (iv) followed by an infusion of 2.5 IU/hour of syntocinon for 4 hours. Routine antibiotic prophylaxis of 1 gram cefazolin was also administered intravenously. Estimated blood loss was 300 mL. Postoperative analgesia included regular oral paracetamol (four times a day) and a continuous infusion of ropivacaine 0.2% + sufentanil 0.5 mcg·mL^{-1} 6.0 mL per hour via the epidural catheter. She was monitored on the high-care unit before returning to the obstetric ward. The patient was discharged with her healthy baby boy four days postpartum.

2.2. Patient 2. A 30-year-old nulliparous woman (1.69 m/ 68 kg) with PD was receiving enzyme therapy for almost 4 years. Besides her PD, her medical history included a nasal septum correction without any anaesthetic problems. Prior to her pregnancy her symptoms included breathlessness on exertion and a mild increase in limb girdle weakness. She was not dependent on nocturnal ventilation. Her lung function tests prior to her pregnancy showed diminished respiratory muscle function with a FVC: 2.86 L (74%) which decreased to a FVC: 2.11 L (54%) towards the end of her pregnancy. Furthermore, ancillary investigations showed

a mild increase of hepatic enzymes, AST 122 U/L and ALAT 129 U/L. Many patients with PD show increased liver function values, which may reflect the presence of ongoing muscle damage, although the levels measured are not indicative of the severity of the disease [6]. For the same reasons as the previous patient, she was planned for an elective caesarean section under combined spinal-epidural anaesthesia at 38 weeks of gestation.

She received the same routine antacid prophylaxis. After securing intravenous access, noninvasive blood pressure, ECG, and oxygen saturation monitoring were established. CSE at the L3-4 interspace was performed in the sitting position and from a solution of 4 mL bupivacaine 0.5% glucose with 1 mL sufentanil 5 mcg·mL^{-1} 1.7 mL, representing 6.8 mg hyperbaric bupivacaine with 1.7 mcg sufentanil, was injected intrathecally. Crystalloid coload of 500 mL and a phenylephrine infusion at 0.23 mcg/kg/min were commenced. The patient was placed supine with a left lateral tilt. She needed 4 increments of 2.5 mL 1% ropivacaine over her epidural to reach a block at the T4 dermatome.

The phenylephrine infusion was increased to 0.37 mcg/ kg/min to maintain a baseline mean BP (85 mmHg). A healthy male infant was delivered uneventfully. Routine antibiotic prophylaxis of 1 gram cefazolin (iv) was administered; oxytocin 5 IU (iv) was given as a slow bolus followed by an infusion of 10 IU over 4 h (iv). Estimated blood loss was 200 mL. Postoperative analgesia included a continuous epidural and oral paracetamol. She was monitored for some hours at the high-care unit before she returned to the obstetric ward. She was discharged in a good condition with her son three days after the caesarean section.

3. Discussion

PD was first linked in 1963 to an inherited deficiency of the lysosomal enzyme acid alpha-glucosidase (GAA). This enzyme is responsible for the breakdown of glycogen to glucose. GAA deficiency leads to the intralysosomal accumulation of glycogen, primarily in muscle cells, causing a progressive loss of muscle function [7].

Until 2006 there was, other than ventilatory support, no treatment for patients with PD. In 2006 enzyme replacement therapy with alglucosidase alfa (Myozyme) was approved for the treatment of babies with infantile-onset PD. This was the first time a specific treatment was available for PD. A recently published Late-Onset Treatment Study (LOTS) showed that alglucosidase alfa treatment, as compared with placebo, has a positive, though modest, effect on walking distance and pulmonary function in patients with late-onset PD and may stabilize proximal limb and respiratory muscle strength [8]. Due to the introduction of ERT, we may increasingly have to deal with patients with Pompe disease who become pregnant. To our knowledge there is only one case report on a patient with Pompe disease undergoing a caesarean section [9].

Little is known about the use of alglucosidase alfa during pregnancy. In animal studies, alglucosidase alfa is not transported across the placental barrier and is, therefore, probably not harmful to the fetus. Furthermore, continuation of ERT during pregnancy has become common practice in other lysosomal storage diseases such as Gaucher disease and Fabry disease [10, 11].

Pregnancy itself is risky for these patients. Due to the mass effect of the uterus and the increased minute ventilation during pregnancy, the respiratory muscle function can be further challenged. The first patient had, prior to her pregnancy, a greater reduction of her respiratory muscle function capacity than the second patient, necessitating the use of noninvasive ventilation during her caesarean section in the supine position.

In addition, in order to avoid the risk of urinary and faecal incontinence, patients with PD should be allowed to undergo an elective caesarean section. If possible, regional anaesthesia is the technique of choice and far superior to general anaesthesia for elective caesarean section both for mother and child [12]. We decided to give regional anaesthesia by means of CSE, so we had the opportunity to minimize the amount of local anaesthesia to the spinal compartment. A lower dose of intrathecal local anaesthetic is likely to reduce the incidence of spinal-induced hypotension and possibly the severity of its maternal effects, at the expense of a slower onset and a shorter duration of anaesthesia and increased risk of intraoperative pain [13]. So, the epidural catheter functioned both as a backup (during the caesarean section) and postoperative analgesia. The backup function was needed in the second patient, preventing the risk of intraoperative pain and the need for a conversion to general anaesthesia.

Acknowledgments

The authors would like to acknowledge the contribution of S. C. A. Wens (Department of Neurology, Erasmus MC University Medical Center, Rotterdam, The Netherlands) and Professor Dr. E. A. P. Steegers (Department of Obstetrics and Gynaecology, Erasmus MC University Medical Center, Rotterdam, The Netherlands). This work was published with the written consent of the patients.

References

[1] P. S. Kishani, R. D. Steiner, D. Bali et al., "Pompe disease diagnosis and management guideline," *Genetics in Medicine*, vol. 8, pp. 267–288, 2006.

[2] M. G. E. M. Ausems, J. Verbiest, M. M. P. Hermans et al., "Frequency of glycogen storage disease type II in The Netherlands: implications for diagnosis and genetic counselling," *European Journal of Human Genetics*, vol. 7, no. 6, pp. 713–716, 1999.

[3] R. Y. Wang, O. A. Bodamer, M. S. Watson, and W. R. Wilcox, "Lysosomal storage diseases: diagnostic confirmation and management of presymptomatic individuals," *Genetics in Medicine*, vol. 13, no. 5, pp. 457–484, 2011.

[4] D. L. Bernstein, M. G. Bialer, L. Mehta, and R. J. Desnick, "Pompe disease: dramatic improvement in gastrointestinal function following enzyme replacement therapy: a report of three later-onset patients," *Molecular Genetics and Metabolism*, vol. 101, no. 2-3, pp. 130–133, 2010.

[5] G. Remiche, A. G. Herbaut, D. Ronchi et al., "Incontinence in late-onset Pompe disease: an underdiagnosed treatable condition," *European Neurology*, vol. 68, pp. 75–78, 2012.

[6] R. P. Morse and N. P. Rosman, "Diagnosis of occult muscular dystrophy: importance of the "chance" finding of elevated serum aminotransferase activities," *Journal of Pediatrics*, vol. 122, no. 2, pp. 254–256, 1993.

[7] H. G. Hers, "Alpha-Glucosidase deficiency in generalized glycogenstorage disease (Pompe's disease)," *The Biochemical journal*, vol. 86, pp. 11–16, 1963.

[8] A. T. van der Ploeg, P. R. Clemens, D. Corzo et al., "A randomized study of alglucosidase alfa in late-onset Pompe's disease," *The New England Journal of Medicine*, vol. 362, no. 15, pp. 1396–1406, 2010.

[9] H. J. Cilliers, S. T. Yeo, and N. P. Salmon, "Anaesthetic management of an obstetric patient with Pompe disease," *International Journal of Obstetric Anesthesia*, vol. 17, no. 2, pp. 170–173, 2008.

[10] G. Kalkum, D. Macchiella, J. Reinke, H. Kölbl, and M. Beck, "Enzyme replacement therapy with agalsidase alfa in pregnant women with Fabry disease," *European Journal of Obstetrics Gynecology and Reproductive Biology*, vol. 144, no. 1, pp. 92–93, 2009.

[11] J. M. Politei, "Treatment with agalsidase beta during pregnancy in Fabry disease," *Journal of Obstetrics and Gynaecology Research*, vol. 36, no. 2, pp. 428–429, 2010.

[12] M. van de Velde, "Anaesthesia for caesarean section," *Current Opinion in Anaesthesiology*, vol. 14, pp. 307–310, 2001.

[13] M. W. M. Rucklidge and M. J. Paech, "Limiting the dose of local anaesthetic for caesarean section under spinal anaesthesia: has the limbo bar been set too low?" *Anaesthesia*, vol. 67, no. 4, pp. 347–351, 2012.

25

Unilateral Hemiparesis with Thoracic Epidural in an Adolescent

Rosalie F. Tassone,[1,2] Christian Seefelder,[1] and Navil F. Sethna[1]

[1] Department of Anesthesiology, Perioperative and Pain Medicine, Children's Hospital Boston, Boston, MA 02115, USA
[2] Division of Pediatric Anesthesiology, Department of Anesthesiology, University of Illinois Medical Center, 1740 West Taylor Street, Chicago, IL 60612, USA

Correspondence should be addressed to Rosalie F. Tassone, rosalie.tassone@post.harvard.edu

Academic Editors: I.-O. Lee, P. Michalek, and S. Ogawa

Objective. Unilateral sensory and motor blockade is known to occur with epidural anesthesia but is rarely reported in children. The differential diagnosis should include the presence of a midline epidural septum. *Case Report*. We describe a case of a 16-year-old adolescent who developed repeated complete unilateral extensive epidural sensory and motor blockade with Horner's syndrome after thoracic epidural catheter placement. This unusual presentation of complete hemibody neural blockade has not been reported in the pediatric population. Maneuvers to improve contralateral uniform neural blockade were unsuccessful. An epidurogram was performed to ascertain the correct location of the catheter within the epidural space and presence of sagittal compartmentalization. *Conclusion*. This case report highlights a less frequently reported reason for unilateral sensory and motor blockade with epidural anesthesia in children. The presence of a midline epidural septum should be considered in the differential diagnosis of unilateral epidural blockade.

1. Introduction

Unilateral blockade is a known occurrence of epidural analgesia. Frequently, it occurs as a result of patient positioning, lateral displacement of the epidural catheter, or an uneven distribution of the local anesthetic. Additionally, a midline epidural septum may result in unilateral epidural blockade. We report a case of recurrent unilateral thoracic epidural analgesia associated with motor and sensory blockade of one side of the body in an adolescent due to midline epidural septum confirmed by epidurogram. Epidural anatomy, diagnosis, and implication for postoperative analgesia are discussed.

2. Case Report

A 16-year-old female, who was 157 cm tall and weighed 54 kg, had a longstanding history of Crohn's disease and presented for an exploratory laparotomy and resection of a small bowel anastomotic stricture. Medications included 6-mercaptopurine, omeprazole, infliximab, lactulose, iron supplements, and mesalamine. The patient and her mother requested epidural analgesia for postoperative pain control. Epidural analgesia had been used with a previous ileocecectomy surgery, and the patient indicated satisfactory postoperative analgesia with apparent unilateral epidural blockade.

After intravenous sedation, the patient was positioned in the left lateral decubitus position and the epidural space was entered using an 18-gauge Tuohy needle and loss of resistance to normal saline at the T9-10 interspace in a midline approach. After negative aspiration for blood and cerebrospinal fluid, a 20-gauge multiorifice epidural catheter was advanced approximately 4 cm in the cephalad direction easily and uneventfully. A test dose of 3 mL of lidocaine 1% with epinephrine 1 : 200,000 was injected without evidence of intravascular or subarachnoid injection.

The patient was then placed in the supine position, and general anesthesia was induced with propofol and vecuronium. The trachea was intubated and anesthesia was maintained with air, oxygen, and isoflurane. Her general anesthetic course was unremarkable.

The epidural catheter was injected with 100 mcg of clonidine and 15 mL of 0.25% bupivacaine. This was followed by an infusion of 0.1% bupivacaine with hydromorphone 10 mcg/mL at 15 mL/hr and was maintained throughout the case.

At the conclusion of surgery, the trachea was extubated and the patient appeared comfortable. In the postanesthesia care unit, it was noted that she had mild left unilateral Horner's sign and weakness of both lower extremities and the epidural infusion rate was decreased to 9 mL/h. She was discharged from the PACU to the ward stable and comfortable.

On postoperative day one, the patient was comfortable but complained of left sided numbness and visual blur. Physical examination revealed left hemibody analgesia, weakness, and Horner's syndrome (Figure 1). The unilateral dilated pupil was sluggishly reactive to light. Muscle strength was weaker in the upper extremity (3/5) than the lower extremity (4/5) with intense brachial plexus weakness. The epidural rate was further reduced to 8 mL/hr. In view of satisfactory analgesia, the patient and her mother elected to continue with epidural analgesia. The patient was turned to the right lateral decubitus position for several hours to determine if the local anesthetic would gravitate to the contralateral side but the sensory and motor examination remained unchanged. The reduction of epidural infusion produced progressive improvement of numbness, weakness, and the Horner's syndrome over the following 48 hours without compromising analgesia. In light of the history of unilateral epidural block with a previous surgery two years earlier, permission was obtained from the patient and her mother to perform an epidurogram. Two milliliters of contrast medium, iohexol180, was injected while observing anteroposterior fluoroscopic views of the thoracolumbar spine. These views showed left unilateral spread of the contrast medium (Figure 2). Contrast medium spread extended cephalad from T10 to C7, suggesting a midline barrier dividing the epidural space. The epidural catheter was removed on the fourth postoperative day and the neurological signs and symptoms and Horner's syndrome completely resolved.

3. Discussion

We describe a case of an adolescent patient with unilateral epidural blockade and radiographic suggestion of a midline epidural septum. The incidence of unilateral epidural blockade in children and adolescents is unknown. In review of the literature, we found only one case report of an incidental finding of an incomplete posterior midline epidural septum. This was noted in a 5.5-month-old infant when an epidurogram was performed to confirm thoracic placement of an epidural catheter that was advanced from the lumbar region [1, 2].

Epidural posterior midline septum (plica dorsalis medianalis), congenital trabeculation or acquired adhesions have been described in the adult literature but notably are rare [3–5]. It is most frequently noted in the obstetric anesthesia literature as an incidental finding when epidural anesthesia is asymmetrical, despite multiple maneuvers to correct the

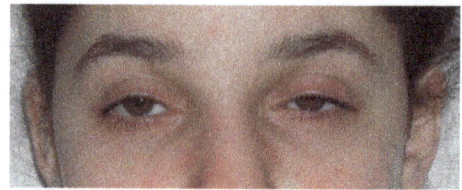

FIGURE 1: Horner's sign.

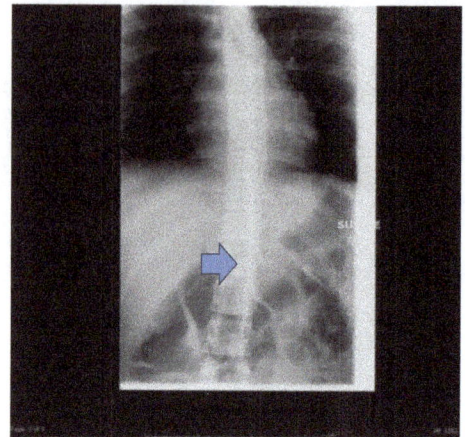

FIGURE 2: Epidurogram revealing unilateral spread of contrast medium.

asymmetry [6]. Although the presence of an epidural posterior and anterior midline septum is proposed to be a diffusion barrier to local anesthetic circumferential spread in the epidural space, the barrier could be incomplete fibrous tissue [1, 5, 7] or fatty tissue [5]. Rarely, a complete impervious epidural midline posterior septum would produce a mechanical barrier that would limit local anesthetic distribution unilaterally leading to ipsilateral anesthesia such as the case in our patient and described in an adult case report [8].

Although rare [5], the existence of an epidural posterior midline connective tissue septum between the dura mater and the ligamentum flavum has been confirmed by radiographic studies and seen frequently during lumbar disc surgery [2], epiduroscopic visualization [9], and CT-epidurography [10].

Another possible cause of unilateral anesthetic blockade in this case could have been subdural placement of the epidural catheter. However, the unilateral anesthetic blockade in our patient was not associated with clinical manifestation of intracranial spread of the local anesthetic such as mental status change, visual and/or bulbar function disturbances due to paralysis of the cranial nerves, nonreactive fully dilated pupil and symmetrical sensory and motor impairments [11]. In addition, the epidurogram in this case was consistent with unilateral epidural spread of the contrast medium rather than the characteristic bilateral pattern reported with subdural spread [7, 11, 12].

The incidence of asymmetrical epidural analgesia in children is unknown. In an earlier report of 202 adults who received a lumbar epidural catheter, the incidence of unilateral epidural analgesia was 5.9%. Replacement of the epidural catheter resulted in bilateral epidural analgesia in all patients [4]. The investigators speculated that the initial catheter was misplaced either in the anterior epidural space or in the paravertebral space via vertebral foramina. The same investigators subsequently examined unilateral epidural analgesia with roentgenographs in a relatively large group of adults who received lumbar epidural catheters and found that in approximately 1.6% of patients the catheter was misplaced in the anterior epidural space and in 1.2% of patients the catheter migrated outside the epidural space via vertebral foramina into the paravertebral space [3]. The use of a therapeutic volume of local anesthetic yielded bilateral epidural analgesia in the group in whom the catheters were within the epidural space. Unilateral epidural analgesia is frequently attributed to catheter placement that is too far anterolateral in the epidural space, nonuniform spread of local anesthetic particularly when small local anesthetic volumes are injected slowly, pooling of local anesthetics in the dependent position, and less frequently to the presence of an epidural midline septum [2]. Migration of the epidural catheter to the paravertebral space may yield paravertebral nerve blockade simulating apparent unilateral epidural analgesia, and the misplacement could be confirmed by obtaining a roentgenograph after injection of contrast medium through the catheter [3, 8, 13].

In summary, we report a case of extensive unilateral epidural sensory and motor blockade most probably due to the presence of a midline posterior and/or anterior septum with adequate postoperative analgesia presumably from eventual spread of the local anesthetics to dural cuffs (root sleeves) and subsequent entry into the cerebral spinal fluid by way of arachnoid granulations [14].

Implication Statement

This case illustrates 3 unusual extensive unilateral epidural spread of local anesthetic in an adolescent, probably due to presence of a complete midline barrier. Epidurogram was useful to confirm the correct location of the epidural catheter and the pattern of spread of the local anesthetic solution.

References

[1] J. C. Finkel, "The epidural dorsomedian septum as a possible cause for unilateral anaesthesia in an infant," *Paediatric Anaesthesia*, vol. 9, no. 5, pp. 456–459, 1999.

[2] W. Luyendijk, "The plica mediana dorsalis of the dura mater and its relation to lumbar peridurography (canalography)," *Neuroradiology*, vol. 11, no. 3, pp. 147–149, 1976.

[3] F. Asato and F. Goto, "Radiographic findings of unilateral epidural block," *Anesthesia and Analgesia*, vol. 83, no. 3, pp. 519–522, 1996.

[4] F. Asato, N. Hirakawa, M. Oda et al., "A median epidural septum is not a common cause of unilateral epidural blockade," *Anesthesia and Analgesia*, vol. 71, no. 4, pp. 427–429, 1990.

[5] Q. Hogan, "Epidural catheter tip position and distribution of injectate evaluated by computed tomography," *Anesthesiology*, vol. 90, no. 4, pp. 964–970, 1999.

[6] D. Portnoy and R. B. Vadhera, "Mechanisms and management of an incomplete epidural block for cesarean section," *Anesthesiology Clinics of North America*, vol. 21, no. 1, pp. 39–57, 2003.

[7] T. Fukushige, T. Kano, and T. Sano, "Radiographic investigation of unilateral epidural block after single injection," *Anesthesiology*, vol. 87, no. 6, pp. 1574–1575, 1997.

[8] A. P. Boezaart, "Computerized axial tomo-epidurographic and radiographic documentation of unilateral epidural analgesia," *Canadian Journal of Anaesthesia*, vol. 36, no. 6, pp. 697–700, 1989.

[9] R. Blomberg, "The dorsomedian connective tissue band in the lumbar epidural space of humans: An anatomical study using epiduroscopy in autopsy cases," *Anesthesia and Analgesia*, vol. 65, no. 7, pp. 747–752, 1986.

[10] E. R. Savolaine, J. B. Pandya, S. H. Greenblatt, and S. R. Conover, "Anatomy of the human lumbar epidural space: new insights using CT-epidurography," *Anesthesiology*, vol. 68, no. 2, pp. 217–220, 1988.

[11] A. J. Haughton and G. A. Chalkiadis, "Unintentional paediatric subdural catheter with oculomotor and abducens nerve palsies," *Paediatric Anaesthesia*, vol. 9, no. 6, pp. 543–548, 1999.

[12] R. A. Stevens and M. D. Stanton-Hicks, "Subdural injection of local anesthetic: a complication of epidural anesthesia," *Anesthesiology*, vol. 63, no. 3, pp. 323–326, 1985.

[13] D. Berkowitz, R. D. Kaye, S. D. Markowitz, and S. D. Cook-Sather, "Inadvertent extra-epidural catheter placement in an infant," *Anesthesia and Analgesia*, vol. 100, no. 2, pp. 365–366, 2005.

[14] M. Cousins and B. Veering, "Epidural neural blockade," in *Neural Blockage in Clinical Anesthesia and Management of Pain*, M. Cousins and L. D. Bridenbaugh, Eds., pp. 243–247, Lippincott-Raven, New York, NY, USA, 3rd edition, 1998.

26

Impossible Airway Requiring Venovenous Bypass for Tracheostomy

Johnathan Gardes and Tracey Straker

Department of Anesthesiology, Montefiore Medical Center, Bronx, New York City, NY 10467, USA

Correspondence should be addressed to Tracey Straker, ts51764@aol.com

Academic Editors: J. J. Derose, M. Kodaka, and M. Marandola

The elective surgical airway is the definitive management for a tracheal stenotic lesion that is not a candidate for tracheal resection, or who has failed multiple-tracheal dilations. This case report details the management of a patient who has failed an elective awake tracheostomy secondary to the inability to be intubated as well as severe scar tissue at the surgical site. A combination of regional anesthesia and venovenous bypass is used to facilitate the surgical airway management of this patient. Cerebral oximetry and a multidisciplinary team approach aid in early detection of an oxygenation issue, as well as the emergent intervention that preserved this patient's life.

1. Introduction

Proper management of the difficult airway presents one of the most important skill sets for the anesthesiologist to master. However, certain situations necessitate one look beyond traditional algorithms. In this case, a multidisciplinary team of otorhinolaryngologists, cardiac surgeons, perfusionists, and anesthesiologists decided to use venovenous bypass as a means to oxygenate a patient whose airway could not be secured because of severe tracheal stenosis.

2. Case Report

A 45-year-old woman with a long history of tracheal stenosis and upper airway obstruction presented for elective tracheostomy placement in the setting of supra- and infraglottic stenosis after failed awake tracheostomy by an otorhinolaryngologist (ORL) (Figures 1 and 2). It was felt by the attending ORL surgeon that the airway could not be secured from above after serial diagnostic scopes. Due to the failed awake tracheostomy, it was felt that surgical airway under bypass was the only option.

Eight years previously, the patient presented for an elective bilateral tubal ligation. At the time, she was otherwise healthy. The intraoperative course was unremarkable and the patient's trachea was extubated on the operating table. However, after moving to the stretcher for transport, she developed acute respiratory distress. She was quickly returned to the operating room (OR) table and her trachea reintubated after several attempts at direct laryngoscopy. At the time, her airway was noted to be acutely swollen and edematous. She remained intubated in the intensive care unit for two weeks during which time several attempts at extubation failed. Finally, she was weaned off support and discharged home. The presumptive diagnosis was an acute allergic reaction to the antibiotic cephazolamine, which she had received intraoperatively.

Two days after discharge the patient returned to the emergency room in acute respiratory distress and could not be intubated. An emergency tracheostomy was performed to secure her airway. The patient remained with the tracheostomy for the next 7 months before she was successfully decannulated. Since that time, the patient has returned to the operating room several times with tracheal stenosis requiring dilation. Her past medical history was also significant for

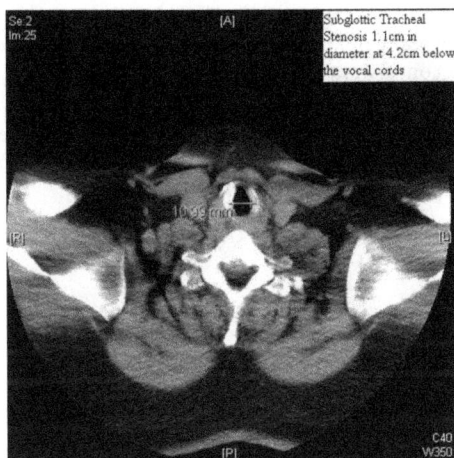

FIGURE 1: CT SCAN of subglottic tracheal stenosis.

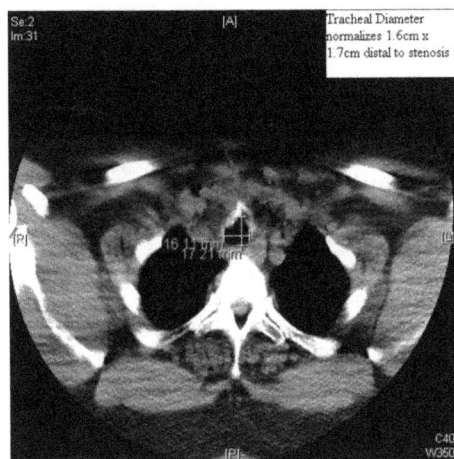

FIGURE 2: CT SCAN of tracheal diameter.

hypothyroidism, morbid obesity, obstructive sleep apnea requiring continuous positive airway pressure (CPAP), and hypertension. Medications included levothyroxine sodium, furoate monohydrate by nasal inhalation and esomeprazole. Allergies to latex and cephalosporins were reported. Review of symptoms was significant for chronic shortness of breath and three pillow orthopnea. The patient had fasted for more than 8 hours. On physical examination, the patient was mildly hypertensive, with a class III airway, mild stridor, and oozing from the site of the prior tracheostomy. All laboratory values and the cardiogram were within normal limits.

Because of the inability to secure the airway, even by tracheostomy, and repeated incidents of desaturation during prior attempts, the team felt that adequate oxygenation could best be managed by venovenous bypass. Venovenous bypass was suggested after consultation with the cardiac anesthesiology team because oxygenation would be maintained and the cardiac function of the patient was normal. The ORL surgeon requested that we do not cannulate any structures in the neck as they would be working in that area. With this request from the ORL service and the fact that arterial venous

bypass provides greater control over hemodynamics, femoral bypass was the chosen area for cannulation.

The anesthetic plan for spinal without sedation was discussed with the patient. The patient was brought into the OR where standard ASA monitors were placed including arterial cannulation and cerebral oximetry. Spinal anesthesia was placed at L4-5 using 24G Gertie Marx spinal needle and 1.2 mL of hyperbaric 7.5% bupivacaine. The patient had a T10 level at 5 minutes with vital signs stable throughout. Of note, the patient started to receive an infusion of vancomycin prior to incision and immediately experienced pruritus and scratchy throat. The antibiotic infusion was promptly discontinued and the patient was given steroids and subcutaneous epinephrine. The symptoms resolved and surgery continued. The patient was heparinized. Just prior to going on femoral venovenous bypass, general anesthesia was induced using midazolam, fentanyl, and etomidate. Once on bypass, vecuronium was given. As the patient was to have a tracheostomy on bypass, general anesthesia was instituted to assure no issues of recall.

Shortly bypass was initiated, cerebral oximetry and pulse oximetry values as well as blood pressure all dropped rapidly, likely from poor brain and upper extremity perfusion caused by the bypass. During cutdown on the patient's vasculature, it was discovered that he had severe tortuosity of the vessels. The cut-down time was extensive and the spinal anesthetic began to wear off. It was thought that one of the differentials for failure of bypass was the creation of a false lumen from the cannulation.

At this point, the otorhinolaryngologist rapidly secured the airway using rigid laryngoscopy and placed an oral endotracheal tube. With proper ventilation, the vital signs all returned to normal and she was taken off bypass and the heparin was reversed. The tracheostomy was then performed by the surgeon under general anesthesia. The remainder of the intraoperative course was unremarkable and the patient was extubated at the end of the case. The patient did well postoperatively and was discharged home.

3. Discussion

The difficult airway algorithm from the American Society of Anesthesiologists details a complex decision tree of basic and advanced airway management choices in both the awake and anesthetized patient who has suspected or known difficult ventilation and/or intubation [1]. The final steps in this algorithm end with invasive or surgical airway access. In this case, the patient had already failed awake surgical airway and was believed to have additional upper airway obstruction and anatomy that would prevent safe intubation either awake or asleep. With the failure of what is usually the final step in the algorithm, the anesthesia team in consultation with other surgical specialists opted for venovenous bypass as a means to oxygenate and anesthetize a patient whose airway could not be secured. While extracorporeal membrane oxygenation (ECMO) has been utilized and reported in the pediatric population fairly extensively, venovenous bypass has only rarely been reported in the literature as a means of oxygenation in the setting of the impossible airway in an adult, often in the setting of a large thyroid or mediastinal tumor or severe tracheal trauma [2, 3]. Rosa and colleagues and Jeon and colleagues both presented cases of cardiopulmonary bypass being safely utilized in this manner for cases of a cervical and thyroid tumor, respectively [4, 5]. Shiraishi and colleagues presented a series of 18 cases of tracheal resection and reconstruction, one of which required percutaneous cardiopulmonary support under minimal sedation [6]. Cardiopulmonary bypass is not without risk and complications as demonstrated by the fall in cerebral oximetry and pulse oximetry in our patient [7].

The ORL surgeon admitted that this case was transferred to him from a colleague, and he had actually never instrumented the patient's airway in the operating room for a direct laryngoscopy. Perhaps had the otorhinolaryngologist actually instrumented the airway previously, better objective data would have been available to avoid the case outcome.

The otorhinolaryngologist was present throughout the procedure and was able to provide a rapid and safe emergency airway intervention that allowed the patient to be adequately oxygenated. While our patient had an uncomplicated postoperative course, the risk of hemorrhage in this population is significant.

Even though the patient was unable to tolerate bypass for the length of the tracheostomy procedure and required alternative means of securing the airway, the presence of the multidisciplinary team provided safe and effective backup. We believe that rare and complex airway situations such as this case should always be approached with a multidisciplinary team of surgeons and anesthesiologists as the alternatives to traditional airway management such as venovenous bypass can be extremely challenging and unpredictable.

References

[1] American Society of Anesthesiologists Task Force on Management of the Difficult Airway, "Practice guidelines for management of the difficult airway: an updated report by the American Society of Anesthesiologists task force on management of the difficult airway," *Anesthesiology*, vol. 98, no. 5, pp. 1269–1277, 2003.

[2] J. Raake, B. Johnson, B. Seger et al., "Extracorporeal membrane oxygenation, extubation, and lung-recruitment maneuvers as rescue therapy in a patient with tracheal dehiscence following slide tracheoplasty," *Respiratory care*, vol. 56, no. 8, pp. 1198–1202, 2011.

[3] C. SenDasgupta, G. Sengupta, K. Ghosh, A. Munshi, and A. Goswami, "Femoro-femoral cardiopulmonary bypass for the resection of an anterior mediastinal mass," *Indian Journal of Anaesthesia*, vol. 54, no. 6, pp. 565–568, 2010.

[4] P. Rosa, E. A. Johnson, and P. J. Barcia, "The impossible airway: a plan," *Chest*, vol. 109, no. 6, pp. 1649–1650, 1996.

[5] H.-K. Jeon, Y. K. So, J. H. Yang, and H. S. Jeong, "Extracorporeal oxygenation support for curative surgery in a patient with papillary thyroid carcinoma invading the trachea," *Journal of Laryngology and Otology*, vol. 123, no. 7, pp. 807–810, 2009.

[6] T. Shiraishi, J. Yanagisawa, T. Higuchi et al., "Tracheal resection for malignant and benign diseases: surgical results and perioperative considerations," *Surgery Today*, vol. 41, no. 4, pp. 490–495, 2011.

[7] M. J. Belmont, M. K. Wax, and F. N. DeSouza, "The difficult airway: cardiopulmonary bypass—the ultimate solution," *Head and Neck*, vol. 20, pp. 266–269, 1998.

27

Myocardial Dysfunction in Acute Traumatic Brain Injury Relieved by Surgical Decompression

Vijay Krishnamoorthy,[1] **Deepak Sharma,**[2] **Sumidtra Prathep,**[1] **and Monica S. Vavilala**[3]

[1] *Department of Anesthesiology and Pain Medicine, University of Washington, WA 98104, USA*
[2] *Departments of Anesthesiology and Pain Medicine, Neurological Surgery (Adj.), University of Washington, WA 98104, USA*
[3] *Departments of Anesthesiology and Pain Medicine, Neurological Surgery (Adj.), Pediatrics (Adj.), and Radiology (Adj.), University of Washington, WA 98104, USA*

Correspondence should be addressed to Vijay Krishnamoorthy; vkrish@u.washington.edu

Academic Editors: I.-O. Lee, C. C. Lu, M. Marandola, H. Shankar, and D. A. Story

Traumatic brain injury (TBI) is a major public health issue and is a leading cause of death in North America. After a primary TBI, secondary brain insults can predispose patients to a worse outcome. One of the earliest secondary insults encountered during the perioperative period is hypotension, which has been directly linked to both mortality and poor disposition after TBI. Despite this, it has been shown that hypotension commonly occurs during surgery for TBI. We present a case of intraoperative hypotension during surgery for TBI, where the use of transthoracic echocardiography had significant diagnostic and therapeutic implications for the management of our patient. We then discuss the issue of cardiac dysfunction after brain injury and the implications that echocardiography may have in the management of this vulnerable patient population.

1. Introduction

Traumatic brain injury (TBI) is a major public health issue and is a leading cause of death in North America [1]. After a primary TBI, the burden of secondary brain insults can predispose patients to a worse outcome than if secondary insults did not occur [2, 3]. One of the earliest secondary insults encountered during the perioperative period is hypotension, which has been directly linked to both mortality and poor disposition after TBI [4, 5]. While recommendations of the 2007 Brain Trauma Foundation recommend maintaining systolic blood pressure (SBP) >90 mmHg [6], it has recently been shown that reduction in SBP to values below 90 mmHg commonly occurs during surgery for TBI. Risk factors for intraoperative hypotension include large lesions and the presence of multiple lesions on CT [7]. Therapy for intraoperative hypotension has traditionally consisted of the administration of intravenous fluids and vasopressors, and vasopressor choice in this setting is often empiric. There are no guidelines specific for treatment of hypotension during the intraoperative period; thus, knowledge of a patient's preexisting cardiac status may impact anesthesiologists' choice of vasopressor for treatment of intraoperative hypotension.

In this report, we present the clinical course of a patient with a traumatic holohemispheric subdural hematoma (SDH), where echocardiographic changes consistent with myocardial dysfunction were observed upon admission to the operating room. The echocardiographic abnormalities were rapidly reversed after craniotomy and surgical decompression. In this case, the use of point of care (POC) intraoperative transthoracic echocardiography (TTE) allowed for timely identification of a cardiac cause of hypotension, and it facilitated appropriate vasopressor choice for treatment. In addition, the phenomenon of reversible cardiac dysfunction after traumatic intracranial hemorrhage, relieved by decompression, is postulated. IRB approval was not required for submission of this case.

2. Case Presentation

The patient was a 76-year-old functionally independent male with a preexisting history remarkable only for hypertension and bipolar disorder. On review of systems, he was found to have a negative cardiac history and no treatment with anticoagulants. He presented to an outside hospital with declining mental status. The patient experienced a ground-level fall and worsening somnolence. At the outside hospital, computed tomography (CT) scan of his head demonstrated a right holohemispheric subdural hematoma (SDH), measuring 1.7 cm at maximal thickness, and with an associated mild 5 mm midline shift (Figure 1). Due to his worsening mental status, the patient's trachea was intubated, and he was transferred to our hospital (regional Level 1 Trauma Center), where he underwent an emergent right craniotomy and SDH evacuation. The patient tolerated the procedure well, and his trachea was extubated at the end of surgery.

On hospital day two, he again became increasingly somnolent and had generalized seizure activity; a stat head CT scan revealed a new acute right-sided subdural hematoma in the same area as the previous traumatic lesion with a new 6 mm midline shift and uncal herniation. Laboratory values were significant for a hematocrit of 35% and an international normalized ratio (INR) of 1.2; and his vital signs were significant for a blood pressure of 140/92 mmHg and a heart rate of 112 bpm. The patient was emergently brought to the operating room for repeat surgical evacuation and hemicraniectomy. General anesthesia was induced with 100 mg propofol, 100 mcg fentanyl, and 100 mg rocuronium administered intravenously. The patient underwent a rapid sequence tracheal intubation with cricoid pressure, and general anesthesia was maintained with intravenous boluses of fentanyl, vecuronium, and isoflurane. After induction of general anesthesia, the patient's systolic blood pressure decreased to 54 mmHg. Multiple intravenous boluses of phenylephrine (totaling 300 mcg) and 750 mL of crystalloid were administered with only minimal improvement and with persistent hypotension (systolic blood pressures less than 90 mmHg). Intraoperative POC TTE was performed by an anesthesiologist with certification in echocardiography: Vijay Krishnamoorthy, which demonstrated a global ejection fraction (EF) of 35% and moderate basal hypokinesis(Figure 2(a)). Based on these echocardiographic findings, the need for an intravenous inotropic vasopressor was identified, and due to ease of availability, 20 mg intravenous ephedrine was administered over five minutes with sustained improvement in systolic blood pressure to greater than 120 mmHg during the next 10 minutes without the need for additional vasopressor support or intravenous fluids. While improvements in EF were noted on TTE after pharmacologic therapy, the EF had not returned to an expected normal level.

Five minutes after surgical decompression of the SDH, a third POC TTE was performed, this time revealing resolution of the previously observed basal hypokinesis and normalization of the EF to 55% (Figure 2(b)). The systolic blood pressure remained above 100 mmHg without the need for any further vasopressor support (Table 1). The remainder of the case proceeded uneventfully, and the patient remained

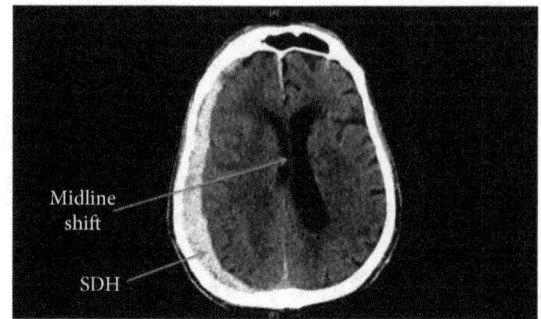

FIGURE 1: Right holohemispheric subdural hematoma (SDH) and midline shift in a 76-year-old male, resulting in neurologic deterioration and emergent surgical decompression management.

TABLE 1: Changes in qualitative ejection fraction (EF) and regional wall motion abnormalities (RWMA) pre and post decompressive craniotomy in a patient with isolated traumatic brain injury.

	Pre decompression	Post decompression
Qualitative EF	35%	55%
RWMA	Basal hypokinesis	None
Blood pressure	88/54 mmHg*	110/62 mmHg
Heart rate	84 bpm	92 bpm
Total crystalloid	1200 mL**	1600 mL
Hematocrit	35%	31%
Anesthesia	Sevoflurane	Sevoflurane
End-tidal sevoflurane	0.5%	1.5%

*: Ephedrine, 20 mg ephedrine administered to restore blood pressure to 124/72 mmHg.
**: Intravenous fluids administered over 1.5 hours, totaling 1600 mL post decompression (400 mL administered after surgical decompression).

intubated and was transferred to the ICU in stable condition. After a 25-day hospital course, the patient was discharged to a skilled nursing facility for further care.

3. Discussion

While intraoperative hypotension during acute decompressive surgery for TBI has previously been described, the etiology of hypotension has not been clearly elucidated. Hence, the traditional approach to intraoperative hypotension during TBI surgery has been empiric and assumed to be a result of the acute cardiopulmonary physiologic stress of brain injury [8], fluid shifts, and effects of anesthetic agents [9, 10]. The therapeutic approach to the treatment of hypotension during decompressive surgery for TBI has involved the administration of intravenous fluids to restore euvolemia, followed by intravenous vasopressors which have alpha-adrenergic effects and those without cerebral effects [11]. In TBI, intravenous phenylephrine has been reported to be the most frequently administered intraoperative vasopressor [12]. Despite this practice, available evidence suggests that vasopressors with inotropic effects such as norepinephrine might be preferable as the vasopressor of choice in acute neurologic injury [13]. This case documents cardiac dysfunction acutely after TBI and suggests that anesthesiologists should

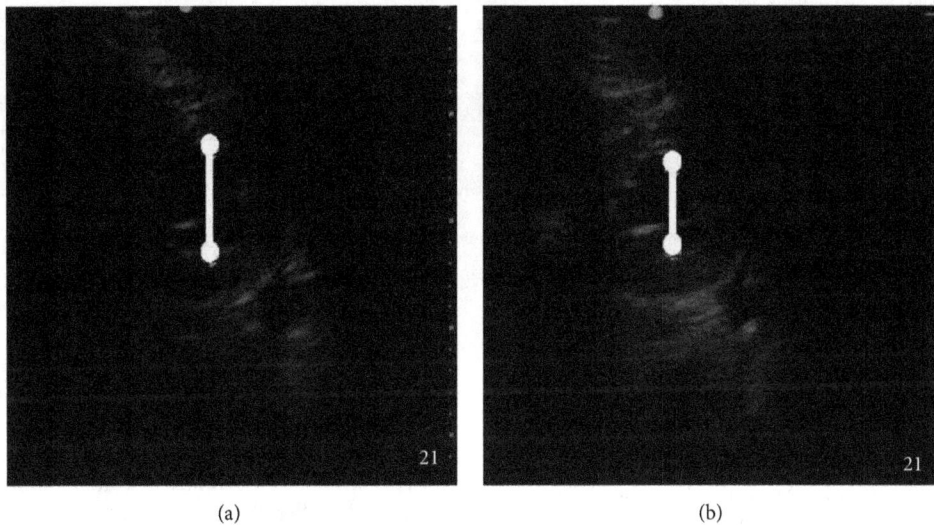

FIGURE 2: Left-ventricular function at end-systole pre decompression (a) and post decompression (b). There is decreased left-ventricular end-systolic internal diameter (line) and improved wall thickening after decompression.

consider point of care evaluation of cardiac function in their decision of vasopressor choice acutely after TBI.

The idea that acute neurologic injury causes acute cardiopulmonary dysfunction is not new. A variety of reports have documented electrocardiographic changes and elevations of cardiac-specific biomarkers in the setting of acute brain injury [14–16], with echocardiographic wall motion abnormalities being observed in patients with subarachnoid hemorrhage [17]. In addition, transient left-ventricular dysfunction (traditionally including apical ballooning) without the presence of preexisting coronary artery disease has been well described after subarachnoid hemorrhage, acute physical stress, or psychological stress, with overactivity of the sympathetic nervous system implicated in the pathogenesis [18, 19]. While these reports suggest that brain-heart interaction may also cause myocardial dysfunction in TBI, direct echocardiographic changes in the perioperative period after TBI have not been previously documented, nor has echocardiographic resolution of myocardial dysfunction following decompression been previously described in the literature. In our case, the critical determinant for improvement in the patient's cardiac function was surgical decompression.

The underlying mechanism of acute cardiopulmonary deterioration secondary to TBI is thought to be secondary to an acute catecholamine excess state [20], with recent evidence suggesting that inflammation may also play a role [21]. This idea is based on the speculation that increased intracranial pressure can cause increased central catecholamine outflow, resulting in both stress cardiomyopathy and isolated acute lung injury, better known as neurogenic pulmonary edema [22]. Interestingly, myocardial biopsies from brain-dead organ donors and survivors of stress-induced cardiomyopathy show mononuclear infiltrates and contraction-band necrosis, which indicate evidence of catecholamine-induced myocardial injury [18, 23].

While stress-induced myocardial dysfunction can transiently decrease cardiac output, a secondary effect of acute heart failure is rapid accumulation of extravascular lung water, thus potentially aggravating hypoxia. Hypoxia has been shown to be an independent predictor of worsened outcomes in TBI, and the combination of hypotension and hypoxia leads to worse outcomes than either factor alone [24]. Thus, it is a possibility that treating hypotension secondary to acute heart failure empirically with intravenous fluids and pure alpha-agonists may lead to a vicious cycle of worsened blood pressure and increasing hypoxia.

Traditionally in the perioperative setting, a craniotomy for a deteriorating patient with TBI is a medical emergency without the time for formal cardiac evaluation, often times leading to the treatment of hypotension without knowing the underlying etiology. While treating intraoperative hypotension is critical to avoiding secondary TBI and improving outcomes, treatment is often undertaken empirically. If the cause of intraoperative hypotension is acute myocardial stunning, perhaps the traditional therapy of fluids and increased afterload with phenylephrine may not be optimal. Instead, consideration of a vasopressor with inotropic activity and a conservative fluid strategy may better improve secondary hemodynamic goals to optimize outcome, especially since phenylephrine has been shown to decrease cardiac output [25], despite often being the vasopressor of choice in the setting of intraoperative management of TBI [12].

In conclusion, we report a case of intraoperative hypotension, where intraoperative POC TTE guided the hemodynamic management of a patient with TBI presenting for emergent decompressive craniotomy. This case highlights the growing role that POC ultrasound technology could add to the anesthesiologists' strategies for management of perioperative hemodynamic and respiratory instability. In addition, the observed cardiac dysfunction in our case likely represents a variant of "stress-induced" cardiomyopathy in

TBI. Finally, to our knowledge, our case is the first to demonstrate the reversibility of cardiac dysfunction in TBI after surgical decompression, setting the stage for further research inquiry into this subject.

References

[1] W. Rutland-Brown, J. A. Langlois, K. E. Thomas, and Y. L. Xi, "Incidence of traumatic brain injury in the United States, 2003," *Journal of Head Trauma Rehabilitation*, vol. 21, no. 6, pp. 544–548, 2006.

[2] E. Jeremitsky, L. Omert, C. M. Dunham, J. Protetch, and A. Rodriguez, "Harbingers of poor outcome the day after severe brain injury: hypothermia, hypoxia, and hypoperfusion," *The Journal of Trauma*, vol. 54, no. 2, pp. 312–319, 2003.

[3] R. M. Chesnut, L. F. Marshall, M. R. Klauber et al., "The role of secondary brain injury in determining outcome from severe head injury," *The Journal of Trauma*, vol. 34, no. 2, pp. 216–222, 1993.

[4] S. N. Zafar, F. H. Millham, Y. Chang et al., "Presenting blood pressure in traumatic brain injury: a bimodal distribution of death," *The Journal of Trauma*, vol. 71, no. 5, pp. 1179–1184, 2011.

[5] J. A. Pietropaoli, F. B. Rogers, S. R. Shackford, S. L. Wald, J. D. Schmoker, and J. Zhuang, "The deleterious effects of intraoperative hypotension on outcome in patients with severe head injuries," *The Journal of Trauma*, vol. 33, no. 3, pp. 403–407, 1992.

[6] S. L. Bratton, R. M. Chestnut, J. Ghajar et al., "Guidelines for the management of severe traumatic brain injury. I. Blood pressure and oxygenation," *Journal of Neurotrauma*, vol. 24, supplement 1, pp. S7–S13, 2007.

[7] D. Sharma, M. J. Brown, P. Curry, S. Noda, R. M. Chesnut, and M. S. Vavilala, "Prevalence and risk factors for intraoperative hypotension during craniotomy for traumatic brain injury," *Journal of Neurosurgical Anesthesiology*, vol. 24, no. 3, pp. 178–184, 2012.

[8] A. Grunsfeld, J. J. Fletcher, and B. R. Nathan, "Cardiopulmonary complications of brain injury," *Current Neurology and Neuroscience Reports*, vol. 5, no. 6, pp. 488–493, 2005.

[9] M. Filipovic, J. Wang, I. Michaux, P. Hunziker, K. Skarvan, and M. D. Seeberger, "Effects of halothane, sevoflurane and propofol on left ventricular diastolic function in humans during spontaneous and mechanical ventilation," *British Journal of Anaesthesia*, vol. 94, no. 2, pp. 186–192, 2005.

[10] D. Bolliger, M. D. Seeberger, J. Kasper et al., "Different effects of sevoflurane, desflurane, and isoflurane on early and late left ventricular diastolic function in young healthy adults," *British Journal of Anaesthesia*, vol. 104, no. 5, pp. 547–554, 2010.

[11] D. Pfister, S. P. Strebel, and L. A. Steiner, "Effects of catecholamines on cerebral blood vessels in patients with traumatic brain injury," *European Journal of Anaesthesiology*, vol. 25, no. 42, pp. 98–103, 2008.

[12] P. Sookplung, A. Siriussawakul, A. Malakouti et al., "Vasopressor use and effect on blood pressure after severe adult traumatic brain injury," *Neurocritical Care*, vol. 15, no. 1, pp. 46–54, 2011.

[13] K. M. Muzevich and S. A. Voils, "Role of vasopressor administration in patients with acute neurologic injury," *Neurocritical Care*, vol. 11, no. 1, pp. 112–119, 2009.

[14] H. Bhagat, R. Narang, D. Sharma, H. H. Dash, and H. Chauhan, "ST elevation—an indication of reversible neurogenic myocardial dysfunction in patients with head injury," *Annals of Cardiac Anaesthesia*, vol. 12, no. 2, pp. 149–151, 2009.

[15] P. James, C. J. Ellis, R. M. L. Whitlock, A. R. McNeil, J. Henley, and N. E. Anderson, "Relation between troponin T concentration and mortality in patients presenting with an acute stroke: observational study," *British Medical Journal*, vol. 320, no. 7248, pp. 1502–1504, 2000.

[16] M. Kaste, J. Hernesniemi, and H. Somer, "Creatine kinase isoenzymes in acute brain injury," *Journal of Neurosurgery*, vol. 55, no. 4, pp. 511–515, 1981.

[17] T. Kono, H. Morita, T. Kuroiwa, H. Onaka, H. Takatsuka, and A. Fujiwara, "Left ventricular wall motion abnormalities in patients with subarachnoid hemorrhage: neurogenic stunned myocardium," *Journal of the American College of Cardiology*, vol. 24, no. 3, pp. 636–640, 1994.

[18] I. S. Wittstein, D. R. Thiemann, J. A. C. Lima et al., "Neurohumoral features of myocardial stunning due to sudden emotional stress," *The New England Journal of Medicine*, vol. 352, no. 6, pp. 539–548, 2005.

[19] J. Ako, K. Sudhir, H. M. O. Farouque, Y. Honda, and P. J. Fitzgerald, "Transient left ventricular dysfunction under severe stress: brain-heart relationship revisited," *American Journal of Medicine*, vol. 119, no. 1, pp. 10–17, 2006.

[20] M. A. Samuels, "The brain-heart connection," *Circulation*, vol. 116, no. 1, pp. 77–84, 2007.

[21] H. A. Mashaly and J. J. Provencio, "Inflammation as a link between brain injury and heart damage: the model of subarachnoid hemorrhage," *Cleveland Clinic Journal of Medicine*, vol. 75, pp. S26–30, 2008.

[22] D. L. Davison, M. Terek, and L. S. Chawla, "Neurogenic pulmonary edema," *Critical Care*, vol. 16, no. 2, article 212, 2012.

[23] M. Berman, A. Ali, E. Ashley et al., "Is stress cardiomyopathy the underlying cause of ventricular dysfunction associated with brain death?" *The Journal of Heart and Lung Transplantation*, vol. 29, no. 9, pp. 957–965, 2010.

[24] G. S. McHugh, D. C. Engel, I. Butcher et al., "Prognostic value of secondary insults in traumatic brain injury: results from the IMPACT study," *Journal of Neurotrauma*, vol. 24, no. 2, pp. 287–293, 2007.

[25] R. H. Thiele, E. C. Nemergut, and C. Lynch III, "The clinical implications of isolated alpha1 adrenergic stimulation," *Anesthesia and Analgesia*, vol. 113, no. 2, pp. 297–304, 2011.

28

Emergence in Elderly Patient Undergoing General Anesthesia with Xenon

Maria Sanfilippo, Ahmed Abdelgawwad Wefki Abdelgawwad Shousha, and Antonella Paparazzo

Department of Anesthesiology and Intensive Care, Sapienza University, Viale del policlinico 155, 00161 Rome, Italy

Correspondence should be addressed to Ahmed Abdelgawwad Wefki Abdelgawwad Shousha; dott.ahmed@gmail.com

Academic Editors: A. Apan, R. S. Gomez, A. Han, and C. Seefelder

Introduction. It is a consensus that the postoperative cognitive function is impaired in elderly patients after general anaesthesia, and such category patient takes more time to recover. Xenon is a noble gas with anesthetic properties mediated by antagonism of N-methyl-D-aspartate receptors. With a minimum alveolar concentration of 0.63, xenon is intended for maintaining hypnosis with 30% oxygen. The fast recovery after xenon anaesthesia was hypothesized to be advantageous in this scenario. *Case Presentation*. We report the case of 99-year-old woman who underwent sigmoid colon carcinoma resection with colorectal anastomosis. We carried out the induction phase by propofol, oxygen, fentanil, and rocuronium bromide, and then we proceeded to a rapid sequence endotracheal intubation consequently. The patient was monitored by IBP, NIBP, ECG, cardiac frequency, respiratory rate, capnometry, TOF Guard, blood gas analysis, and BIS. For maintenance we administrated oxygen, remifentanil, rocuronium bromide, and xenon gas 60–65%. Shortly after the end of surgery the patients started an autonomous respiratory activity, and a high BIS level was also recorded. Decision was made by our team to proceed into the emergence phase. The residual neuromuscular block was antagonized by sugammadex, modified Aldrete score was implicated, and we got our patient fully awake without any cognitive dysfunction or delirium. *Conclusion*. The rapid emergence to full orientation in very elderly patient who had been anesthetized by xenon shows concordance to the high BIS values and the clinical signs of the depth of anesthesia.

1. Introduction

Aging is an irreversible and progressive physiological phenomena characterized by degenerative changes in the structure and functional reserve of organs and tissues [1]. Advances and improvement in medical science have increased life expectancy, and thus perioperative surgery and anesthesia in the elderly patient have become an extremely important issue.

Elderly patients (arbitrarily defined as being over 65 years of age) are vulnerable to the adverse effects of anesthesia because of their reduced margin of safety. Morbidity and mortality increase with advancing age, with a steep increase after the age of 75 years [2]. The frequency of complications related to anesthesia is 0.5% in patients >80 years old [3].

Elderly patients often take more time to recover completely from the central nervous system effects of general

anesthesia, particularly if they were confused or disoriented preoperatively.

Over the last decade there has been renewed interest in the use of xenon as an anaesthetic, and xenon has been licensed as an anaesthetic in Europe since 2005. Xenon potently inhibits N-methyl-D-aspartate (NMDA) noncompetitively, with little effect on GABAA receptors or non-NMDA glutamatergic receptors.

The main beneficial features of xenon anesthesia are fast induction and emergence because of low solubility in blood and tissues, along with remarkably stable hemodynamics even in patients with impaired cardiac function.

Xenon has proven to be a safe and well-tolerated anesthetic in clinical trials [4, 5].

In comparison with nitrous oxide, Goto and colleagues found that emergence from xenon anesthesia is 2 or 3 times faster than that from comparable MACs of nitrous oxide/isoflurane and nitrous oxide/sevoflurane anesthesia. Furthermore, xenon compares favorably with other anesthetic agents [6].

2. Case Presentation

A 99-year-old female (height 1.60 m; weight 45 kg, ASA III) was admitted to our hospital and underwent major abdominal surgery (sigmoid colon carcinoma resection with colorectal anastomosis) under general anesthesia, and the surgery duration was about 220 minutes. Her medical history revealed mild degree heart failure, chronic normocytic anemia, gastritis, and allergy for NSAIDs and penicillin antibiotics.

Her preoperative laboratory tests: hemoglobin 8.8 mg $\cdot dL^{-1}$, hematocrit 30.9%, leukocytes 11,500 mm^{-3} without deviation, platelets 453,000 mm^{-3}, sodium 131 mg $\cdot dL^{-1}$, potassium 4 mg$\cdot dL^{-1}$, magnesium 0.58 mg$\cdot dL^{-1}$, creatinine 0.5 mg$\cdot dL^{-1}$, and total calcium 8.24 mg$\cdot dL^{-1}$.

In the preoperative room we prepared our patient by antibiotics prophylaxis: ciprofloxacin 2 gm; metronidazole 500 mg and an antiemetic agent; ondansetron 4 mg.

Our patient was monitored by pulse oximetry, expiratory capnography, invasive and noninvasive blood pressure, electrocardiogram, bispectral index (BIS), neuromuscular transmission (TOF Guard), and diuresis.

A peripheral venous access (20 G) was established in upper right limb, and also a central venous access was done immediately after the induction phase as it was needed for postoperative chemotherapy afterwards.

We induced our anesthesia by oxygen, propofol 50 mg, fentanil 100 mcg, and rocuronium bromide 30 mg, and then we proceeded to a rapid sequence endotracheal intubation (tube diameter was 6.5 mm),

The maintenance of the anesthesia was achieved by continuous infusion of remifentanil in a dose of 0.2 mcg/kg/min, rocuronium bromide 10 mg, xenon 60–65%, and O_2 35–40%, the fluid replacement was calculated depending on her diuresis, plasma fluid, intraoperative blood loss, and anemia, and she was refunded by ringer lactate 1500 mL, Nacl 0.9% 1000 mL, fresh plasma fluids 1000 mL, and packed red cells 500 mL.

A closed-circuit anesthesia machine (Felix Dual, Taema) was used for xenon gas delivery. The ventilation parameters were the following: "pressure-cycled mechanical ventilation with inhalation pressure indexes of 19 cm H_2O, respiratory frequency 12 incursions per minute, PEEP 5 cm H_2O, FiO$_2$ 35–40%, and inspiratory/expiratory time ratio 1 : 2, and the exhaled tidal volume was around 380 mL."

Blood gas analysis was performed twice: 30 minutes after the start and 30 minutes before the end of surgery.

We registered electrolyte disorders, and they were resolved by administration of KCL 40 mEq and Ca^{++} gluconate in dose of 1 g$\cdot$10 m^{-1} (Tables 1 and 2).

After 5 minutes from the end of the surgery we noticed our patient starting a voluntary respiratory activity with a high BIS level, so we decided to proceed for the emergence

TABLE 1: Hemogasanalysis 30 minutes after the start of the surgery.

Status:	Accepted	
Analysis:	25/01/2013 09:32:29	
Sample Type:	Arterial	
S/N:	08071675	
Measured (37.0°C)		
pH	7.51	
pCO_2	31	mmHg
pO_2	187	mmHg
Na^+	134	mmol/L
K^+	3.1	mmol/L
Ca^{++}	1.08	mmol/L
Glu	125	mg/dL
Lac	0.9	mmol/L
Oximeter		
tHb	9.0	g/dL
O_2Hb	96.2	%
COHb	2.1	%
MetHb	1.8	%
HHb	−0.1	%
sO_2	100.1	%
Derivatives		
TCO_2	25.7	mmol/L
BEecf	1.7	mmol/L
BE (B)	1.9	mmol/L
Ca^{++} (7.4)	1.13	mmol/L
sO_2 (c)	99.7	%
HCO_3^- (c)	24.7	mmol/L
HCO_3^- (std)$_{standard}$	26.4	mmol/L
Hct (c)	27	%
Inserted		
Temp	37.0	°C
O_2/Vent		
FIO_2	35.0	%

phase and extubation reversing the neuromuscular blocking by sugammadex in a dose of 100 mg [7] with careful monitoring for her cardiovascular and respiratory functions. Both modified Aldrete score and BIS values were recorded (Table 3).

After 13 minutes we got the complete recovery of our patient, she was awake without any confusion state, delirium, or cognitive dysfunction, also she had excellent and stabile both hemodynamic and respiratory functions, postoperative pain control was achieved by continuous intravenous infusion of morphine (5 mg over 24 h), and she was transferred to ICU for close monitoring.

3. Conclusion

In our case we got surprised for the rapid emergence of our patient; this corresponds with the low blood gas partition coefficient of xenon (0.115). We also concluded that the BIS values show sufficient concordance with clinical signs of

TABLE 2: Hemogasanalysis 30 minutes after the end of the surgery.

Status:	Accepted	
Analysis:	25/01/2013 13:03:35	
Sample Type:	Arterial	
S/N:	08071675	
Measured (37.0°C)		
pH	7.33	
pCO_2	45	mmHg
pO_2	97	mmHg
Na^+	131	mmol/L
K^+	5.0	mmol/L
Ca^{++}	1.25	mmol/L
Glu	178	mg/dL
Lac	2.3	mmol/L
Oximeter		
tHb	9.7	g/dL
O_2Hb	95.0	%
COHb	2.2	%
MetHb	1.8	%
HHb	1.0	%
sO_2	99.0	%
Derivatives		
TCO_2	25.1	mmol/L
BEecf	−2.2	mmol/L
BE (B)	−2.3	mmol/L
Ca^{++} (7.4)	1.21	mmol/L
sO_2 (c)	97.0	%
HCO_3^- (c)	23.7	mmol/L
HCO_3^- (std)$_{standard}$	23.1	mmol/L
Hct (c)	29	%
Inserted		
Temp	37.0	°C

TABLE 3: BIS: bispectral index.

Time	1 min	5 min	10 min	13 min
BIS	35	92	97	99
Modified Aldrete	5	7	9	10

anesthetic depth and the emergence to full orientation in very elderly patient who had been anesthetized by xenon, and consequently we encourage more studies concerning the use of xenon in general surgery with such category of patients [8–11].

References

[1] S. Muravchik, "Pharmacological changes of aging," in *Proceedings of the 53rd ASA Annual Meeting Refresher Course*, Lectures #19, pp. 1–7, 2002.

[2] R. Raymond, "Anesthetic management of the elderly patient," in *Proceedings of the 53rd ASA Annual Meeting Refresher Course*, Lectures #321, pp. 1–7, 2002.

[3] D. Warner and M. Warner, "Anesthetic risk and the elderly," in *Syllabus on Geriatric Anesthesiology*, pp. 1–4, ASA, 2002.

[4] *Xenon-Based Anesthesia: Theory and Practice Jan-Hinrich Baumert*, Department of Anaesthesiology, UMC, Open Access Surgery, Nijmegen, The Netherlands, 2009.

[5] T. Goto, H. Saito, M. Shinkai, Y. Nakata, F. Ichinose, and S. Morita, "Xenon provides faster emergence from anesthesia than does nitrous oxide- sevoflurane or nitrous oxide-isoflurane," *Anesthesiology*, vol. 86, no. 6, pp. 1273–1278, 1997.

[6] R. D. Sanders, N. P. Franks, and M. Maze, "Xenon: no stranger to anaesthesia," *British Journal of Anaesthesia*, vol. 91, no. 5, pp. 709–717, 2003.

[7] Bridion (Sugammadex) Summary of Product Characteristics available via the electronic Medicines Compendium, July 2009.

[8] M. Coburn, J. H. Baumert, D. Roertgen et al., "Emergence and early cognitive function in the elderly after xenon or desflurane anaesthesia: a double-blinded randomized controlled trial," *British Journal of Anaesthesia*, vol. 98, no. 6, pp. 756–762, 2007.

[9] D. Rörtgen, J. Kloos, M. Fries et al., "Comparison of early cognitive function and recovery after desflurane or sevoflurane anaesthesia in the elderly: a double-blinded randomized controlled trial," *British Journal of Anaesthesia*, vol. 104, no. 2, pp. 167–174, 2010.

[10] M. Derwall, M. Coburn, S. Rex, M. Hein, R. Rossaint, and M. Fries, "Xenon: recent developments and future perspectives," *Minerva Anestesiologica*, vol. 75, no. 1-2, pp. 37–45, 2009.

[11] L. S. Rasmussen, K. Larsen, P. Houx, L. T. Skovgaard, C. D. Hanning, and J. T. Moller, "The assessment of postoperative cognitive function," *Acta Anaesthesiologica Scandinavica*, vol. 45, no. 3, pp. 275–289, 2001.

29

An Unusual Case of Sudden Collapse in the Immediate Postoperative Period in a Young Healthy Female with Myxofibroma of the Maxilla

Manila Singh[1] and Saket Singh[1,2]

[1] Department of Anesthesia and Intensive Care, G.B. Pant Hospital, E-269, East of Kailash, New Delhi, India
[2] Department of C.V.T.S, G.B. Pant Hospital, New Delhi, India

Correspondence should be addressed to Manila Singh; dr.manilasingh@gmail.com

Academic Editors: C. Seefelder, D. A. Story, T. Suzuki, and J.-J. Yang

Benign myxofibromas of heart are well known to cause systemic inflammatory mediator release causing multiple complications ranging from fever and widespread effusions to DIC and shock. We report that in a particular case of maxillary myxofibroma, a shock-like state and widespread serous cavities effusion presented in the immediate postoperative period. The occurrence was possibly due to release of inflammatory mediators by the tumour, disseminated during tumour resection causing diffuse capillary leak, precipitated by fluid resuscitation, leading to decrease in plasma oncotic pressure.

1. Introduction

Odontogenic fibromyxoma is a rare benign tumour arising from odontogenic mesenchyme [1]. Shared field for airway and surgical access [2] is the main anaesthetic challenge along with a smooth postoperative course necessary for maintaining a patent airway as well as the suture line. Any systemic complications related to inflammatory mediator release by the tumour have not been reported before as the available data suggests.

The written informed consent for publication of data was taken postoperatively from the patient and her parents when her condition stabilized on postoperative day two.

2. Case Report

A 13-year-old otherwise healthy female was scheduled to be operated on for myxofibroma of maxilla by a combined team of neurosurgeons and dental surgeons. On routine preanaesthetic check-up, the patient was perceived to be a healthy, 40 kg female, not yet having attained menarche. The patient was receiving dexamethasone 4 mg 12-hourly preoperatively. Routine preoperative biochemical and radiological investigations comprising complete blood count (CBC), LFTs (liver function tests), KFTs (kidney function tests), CXR (chest X-ray), ECG, and PT/INR were within normal limits.

After application of routine monitors, anaesthesia was induced with fentanyl 2 mcg/kg, midazolam 2 mg, and propofol 80 mg. Nasal intubation was facilitated by rocuronium 35 mg and McGill's forceps. Maintenance of anaesthesia was done with inhalational isoflurane and oxygen nitrous mixture with supplementation of relaxant guided by half-hourly TOF count which was kept below two. Hemimaxillectomy using a Weber Fergusson incision with tumour excision was done. Patient was reversed and extubated after a sustained head lift of >5 seconds, and a TOF ratio of 0.9 was demonstrated.

Patient was shifted to the neurosurgical ICU in the immediate postoperative period for overnight monitoring of vitals. Blood gases immediately after shifting and 1 hr thereafter were within normal limits. Pantoprazole infusion was started in the ICU in view of the history of steroid intake preoperatively and continuation of the same postoperatively.

2.5 hrs after arrival, her blood pressure suddenly dropped down from 108/60 mmhg to 66/45 mmhg, and the patient became unconscious. Heart rate was maintained between 110

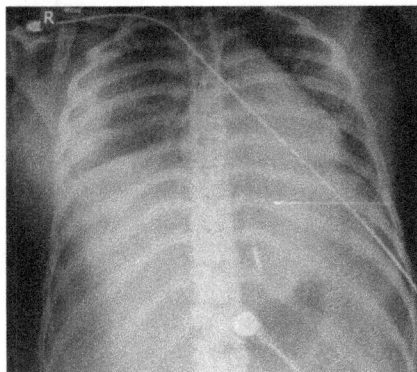

FIGURE 1: Moderate pleural effusion with a large cardiac silhouette suggestive of pericardial effusion.

and 108 per min throughout. Oxygen saturation decreased from 96% to 85%.

RL 1000 ml followed by 500 ml of Haes-steril 6% was administered over 20 minutes to raise the CVP from 6 mmhg to 10–12 mmhg. Patient was ventilated with bag and mask while the intubation tray was kept ready. She became conscious within 5 minutes, and the BP gradually increased to 90/50 mmhg. Decision for intubation, which had the potential to disrupt the suture line as well as being a difficult one owing to the absence of right maxilla and hard palate, was withheld.

Monitoring was continued. Oropharyngeal suction was done, and gauze packs used to pack the maxilla were examined (for any increased bleeding) to have the expected amount of soakage. 50 ml of altered blood was aspirated from Ryle's tube which did not explain the magnitude of hypotension.

After gaining consciousness, the patient complained of diffuse pain per abdomen. On examination, generalised guarding was present per abdomen. Haemoglobin of the patient was 8 gm% after volume infusion, and the patient was transfused 1 unit of packed RBCs. Five mg/kg/min of dopamine infusion was started to support the borderline BP of 86–90 mmhg systolic which increased to >100 mmhg. CVP continued to be 10-11 mmhg after volume infusion. after resuscitation, the SpO$_2$ increased to 89% without O$_2$ supplementation and was maintained at 90–94% with O$_2$ supplementation.

A chest X-ray was ordered next which showed signs of pleural effusion (Figure 1). Ultrasound and CT whole abdomen revealed gross ascites and a hemorrhagic ovarian cyst (4.5 cm × 5 cm) (Figure 2), and echocardiography revealed pericardial effusion. Blood investigations revealed hypoalbuminemia (serum albumin −2.5 mg/dl). Haemoglobin increased to 10 gm% after transfusion. Ascitic fluid biochemistry revealed a SAAG of 1 indicating absence of a cardiac, gastrointestinal, or renal cause of ascites.

Over the next 24 hrs, PaO$_2$ of the patient dropped down from 54 mmhg to 46 mmhg. Dopamine was increased to 8 μ/kg/min to maintain a systolic blood pressure over 90 mmhg. Noninvasive BiPAP of 15 and 7 mmhg was started to which the patient responded well, and the SpO$_2$ increased

to 95% while the PaO$_2$ increased to 57 mmhg over the next 1 hr.

Contrast enhanced computed tomography (CECT) and repeat echocardiography were done which revealed a cardiac tamponade due to moderate pericardial effusion and bilateral pleural effusion with collapse of lower lobes and large volume ascites (Figure 3). Ascites was drained under ultrasound guidance, and over 4 litres of fluid was drained over 2 days in 6 divided sessions. Dopamine infusion had to be increased to 9 μ/kg to maintain the BP over 90/50 mmhg. A pigtail catheter was inserted, and 150 ml of pericardial fluid was drained immediately (Figure 4). USG guided pleural tapping was also done, and up to 300 ml of fluid was removed from each side. Ascitic and pleural fluids were negative for AFB.

By the next day, dopamine was tapered and stopped. Pleural and pericardial fluid adenine deaminase (ADA) was of a borderline value of 35 IU excluding tuberculosis as the cause of such widespread serous cavities effusion.

Based on serum-ascites albumin gradient (SAAG) value and USG findings, serum α fetoprotein, C-reactive protein (CRP), β human chorionic gonadotropin (HCG) and cancer antigen-125 (CA-125) were done as advised by the gynaecology team. CA125 was found to be markedly raised, with an absolute value of 241 U/ml (normal < 35 IU/ml) [3]. CRP was 38 mg/L. Serum alfa fetoprotein (AFP) and β HCG were within normal limits.

A suspicion of a gynaecological malignancy was made, and it was decided to transfer the patient to gynaecology unit for management after recovery.

Over the next 2 days, blood gases improved remarkably, and the patient was gradually weaned off NIV. Repeat CXR (Figure 5) showed no signs of reaccumulation of pleural or pericardial effusion. MRI of abdomen and pelvis showed no significant finding. Abdomen was soft, and no pain per abdomen or guarding was present. Oxygen supplementation was stopped over the next 4-5 hrs. PaO$_2$ on room air was 70 mmhg. All other blood investigations were within normal limits, and serum albumin levels had normalised. Over the next week, CA-125 levels decreased to 32 U/ml and the size of the cyst on repeat pelvic ultrasound 8 days later showed a decrease in size to 3.5 cm. CRP levels also decreased to 15 mg/L. Interleukin-6 (IL-6) levels done (samples taken on days one and five) were reported to be 10 μg/ml (increase) and 2 μ/ml (normal), respectively (report received 12 days later).

On routine follow up the patient had no signs of gynaecological or peritoneal malignancy which were earlier pointing towards a Meigs syndrome-like picture.

3. Discussion

Odontogenic myxoma (OM) is a rare benign tumour arising from tooth forming mesenchyme [4, 5]. Primary anaesthetic concern is maintaining a patent and protected airway while allowing for unhindered surgical access. With airway being the main concern, patient is extubated only after full neuromuscular reversal and no active bleeding is present in the surgical site, which might compromise the airway.

In our patient, all of the above-mentioned precautions were taken care of. Myxomas present elsewhere are known

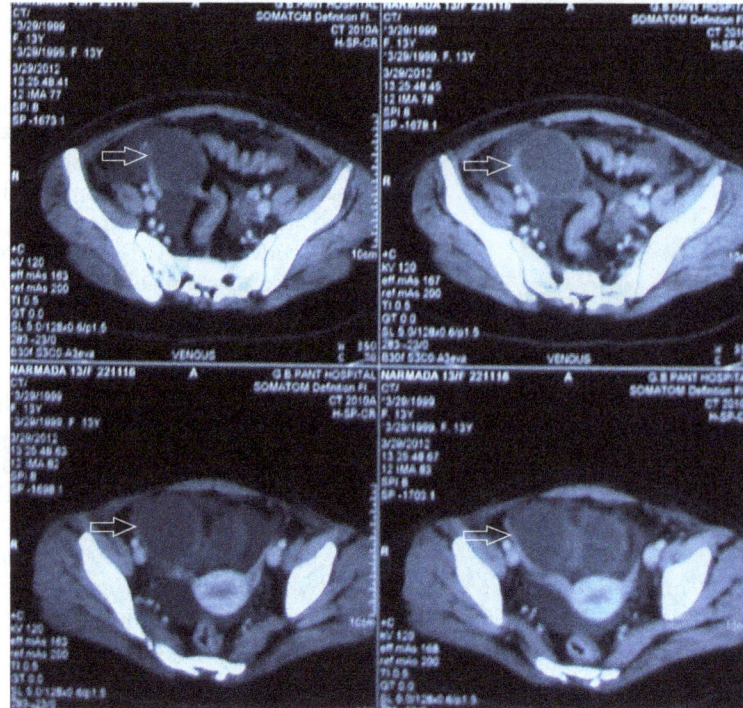

FIGURE 2: CT sections showing a hemorrhagic ovarian cyst.

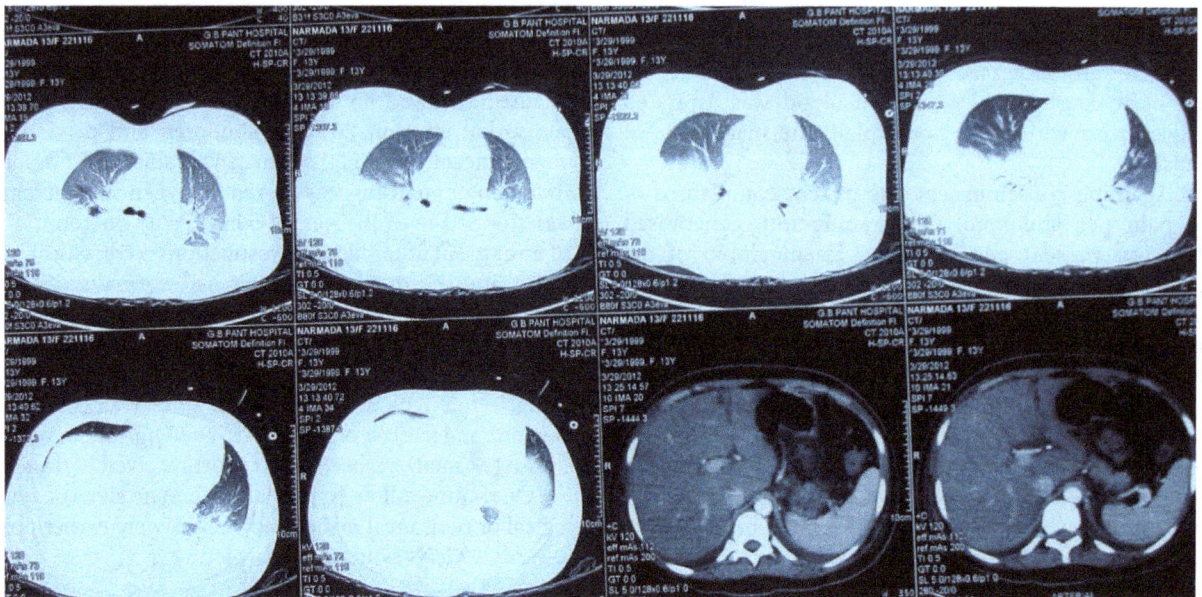

FIGURE 3: CT sections showing bilateral pleural effusion with atelectatic lower zones.

to cause serous cavity effusions [6, 7]. Suspicion of Meigs syndrome [8, 9] was negated by a finding of a small hemorrhagic ovarian cyst without any myxoid component [10, 11]. Suspicion of pseudo-meigs syndrome [12] was made by raised CA-125, massive ascites, and pleural, and pericardial effusions with small hemorrhagic ovarian cyst. Negative pleural and ascitic fluid cytology for malignant cells, premenarchal age group, and spontaneous resolution of all the findings without any surgical or medical intervention went against the diagnosis of any pelvic or abdominal malignancy. Benign hemorrhagic ovarian cysts are not known to cause such massive serous cavities effusion.

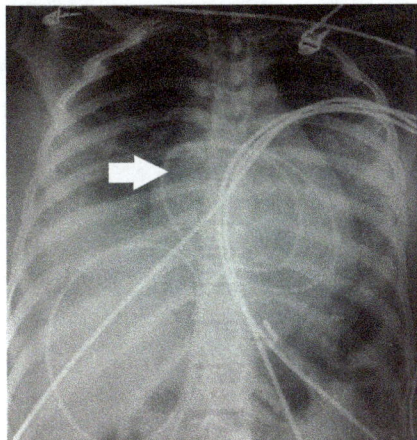

FIGURE 4: CXR film showing pigtail catheter in situ (arrow).

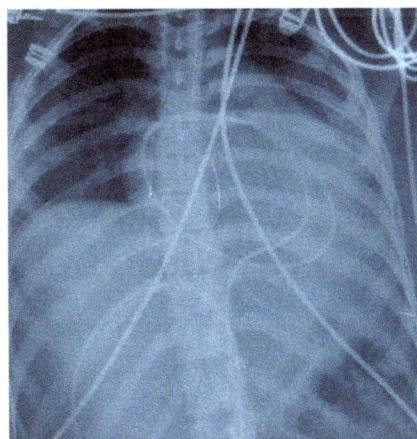

FIGURE 5: Repeat CXR film showing no increase in pleural or pericardial effusions.

It was later concluded that the postoperative events were not due to any ovarian pathology, but due to mediators produced by the primary tumour itself. The incidental finding of raised CA-125 was due to hemorrhagic ovarian cyst as it decreased spontaneously. As IL-6 was raised in the sample taken during the event and subsided thereafter coinciding with relief of symptoms, it can be proposed that the primary tumour released factors responsible for clinical findings. IL-6 is known to cause capillary leakage syndrome and might be responsible along with other mediators for the hemodynamic collapse and serous cavity effusions in concert with fluid resuscitation [3].

In summary, we suggest that odontogenic myxofibroma patients be monitored postoperatively for occurrence of inflammatory mediator related complications apart from the usual airway complications.

References

[1] P. Infante-Cossío, R. Martínez-de-Fuentes, A. García-Perla-García, E. Jiménez-Castellanos, and L. Gómez-Izquierdo, "Myxofibroma of the maxilla: reconstruction with iliac crest graft and dental implants after tumor resection," *Medicina Oral, Patología Oral y Cirugía Bucal*, vol. 16, no. 4, pp. e532–e536, 2011.

[2] R. M. Kellman and W. D. Losquadro, "Comprehensive airway management of patients with maxillofacial trauma," *Craniomaxillofacial Trauma and Reconstruction*, vol. 1, no. 1, pp. 39–47, 2008.

[3] S. A. Vasilev, J. B. Schlaerth, J. Campeau, and C. P. Morrow, "Serum CA 125 levels in preoperative evaluation of pelvic masses," *Obstetrics and Gynecology*, vol. 71, no. 5, pp. 751–756, 1988.

[4] J. P. Sapp, L. R. Eversole, and G. P. Wysocki, *Contemporary Oral and Maxillofacial Pathology*, Mosby, St. Louis, Mo, USA, 2nd edition, 2002.

[5] P. A. Reichart and H. P. Philipsen, *Odontogenic Tumors and Allied Lesions*, Quintessence Publishing, London, UK, 2004.

[6] Y. Seino, U. Ikeda, and K. Shimada, "Increased expression of interleukin 6 mRNA in cardiac myxomas," *British Heart Journal*, vol. 69, no. 6, pp. 565–567, 1993.

[7] M. Jourdan, R. Bataille, J. Seguin, X. G. Zhang, P. A. Chaptal, and B. Klein, "Constitutive production of interleukin-6 and immunologic features in cardiac myxomas," *Arthritis and Rheumatism*, vol. 33, no. 3, pp. 398–402, 1990.

[8] A. Morán-Mendoza, G. Alvarado-Luna, G. Calderillo-Ruiz, A. Serrano-Olvera, C. M. López-Graniel, and D. Gallardo-Rincón, "Elevated CA125 level associated with Meigs' syndrome: case report and review of the literature," *International Journal of Gynecological Cancer*, vol. 16, no. 1, pp. 315–318, 2006.

[9] A. Krüttgen and S. Rose-John, "Interleukin-6 in sepsis and capillary leakage syndrome," *Journal of Interferon and Cytokine Research*, vol. 32, no. 2, pp. 60–65, 2012.

[10] K. K. Samanth and W. C. Black III, "Benign ovarian stromal tumors associated with free peritoneal fluid," *The American Journal of Obstetrics and Gynecology*, vol. 107, no. 4, pp. 538–545, 1970.

[11] F. T. Fischbach and M. B. Dunning III, *Manual of Laboratory and Diagnostic Tests*, Lippincott Williams and Wilkins, Philadelphia, Pa, USA, 8th edition, 2009.

[12] L. Kazanov, D. S. Ander, E. Enriquez, and F. M. Jaggi, "Pseudo-Meigs' syndrome," *The American Journal of Emergency Medicine*, vol. 16, no. 4, pp. 404–405, 1998.

30

Anesthesia Management of a 20-Month-Old Patient with Giant Unilateral Wilms Tumor

Nune Matinyan, Alexander Saltanov, Leonid Martynov, and Anatolij Kazantsev

N. N. Blokhin Cancer Research Center, Pediatric Oncology and Hematology Research Institute, Moscow 115478, Russia

Correspondence should be addressed to Leonid Martynov; leonid.martynov@gmail.com

Academic Editor: Maurizio Marandola

Wilms tumour (WT) (or nephroblastoma) is one of the most common malignant kidney tumors in children. On subsequent stages clinically it is often characterized by abdominal hypertension syndrome, which, in turn, leads to development of respiratory insufficiency. Other symptoms comprise renal deficiency, hypertension, and abnormalities of hemostasis and hemogram. Treatment includes rounds of preoperative chemotherapy and subsequent surgery. We report a case of perioperative management for nephrectomy in 20-month-old patient with a giant unilateral WT. The complexity of anesthesia was determined by the size of tumor, increased intra-abdominal pressure, respiratory deficiency, and hypercoagulation.

1. Introduction

WT incidence accounts for 1/10,000 children. On presentation typical symptoms may include abnormally large abdomen, fever, nausea and vomiting, hypertension, tachycardia, and tachypnea. Diagnostic evaluation includes ultrasound and computed tomography (CT) scans, complete blood count (CBC), biochemistry, urinalysis, and coagulation tests. Treatment consists of rounds of polychemotherapy with subsequent surgery. Anesthesia management in these patients is complicated by respiratory and renal insufficiency, coagulation disorders, and anemia [1]. We report a successful case of anesthesia management for nephrectomy in 20-month-old patient with a giant unilateral nephroblastoma. The complexity of the perioperative period was determined by the size of tumor, increased intra-abdominal pressure, respiratory deficiency, and hypercoagulation. Lung-protective ventilation and administration of minimal doses of opioids due to the epidural anesthesia implementation provided surgical team with optimal conditions for secure tumor extraction, followed by extubation and awakening on the operating table. Postoperative analgesia was performed using an epidural catheter. After 3 days in intensive care unit patient was transferred to Oncology Department for adjuvant postsurgery chemotherapy.

2. Case Report

A 20-month-old female was admitted to our hospital with complaints of palpable unilateral abdominal mass, abdominal pain, fever, tachycardia, and tachypnea. Abdominal CT scans revealed right kidney subtotally replaced by tumor with dimensions $100 \times 120 \times 140$ mm. Lungs CT revealed bilateral multilobar pneumonia, multiple atelectasis, and hypoventilation. Diagnostic evaluation was confirmed by punction biopsy: nephroblastoma cells. After antibacterial therapy and 3 rounds of chemotherapy without convincing tumor reduction, which took 3 weeks, decision to perform the surgery for tumor resection was made. Day prior to surgery physical exam revealed tachycardia 164 beats per minute, tachypnea 60 breaths per minute, and blood pressure 135/65 mmHg. Abdominal CT scans revealed right kidney subtotally replaced by tumor with dimensions $150 \times 130 \times 220$ mm (Figure 1). Lab results showed hemoglobin: 85 g/L, platelet count: 864.000/mcL, total leucocyte count: 15,9 $\times 10^9$/L, hypoproteinemia: 48 g/L, and hypoalbuminemia: 21.0 g/L. Patient was staged ASA V due to progressing respiratory deficiency and lack of pathomorphosis after polychemotherapy; she was not expected to survive without the operation.

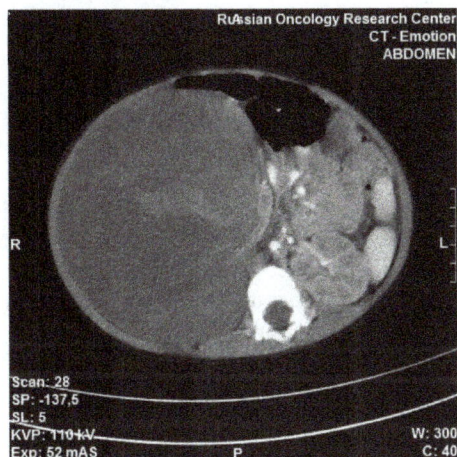

FIGURE 1: Preoperative abdominal computed tomography: right kidney subtotally replaced by tumor.

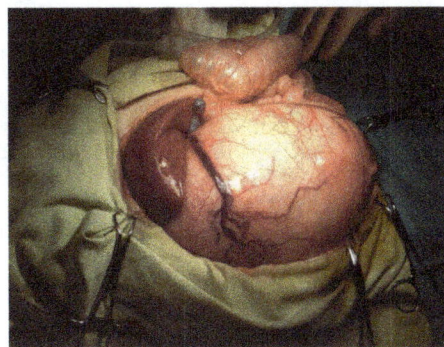

FIGURE 2: Partial tumor mobilization.

Patient presented to the operating theater in sitting position with tachycardia (160 beats per minute), tachypnea (63 breaths per minute). and SpO2 89%. ECG, capnometry and capnography, BIS monitoring, and noninvasive blood pressure monitoring were started. Peripheral intravenous catheter was installed; two unsuccessful attempts to place a radial artery catheter for invasive arterial pressure monitoring were made.

Forced air warming and fluid warmer were used in order to maintain intraoperative normothermia.

Induction of anesthesia was started in Fowler (reverse Trendelenburg) position with sevoflurane 8%, nasogastric tube was installed, fentanyl 50 μg (4.5 μg/kg) and rocuronium 7 mg (0.63 mg/kg) were administered. After 150 s direct laryngoscopy and endotracheal intubation with 4.0 cuffed endotracheal tube were performed, and transesophageal Doppler monitoring was established. Ventilation was straitened after intubation, SatO2 89–92% with FiO2 100%.

Considering the large size of the tumor and the possibility of blood loss due to involvement of major blood vessels, vena subclavia sinistra and vena femoralis dextra were catheterized under ultrasound guidance for intraoperative fluid administration. Continuous infusion with rate of 1.6 mg/hour of rocuronium was established for intraoperative neuromuscular blockade.

Epidural space on T9-T10 level was identified using loss-of-resistance technique and epidural catheter 19 G was installed. A test dose of 0.5 mL lidocaine 2% was injected into the catheter to exclude subarachnoidal placement. To maintain intraoperative analgesia continuous infusion 1,6 mL per hour (0.15 mL/kg/hr) of triple component mixture of ropivacaine (2 mg/mL), fentanyl (2 μg/mL), and epinephrine (2 μg/mL) for intraoperative analgesia was started before the incision [2]. Fentanyl 50 μg (4.5 μg/kg) was administered just before the incision; additional opioids administration was not required during subsequent surgery.

Anesthesia was maintained with sevoflurane 1.8–2.3%. Patient was ventilated with pressure control mode.

Complete blood count and blood gases analyses were performed before the incision: hemoglobin: 76 g/L, platelet count: 607.000/mcL, total leucocyte count: 13,3 × 10^9/L, pH: 7.474, PCO2: 30.2 mmHg, and PO2: 76 mmHg. Blood pressure was 75/30 mmHg and heart rate was 110 beats per minute.

The abdomen was explored through a midline incision. As expected, solid mass occupying the whole right half of the abdomen was visualized. The medial margin of the tumor was soldered with greater curvature of the stomach; the lower margin of the tumor was soldered with right adnexa. Stomach, right salpinx, and ovary were separated from the tumor. After incision and partial mobilization of the tumor (Figure 2), ventilation, saturation, and cardiac output were gradually improving. Cardiac output increased from 1.0 to 1.4 L/min according to transesophageal Doppler. Patient's mechanical ventilation was greatly facilitated and pressure control mode with Pinsp 14 and PEEP 5 was selected. At this point we could adjust FiO2 from 100% to 50% and patient was positioned supine (from Fowler). Inferior vena cava was separated from the tumor; right renal vein and right renal artery were mobilized and crossed. The upper margin of the tumor was soldered with the right dome of the diaphragm, grown into the S6 segment of the liver and into the right adrenal gland. Mobilization of the tumor was accompanied with resection of the right dome of the diaphragm, S6 segment of the liver, and right adrenal gland. Nephrectomy on the right side was performed. Biopsy of two para-aortic lymph nodes was taken. After installation of the drains the surgical wound was closed. Patient was awakened and extubated on the operating table. Surgery time was 340 min.

Resected specimen weighted 2200 gr (Figure 3); subsequent histological analysis matched the diagnosis of WT (nephroblastoma).

Total intraoperative IV fentanyl consumption was 1.5 μg/kg/hour.

Intraoperative blood loss was 150 mL, diuresis: 100 mL. Intraoperative infusion comprised 200 mL of red blood cells, 300 mL of balanced isotonic sodium solution, and 80 mL of gelatin 4% solution.

Blood gases analysis was performed at the end of the surgery, pH: 7.3, PCO2: 42.2 mmHg, and PO2: 214 mmHg.

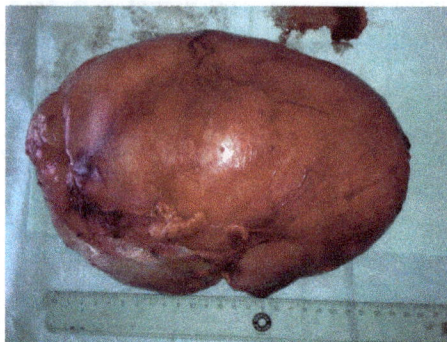

FIGURE 3: Resected specimen.

Postoperative course was favorable and uncomplicated, after 3 days in intensive care unit patient was transferred to Oncology Department for postsurgery chemotherapy. The patient remained fit at a follow-up examination, 3 months after surgery.

3. Discussion

Anesthesia management of pediatric patients with large abdominal mass is always complex and challenging. Due to asymptomatic course of early stages of diseases and the need for lengthy preoperative chemotherapy surgery is often performed in later stages of the disease. Due to rapid mass growth there is no time for development of coping mechanisms and infants with WT may present with tachypnea or dyspnea, hypertension, tachycardia, hypoproteinemia, and hypercoagulation. In our case respiratory insufficiency developed due to bilateral multilobar pneumonia and hypoventilation associated with high intra-abdominal pressure.

In our case plan of anesthesia was induction with sevoflurane, endotracheal intubation, epidural catheter placement for perioperative and prolonged postoperative analgesia, and awakening and extubation on operating table [3]. Lowest possible doses of opioids were used in order not to compromise respiratory function in the early postoperative period [4].

Epidural analgesia with three-component mixture in a patient with the V ASA grade provided smooth intraoperative period without the expressed hypotension. Lipophilic adjuvant opioid fentanyl provided a quick and adequate analgesic effect at the segmental level. Low concentrations of ropivacaine provided adequate analgesia without severe neuromuscular block and hypotension. And adding epinephrine intensified analgesia due to the action on the alpha-2 adrenergic receptors and also inhibited absorption of the mixture. Resorting to epidural analgesia of this kind during emergency surgery in a patient with V ASA grade allowed not only the adequate analgesia, but also rapid recovery of vital functions in the immediate postoperative period (extubation on the operating table) [2, 3, 5].

Transesophageal dopplerography provided intraoperative preload and cardiac output monitoring. Sufficient intraoperative infusion allowed avoiding a severe drop in blood pressure at the moment of mobilization of the giant tumor.

BIS monitoring allowed administering the optimal dose of inhalational anesthetic for maintenance of anesthesia. Prompt recovery was achieved due to intraoperative normoventilation, stable hemodynamic, maintenance of normothermia, and the use of low-dose IV opioid (fentanyl 1.5 mkg/kg/hour).

In conclusion, in this successful case anesthesiologist's goal was to secure adequate perioperative anesthesia management, providing optimal conditions for the surgical team, to conduct adequate postoperative analgesia, provision of early activation, and rehabilitation.

References

[1] A. M. Davidoff, "Wilms Tumor," Advances in Pediatrics, vol. 59, no. 1, pp. 247–267, 2012.

[2] G. Niemi, "Advantages and disadvantages of adrenaline in regional anaesthesia," Best Practice & Research: Clinical Anaesthesiology, vol. 19, no. 2, pp. 229–245, 2005.

[3] J. K. Goeller, T. Bhalla, and J. D. Tobias, "Combined use of neuraxial and general anesthesia during major abdominal procedures in neonates and infants," Paediatric Anaesthesia, vol. 24, no. 6, pp. 553–560, 2014.

[4] D. H. Jablonka and P. J. Davis, "Opioids in pediatric anesthesia," Anesthesiology Clinics of North America, vol. 23, no. 4, pp. 621–634, 2005.

[5] A. Moriarty, "Pediatric epidural analgesia (PEA)," Paediatric Anaesthesia, vol. 22, no. 1, pp. 51–55, 2012.

31

Delayed Onset Malignant Hyperthermia after Sevoflurane

K. Sanem Cakar Turhan,[1] Volkan Baytaş,[2] Yeşim Batislam,[1] and Oya Özatamer[1]

[1] *Department of Anaesthesiology and Reanimation, Ankara University Medical School, Ankara, Turkey*
[2] *Department of Anaesthesiology and Reanimation, Ankara Güven Hospital, Ankara, Turkey*

Correspondence should be addressed to Yeşim Batislam; ybatislam@gmail.com

Academic Editors: U. Buyukkocak and R. S. Gomez

Malignant hyperthermia is a hypermetabolic response to inhalation agents (such as halothane, sevoflurane, and desflurane), succinylcholine, vigorous exercise, and heat. Reactions develop more frequently in males than females (2 : 1). The classical signs of malignant hyperthermia are hyperthermia, tachycardia, tachypnea, increased carbon dioxide production, increased oxygen consumption, acidosis, muscle rigidity and rhabdomyolysis. In this case report, we present a case of delayed onset malignant hyperthermia-like reaction after the second exposure to sevoflurane.

1. Introduction

Malignant hyperthermia is characterized by a hypermetabolic response to triggering agents. In this case report, we present delayed onset malignant hyperthermia-like reaction after the second exposure to sevoflurane [1].

2. Case

An 8-day-old boy was scheduled for choanal atresia evaluation under general anesthesia. Anesthesia induction maintenance was done with sevoflurane 7-8%, after intubation remifentanil 2 μg was given. No muscle relaxant was used. Anesthesia lasted 35 minutes without any problem. One week after this procedure, the patient was scheduled for bilateral nasopharyngeal tube application under general anesthesia with sevoflurane. The procedure ended without any problem. During his followup, the temperature increased to 42.5°C, heart rate increased to 250/min, and respiratory distress developed. Creatinine phosphokinase levels reached 929 IU/L, and hyperpotassemia developed. Blood gas analysis revealed hypoxemia (SO$_2$ < 85%), respiratory acidosis (PaCO$_2$ > 60 mm Hg) and metabolic acidosis (base deficit > 10 mEq/L). The clinical condition of the patient was thought to be due to malignant hyperthermia, and dantrolene sodium was given orally. After dantrolen sodium, the body temperature minimally decreased, and as the respiratory distress continued, the patient was intubated and mechanical ventilation was started. Dantrolen sodium 2.5 mg/kg was given intravenously with 6-hours intervals for 2 days and his temperature decreased. Following 10-hours period of intubation, the patient was extubated and CPAP was done.

There was no family history of malignant hyperthermia or disease increasing the susceptibility to malignant hyperthermia in this patient. He was born with cesarean section after 39 weeks of gestation and his birth weight was 4050 and APGAR score was 6/8. Any systemic problems and fetal anomalies were not seen during pregnancy. There were 3 abortuses with unknown etiologies before this pregnancy. After the delivery as the baby had syndromic facial appearance and inadequate spontaneous respiration, he was followed up in the newborn service and positive pressure ventilation was done. Physical examination revealed dysmorphic face, micrognathia, high-arched palate, low-set ears, popeyed appearance, hypertelorism, low-slanting palpebral fissures, cryptochidism, clinodactyly, and craniosynostosis. There was bilateral hearing loss.

3. Discussion

Malignant hyperthermia is a hypermetabolic response to potent inhalation agents (such as halothane, sevoflurane, and desflurane), succinylcholine, vigorous exercise, and heat. Reactions develop more frequently in males than females

(2:1). The classical signs of malignant hyperthermia are hyperthermia, tachycardia, tachypnea, increased carbondioxide production, increased oxygen consumption, acidosis, muscle rigidity, and rhabdomyolysis [1].

The gold standard for diagnosis of susceptibility to malignant hyperthermia is caffeine-halothane contracture test. However, as this test is not widely available, the diagnosis of malignant hyperthermia can only be made by clinical presentation. Dantrolene sodium is a specific antagonist of the pathophysiologic changes of malignant hyperthermia and when given in the early period it is lifesaving [1, 2].

Malignant hyperthermia was suspected with the presence of respiratory acidosis, sinus tachycardia, metabolic acidosis, increased serum creatinine kinase levels, hyperpotassemia, and hyperthermia in our patient and dantrolen sodium was given for treatment. The improvement of the clinical signs after administration of dantrolen sodium suggested that our diagnosis of malignant hyperthermia is correct. However, to confirm the diagnosis, caffeine-halothane contracture test could not be done as this test is not available in our institution.

In our patient, serum creatinine kinase levels increased only moderately and we thought that moderate increase of serum creatinine kinase level may be due to immediate treatment with dantrolene sodium and rapid improvement of the clinical signs. Also, the young age of the patient may be another factor. As the muscle mass in older children and the adults is relatively greater, serum creatinine kinase levels are expected to be higher in older patients.

Although sevoflurane is known as a less potent agent triggering malignant hyperthermia, malignant hyperthermia after sevoflurane exposure was reported in the literature. Malignant hyperthermia after sevoflurane exposure is thought to be related to calcium release from sarcoplasmic reticulum [3].

Hsu et al. have reported malignant hyperthermia in a boy aged 3 years and 9 months who was scheduled for Hotz's operation under general anesthesia with sevoflurane and the symptoms of this patient have improved after discontinuation of sevoflurane. Molecular genetic testing identified a novel ryanodine receptor (RYR1) mutation in this patient and this confirmed the malignant hyperthermia susceptibility in this patient [2].

Bonciu et al. have reported malignant hyperthermia in a 7-years old boy who was scheduled for tympanoplasty under general anesthesia with sevoflurane. The patient had a history of anesthesia induction with sevoflurane without any complication. But the maintenance had been done with propofol. It was reported that the clinical symptoms were improved with discontinuation of sevoflurane and increasing the minute ventilation [4].

The late onset of malignant hyperthermia is a rare clinical entity. Chen et al. have reported malignant hyperthermia in a 5-years old boy after second exposure to sevoflurane. This patient had general anesthesia with sevoflurane for 2 times with an interval of 2 days [3].

Greenberg et al. have reported malignant hyperthermia in a 6-months old baby with 5q chromosomal deletion scheduled for cleft palate repair under general anesthesia with sevoflurane. The patient had a history of magnetic resonance imaging under general anesthesia with sevoflurane 2 weeks before the surgery and he had had increased temperature and tachycardia but these symptoms reversed spontaneously. After the second exposure to sevoflurane tachycardia, increased temperature, and hypercarbia were seen and these symptoms reversed with treatment with dantrolene sodium. Greenberg et al. reported that this is the first case of malignant hyperthermia in a patient with 5q chromosomal deletion in the literature [5].

During his first anesthesia experience, our patient had general anesthesia with sevoflurane and no complication were seen. But 1 week later, after his second exposure to sevoflurane, clinical symptoms of malignant hyperthermia was seen during postoperative period. The late onset of malignant hyperthermia after the second exposure is a rare condition. We thought that this may be related to latent effect of volatile anesthetics on skeletal muscles.

Claussen et al. have reported malignant hyperthermia following general anesthesia with sevoflurane in a 5-year-old boy who had been anaesthetized two times with halothane without any complication. The timely administration of dantrolene rapidly reversed the life-threatening signs and prevent progression of the disease in this patient [6]. In a similar manner, in our patient we have administered dantrolen sodium in the early period and the symptoms reversed.

Reed et al. have reported on two boys aged 2 and 6 years, respectively, with dysmorphic face, ptosis, downslanting palpebral fissures, hypertelorism, epicanthic folds, low-set ears, malar hypoplasia, micrognathia, high-arched palate, clinodactyly, palmar simian line, pectus excavatum, winging of the scapulae, lumbar lordosis, and mild thoracic scoliosis who present congenital hypotonia, slightly delayed motor development diagnosed as King-Denborough syndrome. Reed et al. have emphasized the fact that patients with King Denborough syndrome may undergo general anesthesia for cryptrochidism and skeletal deformities and the objective must be increasing the awareness of this disorder as these patients are predisposed to developing malignant hyperthermia [7].

The preoperative physical examination in our patient also revealed dysmorphic face, micrognathia, high-arched palate, low-set ears, popeyed appearence, hypertelorism, low-slanting palpebral fissures, cryptochirdism, clinodactyly, craniosynostosis, and bilateral hearing loss but definite diagnosis was not done by the genetic department. However malignant hyperthermia during the postoperative period following general anesthesia together with the syndromic appearance made us think this may be King Denborough syndrome.

Kinouchi et al. reported two cases of malignant hyperthermia triggered by sevoflurane and these patients had no familial susceptibility to malignant hyperthermia. Postoperatively, one of these patients was noted to have downslanting palpebral fissures, micrognathia, low-set ears, and a single crease of the fifth finger and diagnosed as King syndrome which is reported to have association with malignant hyperthermia [8].

Although there was no definite diagnosis in the preoperative period, the development of malignant hyperthermia during the postoperative period has made us think of this syndrome as King-Denborough syndrome. The King-Denborough syndrome (KDS) is a congenital myopathy associated with susceptibility to malignant hyperthermia, skeletal abnormalities, and dysmorphic features with characteristic facial appearance. As there is susceptibility to malignant hyperthermia in these patients, it is important to evaluate the clinical signs of King-Denborough syndrome during the preoperative period especially in the newborn.

References

[1] H. Rosenberg, M. Davis, D. James, N. Pollock, and K. Stowell, "Malignant hyperthermia," *Orphanet Journal of Rare Diseases*, vol. 2, no. 1, article 21, pp. 1–14, 2007.

[2] S. C. Hsu, W. T. Huang, H. M. Yeh, and Y. J. A. Hsich, "Suspected malignant hyperthermia during sevoflurane anesthesia," *Journal of the Chinese Medical Association*, vol. 20, no. 11, pp. 507–510, 2007.

[3] P. Chen, Y. Day, B. Su, P. Lee, and C. Chen, "Delayed onset of sevoflurane-induced juvenile malignant hyperthermia after second exposure," *Acta Anaesthesiologica Taiwanica*, vol. 45, no. 3, pp. 189–193, 2007.

[4] M. Bonciu, A. de la Chapelle, H. Delpech, T. Depret, R. Krivosic-Horber, and M. R. Aimé, "Minor increase of endtidal CO_2 during sevoflurane-induced malignant hyperthermia," *Paediatric Anaesthesia*, vol. 17, no. 2, pp. 180–182, 2007.

[5] M. Greenberg, A. Faierman, B. Fisher, and B. Harris, "A malignant hyperthermia-like reaction in a six-month-old female with a 5q chromosomal deletion," *Canadian Journal of Anesthesia*, vol. 52, no. 7, pp. 772–773, 2005.

[6] D. Claussen, K. Wuttig, J. Freudenberg, and A. Claussen, "Malignant hyperthermia and sevoflurane-a case report," *Anästhesiologie, Intensivmedizin, Notfallmedizin, Schmerztherapie*, vol. 32, no. 10, pp. 641–644, 1997.

[7] U. C. Reed, M. B. D. Resende, L. G. Ferreira et al., "King-Denborough syndrome: report of two Brazilian cases," *Arquivos de Neuro-Psiquiatria*, vol. 60, no. 3B, pp. 739–741, 2002.

[8] K. Kinouchi, M. Okawa, K. Fukumitsu, K. Tachibana, S. Kitamura, and A. Taniguchi, "Two pediatric cases of malignant hyperthermia caused by sevoflurane," *Masui*, vol. 50, no. 11, pp. 1232–1235, 2001.

32

Combined Spinal-Epidural Analgesia for Laboring Parturient with Arnold-Chiari Type I Malformation

Clark K. Choi and Kalpana Tyagaraj

Department of Anesthesiology, Maimonides Medical Center, 4802 10th Avenue, Brooklyn, NY 11219, USA

Correspondence should be addressed to Kalpana Tyagaraj; kalpana_tyagaraj@msn.com

Academic Editors: R. S. Gomez, C.-H. Hsing, T. Suzuki, and E. A. Vandermeersch

Anesthetic management of laboring parturients with Arnold-Chiari type I malformation poses a difficult challenge for the anesthesiologist. The increase in intracranial pressure during uterine contractions, coughing, valsalva maneuvers, and expulsion of the fetus can be detrimental to the mother during the process of labor and delivery. No concrete evidence has implicated high cerebral spinal fluid pressure on maternal and fetal complications. The literature on the use of neuraxial techniques for managing parturients with Arnold-Chiari is extremely scarce. While most anesthesiologists advocate epidural analgesia for management of labor pain and spinal anesthesia for cesarean section, we are the first to report the use of combined spinal-epidural analgesia for managing labor pain in a pregnant woman with Arnold-Chiari type I malformation. Also, we have reviewed the literature and presented information from case reports and case series to support the safe usage of neuraxial techniques in these patients.

1. Introduction

Arnold-Chiari type I malformation (ACM-I) is a congenital neurological anomaly associated with prolapse of the cerebellar tonsils into the magnum foramen [1, 2]. Approximately 30% to 50% of the ACM-I patients have associated syringomyelia. Incidence of ACM-I ranges between 0.56% and 0.77% on magnetic resonance imaging (MRI) studies, of which 15% to 30% are asymptomatic. This abnormality is mostly predisposed to women, with a female-to-male ratio of 3:1. Symptoms including headaches, neck and shoulder pain, paresthesia, loss of pain and temperature sensation in the upper extremities, and unsteady gait are the usual manifestations seen during early adolescence into adulthood. Severity of the symptoms ranges from mild when tonsillar herniation is larger than 5 mm to severe if it is more than 12 mm on the sagittal MRI view [3].

A combined spinal-epidural (CSE) technique was used to provide labor analgesia for our parturient with ACM-I. We also conducted a literature search for our case presentation using a public accessible medical database MEDLINE. Individual key words were entered into the query: "Arnold-Chiari," "vaginal delivery," "pregnancy," "combined spinal-epidural analgesia," "epidural analgesia," "spinal analgesia," "cesarean section," "perioperative outcomes," and their combinations. Only articles in English language were selected. The database search yielded limited number of articles, mainly case reports and case series (Table 1).

2. Case Presentation

A 17-year-old female, G1P0, with history of hypothyroidism and ACM-I diagnosed during childhood, presented with symptoms of occasional headache and neck pain. She denied any visual disturbances or abnormal pain and temperature sensation in both upper extremities. She was consulted by a multidisciplinary team, including the anesthesiologist, perinatologist, and neurologist, for a planned labor induction with instrument-assisted vaginal delivery. MRI of the brain showed a 7 mm cerebellar tonsil herniation into the foramen magnum without syringomyelia (Figure 1).

Physical examination showed a 62 kg afebrile woman, in mild distress from uterine contractions, with a blood pressure

TABLE 1: Summary of anesthetic management of patients with Arnold-Chiari type I malformation.

Authors and references	Age (years)	Symptoms	Tonsillar herniation (mm)	Syrinx	Surgery before labor	Gravida and para	Gestation age (wks)	Delivery method	Apgar at 1 min and 5 min	Neuraxial method	Maternal postpartum symptoms
Landau et al. [3]	31	Headache, vertigo, nausea, nystagmus, lower extremity, and hyperreflexia	Descended to C3	No	Yes	G2P1	37	CS	9, 10	Spinal	No change
	30	Arm and leg tingling	Not reported	No	No	G1P0	Not reported	CS	Not reported**	Continuous spinal	PDPH requiring blood patch
	32	Arm and leg tingling	Not reported	No	No	G2P1	Not reported	CS	Not reported**	Spinal	No change
	35	Arm and leg tingling and headache	Not reported	No	No	G3P2	Not reported	CS	Not reported**	Spinal	No change
	20	None	Undiagnosed	Undiagnosed	No	G1P0	Not reported	NSVD	Not reported**	Epidural	No change
Chantigian et al. [4]	39	Headache, right arm paresthesia, and numbness	Not reported	No	No	G3P2	Not reported	NSVD	Not reported**	Epidural	No change
	21	Headache	Not reported	No	No	G2P1	Not reported	NSVD	Not reported**	Epidural	No change
	25	None	Undiagnosed	Undiagnosed	No	G1P0	Not reported	NSVD	Not reported**	Epidural	No change
	21	None	Undiagnosed	Undiagnosed	No	G1P0	Not reported	NSVD	Not reported**	Epidural	No change
	25	None	Undiagnosed	Undiagnosed	No	G2P1	Not reported	NSVD	Not reported**	Epidural	No change
Kuczkowski [5]	35	Headache, vertigo, and upper extremity paresthesia	Not reported	No	No	G1P0	37	CS	Not reported**	Spinal	No change
Hullander et al. [6]	31	None	Undiagnosed	Undiagnosed	No	G1P0	Not reported	CS	Not reported**	Epidural and spinal	Headache and neck pain requiring blood patch
	30	Headache, dizziness, vision changes, upper extremities paresthesia, and dyspnea	8	Yes	No	G2P1	32	NSVD	Not reported*	Epidural	No change
	27	Headache, tinnitus, and dizziness	4	No	Yes	G2P1	Not reported	NSVD	Not reported**	Epidural	No change
Mueller and Oró [7]	31	Headache, blurred vision, hoarseness, dizziness, neck pain, upper extremities paresthesia, tinnitus, and dyspnea	10	No	Yes	Not reported	Not reported	NSVD	Not reported**	Epidural	No change
	32	Headache, neck pain, dizziness, hoarseness, dysphagia, and upper extremity paresthesia	13	No	Yes	G1P0	Not reported	NSVD	Not reported**	Epidural	Neck pain, spasm

TABLE 1: Continued.

Authors and references	Age (years)	Symptoms	Tonsillar herniation (mm)	Syrinx	Surgery before labor	Gravida and para	Gestation age (wks)	Delivery method	Apgar at 1 min and 5 min	Neuraxial method	Maternal postpartum symptoms
Semple and McClure [8]	30	Ataxia, upper extremity paresthesia, and preeclamptic	Not reported	No	No	Not reported	30	CS	8, 9	Epidural	No change
Nel et al. [9]	31	Headache, reduced pain and temperature, and wasting on left hand	Not reported	Yes	No	G2P1	38	CS	Not reported**	Epidural	No change
Parker et al. [10]	26	Headaches, peripheral paresthesias, and weakness	Not reported	Yes	No	G1P0	38	CS	Not reported**	Epidural	No change
	30	None	Not reported	Yes	No	G1P0	39	CS	Not reported**	Epidural	No change
Newhouse and Kuczkowski [11]	20	Headache, chest pain, and hand and foot numbness	Not reported	Yes	No	G1P0	35	NSVD	8, 9	Epidural	No change
Our patient	17	Headache and neck pain	7	No	No	G1P0	39	NSVD	9, 9	CSE	No change

NSVD: normal spontaneous vaginal delivery; CS: cesarean section; CSE: combined spinal-epidural; PDPH: postdural puncture headache. *Neonate required hospitalization for pneumonia and respiratory distress. **Healthy neonate.

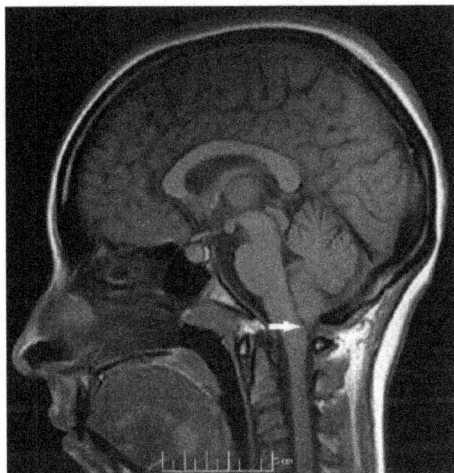

FIGURE 1: Sagittal magnetic resonance image of Arnold-Chiari type I malformation. White arrow denotes the 7 mm tonsillar herniation from the cerebellum. No syringomyelia is seen.

of 134/89 mmHg, pulse of 62/min, respiratory rate of 12/min, and pulse oximetry saturation of 99%. Baseline laboratory values were hemoglobin 11.9 g/dL and platelets 206×10^9/L. With a single attempt, CSE was achieved using a 17-gauge Tuohy needle and a 5-inch 27-gauge Whitacre spinal needle at the midline of the L3-L4 interspinous space while the patient was in a sitting position. Analgesia was obtained with fentanyl 15 μg and bupivacaine 1.5 mg intrathecally. Aspiration of the epidural catheter and test dose of lidocaine 1.5% with epinephrine 1 : 200,000 were negative. A continuous epidural infusion of bupivacaine 0.1% and fentanyl 0.0002% was initiated at the rate of 10 mL/h. A 5 mL bolus of bupivacaine 0.25% was injected epidurally 90 minutes before the onset of fetal expulsion and subsequently augmented with another bolus to provide a denser block to minimize the urge to push.

Fetal heart rate (FHR) and uterine contractions were continuously monitored by an external cardiotocograph. Category I FHR tracing was noted throughout the first and second stages of labor. Maternal and fetal hemodynamics were stable during the entire labor and delivery process. Labor progressed smoothly and lasted for 9 hours. The patient gave birth to a 2,995 g healthy girl using vacuum-assisted extraction. Apgar scores at 1 and 5 minutes were 9 and 9, respectively. Estimated blood loss was 200 mL. The patient had an uneventful postpartum course without any neurological sequelae. She was discharged home three days later.

3. Discussion

Attempts to demonstrate the efficacy and safety of neuraxial technique (epidural versus spinal) in a pregnant woman with ACM-I have been the subject of controversy. The risks of accidental dural puncture with the epidural needle can lead to tentorial herniation, decreased cerebral perfusion pressure, and brain shifts. Intentional intrathecal puncture using spinal

needle can also present with similar manifestations but the magnitude of the effect and incidence is relatively less than the epidural needle-induced dural puncture due to the larger size of the dural puncture. Selection of smaller size epidural and spinal needles is an important factor to improve safety, but, ultimately, the danger can be significantly minimized with an experienced and trained anesthesiologist to avoid inadvertent dural puncture as well as multiple needle attempts.

The safety of providing intrathecal analgesia for immediate pain relief during labor and anesthesia for cesarean section (CS) can be effectively implemented provided that there are no acute worsening of clinical signs and symptoms of intracranial pressure (ICP). In our case presentation, we selected the use of CSE to provide immediate pain relief intrathecally for our patient and the epidural catheter to administer intermittent extradural boluses for analgesia during the course of labor and delivery as well as for anesthesia for emergent CS due to obstetrical and fetal concerns. Had our patient developed severe or new onset of neurological symptoms during pregnancy, neuraxial technique would be contraindicated. Even without any absolute contraindications, there are currently no firm guidelines to suggest preference for general anesthesia over neuraxial techniques except many believe that the patients with ACM-I have inherent high ICP; therefore, neuraxial techniques are unsuitable choice for analgesia and anesthesia [12–17]. General anesthesia is not without any risks as airway management by rapid sequence induction and intubation from direct laryngoscopy to protect parturients from aspiration can potentially increase ICP. Difficult intubation, as encountered in some of the obese pregnant patients, can cause rapid desaturation leading to hypoxia and hypercarbia which further enhance the effect on ICP. Landau et al. described a case of successful spinal anesthesia after surgical decompression of a parturient with ACM-I [3]. Moreover, spinal anesthesia for CS has been successfully performed for undiagnosed parturients with ACM-I and also those without neurosurgery [4–6].

The choice for the mode of delivery (vaginal versus CS) is also a controversial issue. The contractile force of the uterus on cerebral spinal fluid (CSF) can cause an increase in ICP and unsuspected herniation. The hydrodynamic effect on CSF pressure during labor was investigated by several researchers in the 1960s [18–21]. Changes in the intra-abdominal and intrathoracic pressure secondary to sensation of pain were factors causing elevated CSF pressure during uterine contractions. Pain can induce elevated CSF but whether it contributes to a significant impact on unfavorable maternal and fetal outcomes is unclear. Mueller and Oró reported three case presentations of normal spontaneous vaginal delivery in parturients with ACM-I without receiving epidural block during labor [7]. Semple and McClure [8] and Nel et al. [9] used epidural anesthesia for CS without a clear obstetric indication other than the fear of increased ICP from straining in the second stage of delivery except from one case report described by Parker et al. [10]. Newhouse et al. managed successfully a parturient with ACM-I and sickle cell disease presented with acute pain crisis using epidural analgesia via vacuum-assisted vaginal delivery without neurological complications [11].

Key points in the anesthetic management of laboring parturients with ACM-I include (1) early CSE analgesia to decrease painful uterine contractions to limit intra-abdominal and intrathoracic excursions to dampen elevated CSF pressure; (2) slow titration of bolus through the epidural to prevent undue extradural pressure; (3) vacuum-assisted vaginal delivery in the second stage of labor to minimize increase in ICP during fetal expulsion and maternal valsalva maneuvers; and (4) minimization of wide variations of maternal hemodynamics to preserve adequate cerebral perfusion pressure.

In summary, CSE labor analgesia can provide safe and effective pain relief to parturient with ACM-I. We emphasize the importance of multidisciplinary approach to tailor an individualized care plan for favorable maternal and fetal outcomes.

References

[1] G. K. Bejjani, "Definition of the adult Chiari malformation: a brief historical overview," *Neurosurgical Focus*, vol. 11, no. 1, pp. 1–8, 2001.

[2] G. K. Bejjani and K. P. Cockerham, "Adult Chiari malformation," *Contemporary Neurosurgery*, vol. 23, no. 26, pp. 1–7, 2001.

[3] R. Landau, R. Giraud, V. Delrue, and C. Kern, "Spinal anesthesia for cesarean delivery in a woman with a surgically corrected Type I Arnold Chiari malformation," *Anesthesia and Analgesia*, vol. 97, no. 1, pp. 253–255, 2003.

[4] R. C. Chantigian, M. A. Koehn, K. D. Ramin, and M. A. Warner, "Chiari I malformation in parturients," *Journal of Clinical Anesthesia*, vol. 14, no. 3, pp. 201–205, 2002.

[5] K. M. Kuczkowski, "Spinal anesthesia for Cesarean delivery in a parturient with Arnold-Chiari type I malformation," *Canadian Journal of Anesthesia*, vol. 51, no. 6, p. 639, 2004.

[6] R. M. Hullander, T. D. Bogard, D. Leivers, D. Moran, and D. M. Dewan, "Chiari I malformation presenting as recurrent spinal headache," *Anesthesia and Analgesia*, vol. 75, no. 6, pp. 1025–1026, 1992.

[7] D. M. Mueller and J. Oró, "Chiari I malformation with or without syringomyelia and pregnancy: case studies and review of the literature," *American Journal of Perinatology*, vol. 22, no. 2, pp. 67–70, 2005.

[8] D. A. Semple and J. H. McClure, "Arnold-Chiari malformation in pregnancy," *Anaesthesia*, vol. 51, no. 6, pp. 580–582, 1996.

[9] M. R. Nel, V. Robson, and P. N. Robinson, "Extradural anaesthesia for Caesarean section in a patient with syringomyelia and Chiari type I anomaly," *British Journal of Anaesthesia*, vol. 80, no. 4, pp. 512–515, 1998.

[10] J. D. Parker, J. C. Broberg, and P. G. Napolitano, "Maternal Arnold-Chiari type I malformation and syringomyelia: a labor management dilemma," *American Journal of Perinatology*, vol. 19, no. 8, pp. 445–449, 2002.

[11] B. J. Newhouse and K. M. Kuczkowski, "Uneventful epidural labor analgesia and vaginal delivery in a parturient with Arnold-Chiari malformation type I and sickle cell disease,"

Archives of Gynecology and Obstetrics, vol. 275, no. 4, pp. 311–313, 2007.

[12] M. Agustí, R. Adàlia, C. Fernández, and C. Gomar, "Anaesthesia for caesarean section in a patient with syringomyelia and Arnold-Chiari type I malformation," *International Journal of Obstetric Anesthesia*, vol. 13, no. 2, pp. 114–116, 2004.

[13] L. Jayaraman, N. Sethi, and J. Sood, "Anaesthesia for caesarean section in a patient with lumbar syringomyelia," *Revista Brasileira de Anestesiologia*, vol. 61, no. 4, pp. 469–473, 2011.

[14] K. Murayama, K. Mamiya, K. Nozaki et al., "Cesarean section in a patient with syringomyelia," *Canadian Journal of Anesthesia*, vol. 48, no. 5, pp. 474–477, 2001.

[15] R. F. Ghaly, K. D. Candido, R. Sauer, and N. N. Knezevic, "Anesthetic management during cesarean section in a woman with residual Arnold-Chiari malformation type I, cervical kyphosis, and syringomyelia," *Surgical Neurology International*, vol. 3, article 26, 2012.

[16] D. J. Penney and J. M. B. Smallman, "Arnold-Chiari malformation and pregnancy," *International Journal of Obstetric Anesthesia*, vol. 10, no. 2, pp. 139–141, 2001.

[17] G. B. Sicuranza, P. Steinberg, and R. Figueroa, "Arnold-Chiari malformation in a pregnant woman," *Obstetrics and Gynecology*, vol. 102, no. 5, pp. 1191–1194, 2003.

[18] A. Vasicka, H. Kretchmer, and F. Lawas, "Cerebrospinal fluid pressures during labor," *American Journal of Obstetrics and Gynecology*, vol. 84, pp. 206–212, 1962.

[19] E. L. Hopkins, C. H. Hendricks, and L. A. Cibils, "Cerebrospinal fluid pressure in labor," *American Journal of Obstetrics and Gynecology*, vol. 93, no. 7, pp. 907–916, 1965.

[20] G. F. Marx, Y. Oka, and L. R. Orkin, "Cerebrospinal fluid pressures during labor," *American Journal of Obstetrics and Gynecology*, vol. 84, pp. 213–219, 1962.

[21] G. F. Marx, M. T. Zemaitis, and L. R. Orkin, "Cerebrospinal fluid pressures during labor and obstetrical anesthesia," *Anesthesiology*, vol. 22, pp. 348–354, 1961.

33

Ultrasound-Guided Popliteal Nerve Block in a Patient with Malignant Degeneration of Neurofibromatosis 1

Arjun Desai, Brendan Carvalho, Jenna Hansen, and Jonay Hill

Department of Anesthesia, H3580, Stanford University School of Medicine, Stanford, CA 94305, USA

Correspondence should be addressed to Arjun Desai, adesai5@gmail.com

Academic Editors: A. Apan, U. Buyukkocak, P. Michalek, and E. A. Vandermeersch

A 41-year-old female patient with neurofibromatosis 1 presented with new neurologic deficits secondary to malignant degeneration of a tibial lesion. Ultrasound mapping of the popliteal nerve revealed changes consistent with an intraneural neurofibroma. Successful popliteal nerve blockade was achieved under ultrasound guidance.

1. Introduction

Neurofibromatosis 1 (NF) or von Recklinghausen disease is a systemic genetic disorder that commonly presents with cutaneous neurofibromas, café-au-lait spots, and hallmark plexiform neurofibromas [1]. NF presents several difficulties for anesthesiologists including potential airway difficulty, abnormal spinal anatomy, and peripheral neurofibromas [2].

The role of CT and MRI are well established for mapping anatomical variations in airway and spinal regions in patients with neural sheath tumors. Recently, ultrasound (US) has become a useful adjunct diagnostic modality in occult NF [3]. With widespread use of US in regional anesthesia, sonographic characteristics of neurofibromas are increasingly described in the literature [4]. However, there is a lack of information regarding the efficacy and safety of providing regional anesthesia in the setting of peripheral nerve sheath tumors. We present a case of successful popliteal nerve blockade under ultrasound guidance in a patient with NF by administering local anesthetic proximal to a lesion consistent with intraneural neurofibromatosis.

2. Case Report

A 41-year-old Caucasian female patient with a past medical history significant for NF presented for open biopsy of her left tibia. The patient detailed a one and a half year progressive weakness and pain in her left ankle. Initial plain film radiographic examination in August 2010 showed a

3 × 1.5 × 2 cm destructive lesion of the cortical bone in the distal tibia. MRI analysis of the lesion in September 2010 showed a larger enhancing 5.7 × 4.6 cm lesion. At that time the patient underwent Tru-Cut soft tissue biopsy of the mass with pathology confirming a nerve sheath tumor. However, there was insufficient tissue to determine malignancy and further tests were required. After a brief loss to follow up for insurance and financial difficulties, another MRI examination in January 2011 revealed an even larger 6.5 × 5.1 cm T2 hyperintense lesion eroding through the tibia with a 2.4 cm proximal periosteal extension. The patient's condition had also deteriorated, and she now required crutch support for ambulation. She reported decreased sensation to cold, light touch, and pinprick over the left first and second toes. Concern for malignant degeneration of her NF disease in the left ankle warranted a more extensive open biopsy for definitive diagnoses.

Preoperative anesthetic evaluation revealed no other significant medical problems, no known drug allergies, no prior general anesthetics, and a family history of pseudocholinesterase deficiency. She had several previous cutaneous nodule excisions for cosmesis completed under a combination of local anesthesia and sedation at outside institutions. The patient was prescribed temazepam (Restoril, Mallinckrodt Pharmaceuticals Group, MO) orally for insomnia as necessary, as well as hydrocodone-acetaminophen (Vicodin, Abbott Laboratories, IL) and ibuprofen (Motrin, McNeil Consumer Healthcare Division, PA) orally as required for ankle related pain. On general examination, she had multiple cutaneous neurofibromas diffusely distributed throughout her body. Her BMI was 29 and her airway examination was unremarkable.

2.1. Popliteal Nerve Regional Anesthetic Blockade. Prior to the nerve blockade, standard monitors (noninvasive blood pressure cuff, pulse oximeter, and 3-lead ECG) were applied. Supplemental oxygen (3 L/minute) was administered via nasal cannula. Adequate sedation was achieved with intravenous midazolam 2 mg (Versed, Roche, NY), and fentanyl 150 mcg after timeout was completed. The patient was placed in supine position with left foot elevation and left knee flexion, and the skin sterilized with ChloraPrep (Cardinal Health, OH).

The US transducer (linear, 12-3 MHz, L12-3 Phillips) was placed transversely at the inferior aspect of the popliteal fossa. Cephalad and caudad orientation of the probe demonstrated relevant anatomy including the popliteal artery, vein, sciatic nerve, and its bifurcation into the common peroneal and tibial nerves. Of specific interest, sonographic "target signs" [5] consistent with previous descriptions of intraneural fibromas [6] were demonstrated in the sciatic, common peroneal, and tibial nerves [7]. The lesions appeared solitary, ovoid and contiguous with the nerve, had a hypoechoic echotexture with well-defined margins, and demonstrated subtle distal acoustic enhancement (Figure 1). With popliteal artery in view, we were able to demonstrate true and faux (neurofibroma) arterial structures using doppler analysis (Figure 2). Tracing the path of the sciatic nerve proximally, we identified a portion of the nerve with no neurofibromatous changes on ultrasound. We also carefully selected an area of the inferior thigh void of cutaneous neurofibromas for needle insertion. The skin was infiltrated with 2 mL 2% lidocaine, and a 10 cm 22-gauge Stimuplex needle (B. Braun, PA) was utilized. A real-time view of the Stimuplex needle tip, popliteal artery, and sciatic nerve was maintained at all times during the block. A total of 30 mL 0.5% ropivacaine (APP Pharmaceuticals, IL) with 1 : 400.000 epinephrine was injected with intermittent negative aspiration for blood. The local anesthetic spread circumferentially around the sciatic nerve as noted on ultrasound examination (Figure 3). The patient reported no paresthesias or discomfort during the procedure.

Within ten minutes, the patient reported subjective numbness, warmth, and heaviness of her left calf and foot. On examination she had complete sensation loss to sharp touch and cold in the sciatic distribution of her left lower extremity. Intraoperatively, sedation was provided with midazolam 2 mg IV followed by a propofol infusion (25–50 mcg/kg/min). She maintained spontaneous ventilation via laryngeal mask airway. The patient did not respond to the incision and remained hemodynamically stable for the duration of surgery. She received ondansetron 4 mg (Zofran, GlaxoSmithKline, NC) intravenously twenty minutes prior to the completion of surgery for nausea prophylaxis.

The patient was alert, awake, and oriented in the post-anesthesia care unit. She complained of no pain (verbal pain score 0/10) and had residual sensory loss and motor

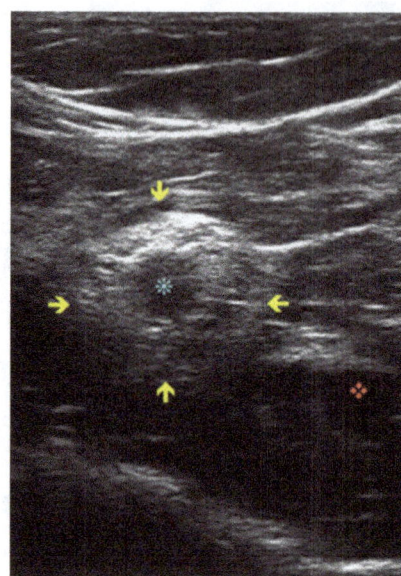

▣	Sciatic nerve	▣	Stimuplex needle
▣	Neurofibroma	▣	Local anesthetic
▣	Popliteal artery		

FIGURE 1: Ultrasound image of popliteal fossa including the sciatic nerve with intraneural neurofibroma and popliteal artery.

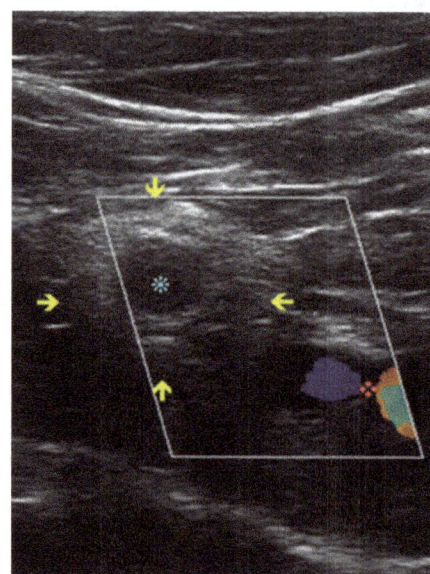

▣	Sciatic nerve	▣	Stimuplex needle
▣	Neurofibroma	▣	Local anesthetic
▣	Popliteal artery		

FIGURE 2: Ultrasound image with doppler flow analysis of popliteal fossa including the sciatic nerve with intraneural neurofibroma and popliteal artery. Doppler analysis correctly identifies blood flow in the popliteal artery and lack of flow in the intraneural inclusion of the sciatic nerve.

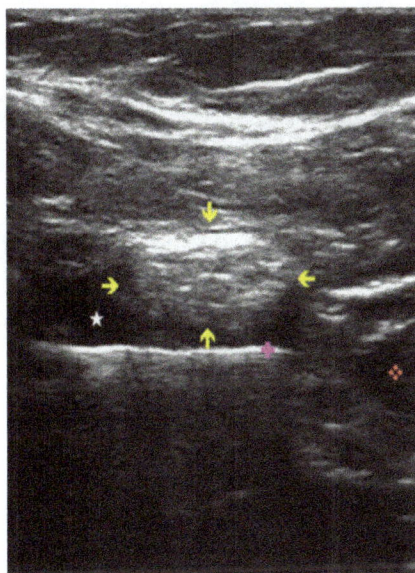

Sciatic nerve   Stimuplex needle

Neurofibroma   Local anesthetic

Popliteal artery

FIGURE 3: Ultrasound image of the popliteal fossa including the sciatic nerve with no intraneural inclusion, perineural infiltration of local anesthetic, Stimuplex needle, and popliteal artery.

weakness of 1/5 in the left lower extremity. The patient denied symptoms of nausea and was discharged home later that afternoon. On post-operative day one, the patient was contacted at home via telephone for followup. The patient stated baseline motor and sensory functions returned approximately eight hours after the operation. Her pain was adequately addressed at home with hydrocodone-acetaminophen (Vicodin, Abbot Laboratories, IL) orally every six hours as needed. Her pain at rest was 1-2/10, and with activity increased to 3-4/10. She had no hematoma or tenderness at the site of the regional blockade. The patient reported an overall favorable anesthetic and postoperative pain experience.

3. Discussion

NF poses many potential challenges to the performance of general, neuraxial, and regional anesthesia [8]. Anesthesiologists must tailor their anesthetic technique on a perpatient basis, balancing the risks and benefits of specific procedures in NF patients.

Neuraxial (epidural and spinal) anesthesia may be relatively contraindicated in many patients with NF. Clinically silent neurofibromas may involve spinal cord and nerve roots in up to 40% of patients [9]. Risks associated with neuraxial anesthesia range from hematoma, paralysis, or even death with acute spinal decompression [10]. Despite these dangers, the literature shows that preintervention anatomic mapping via CT and MRI can lead to safe and effective clinical interpretations and outcomes [7, 11].

Although neuraxial anesthesia has been studied extensively in NF patients, we found limited published reports of outcomes for regional anesthesia procedures [4]. There are however increasing sonographic descriptions of neurofibromas in the regional anesthesia literature. In addition, real-time US imagery allows accurate lesion localization and may possibly reduce the risks. In this paper we were able to demonstrate previously described ultrasonographic characteristics of neurofibromas. In particular, we demonstrate the "target sign" [5, 12] and replicate images consistent with published descriptions of solitary, ovoid, and hypoechoic intraneural lesions with well-defined margins and subtle distal acoustic enhancements [5–7]. The hypoechoic foci are believed to be caused by collagen deposits [13]. Beggs et al. also details subtle differences between neurilemomas (where the nerve travels peripherally to the lesion) and neurofibromas (where the nerve runs into the middle of the lesion). Building on these concepts, the use of US as both a diagnostic tool for NF and a therapeutic guide for interventional procedures is becoming increasingly evident.

Establishing the sonographic characteristics of neural sheath tumors enabled us to diagnose the NF lesions and differentiate them from other soft tissue structures such as lymph nodes [14] (Figure 2). US also allowed us to insert the needle in an area void of neural tumors. The doppler function highlighted vasculature structures, differentiating vascular from relevant nerve anatomy or tumor structures (Figure 1).

Despite well-described sonographic details of peripheral nerve sheath tumors, the efficacy and outcomes of regional blockade in patients with NF1 is limited [4]. Manickam et al. [14] describe the utility of a thorough sonographic survey. After defining an intraneural lesion with US in their patient, the team confirmed multiple similar lesions along the proximal course of the nerve. Their patient however chose to avoid regional anesthesia and had an uncomplicated general anesthetic. Rocco and Rosenblatt [4] reported performing successful regional blockade in a patient with an intraneural lesion in the popliteal fossa. The authors performed this block after a detailed sonographic survey to avoid direct contact with the tumor.

In our case, we used US to identify lesions and provide sonopathology of the NF tumors. We then performed a detailed sonographic survey to define lesion-free nerve that would minimize injury to the neurofibroma and reduce any associated risks. The block efficacy appeared to be unaffected by the NF tumors. The onset, duration, and resolution of regional anesthesia in our NF patient were as expected in a healthy patient.

In conclusion, we report successful popliteal nerve block using US guidance in a patient with NF. US guidance allows a unique opportunity to visualize and therefore avoid puncture of lesions in patients with NF and other types of neuralsheath tumors. Although this paper demonstrates that regional anesthesia can be offered to and successfully performed in patients with NF, more research is necessary to show efficacy and safety of peripheral nerve blockade in these patients. Potential issues that may be unique to NF patients include alterations in nerve conduction, spread of local anesthetic, and onset and duration of blockade. We recommend that any decision to use a regional anesthetic technique should be individualized. Further studies of the safety and efficacy of regional anesthesia in this patient population are necessary to establish consensus for routine practice of a regional anesthetic technique in this setting.

References

[1] R. P. Morse, "Neurofibromatosis type 1," *Archives of Neurology*, vol. 56, no. 3, pp. 364–365, 1999.

[2] N. P. Hirsch, A. Murphy, and J. J. Radcliffe, "Neurofibromatosis: clinical presentations and anaesthetic implications," *British Journal of Anaesthesia*, vol. 86, no. 4, pp. 555–564, 2001.

[3] V. N. Sehgal, S. Sharma, and R. Oberai, "Evaluation of plexiform neurofibroma in neurofibromatosis type 1 in 18 family members of 3 generations: ultrasonography and magnetic resonance imaging a diagnostic supplement," *International Journal of Dermatology*, vol. 48, no. 3, pp. 275–279, 2009.

[4] M. L. Rocco and M. A. Rosenblatt, "Ultrasound-guided peripheral nerve block in a patient with neurofibromatosis," *Regional Anesthesia and Pain Medicine*, vol. 36, no. 1, pp. 88–89, 2011.

[5] J. Lin, J. A. Jacobson, and C. W. Hayes, "Sonographic target sign in neurofibromas," *Journal of Ultrasound in Medicine*, vol. 18, no. 7, pp. 513–517, 1999.

[6] D. L. Reynolds, J. A. Jacobson, P. Inampudi, D. A. Jamadar, F. S. Ebrahim, and C. W. Hayes, "Sonographic characteristics of peripheral nerve sheath tumors," *American Journal of Roentgenology*, vol. 182, no. 3, pp. 741–744, 2004.

[7] J. Lin and W. Martel, "Cross-sectional imaging of peripheral nerve sheath tumors: characteristic signs on CT, MR imaging, and sonography," *American Journal of Roentgenology*, vol. 176, no. 1, pp. 75–82, 2001.

[8] M. Dounas, F. J. Mercier, C. Lhuissier, and D. Benhamou, "Epidural analgesia for labour in a parturient with neurofibromatosis," *Canadian Journal of Anaesthesia*, vol. 42, no. 5 I, pp. 420–424, 1995.

[9] S. D. Thakkar, U. Feigen, and V. F. Mautner, "Spinal tumours in neurofibromatosis type 1: an MRI study of frequency, multiplicity and variety," *Neuroradiology*, vol. 41, no. 9, pp. 625–629, 1999.

[10] M. D. Esler, J. Durbridge, and S. Kirby, "Epidural haematoma after dural puncture in a parturient with neurofibromatosis," *British Journal of Anaesthesia*, vol. 87, no. 6, pp. 932–934, 2001.

[11] D. S. Ginsburg, E. Hernandez, and J. W. C. Johnson, "Sarcoma complicating von Recklinghausen disease in pregnancy," *Obstetrics and Gynecology*, vol. 58, no. 3, pp. 385–387, 1981.

[12] M. Kara, A. Yilmaz, S. Özel, and L. Özçakar, "Sonographic imaging of the peripheral nerves in a patient with neurofibromatosis type 1," *Muscle and Nerve*, vol. 41, no. 6, pp. 887–888, 2010.

[13] I. Beggs, "Sonographic appearances of nerve tumors ," *Journal of Clinical Ultrasound* , vol. 27, no. 7, pp. 363–368, 1999.

[14] B. P. Manickam, A. Perlas, V. W. S. Chan, and R. Brull, "The role of a preprocedure systematic sonographic survey in ultrasound-guided regional anesthesia," *Regional Anesthesia and Pain Medicine*, vol. 33, no. 6, pp. 566–570, 2008.

34

Anesthetic Implications for Cesarean Section in a Parturient with Complex Congenital Cyanotic Heart Disease

Huili Lim, Chuen Jye Yeoh, Jerry Tan, Harikrishnan Kothandan ⓘ, and May U. S. Mok

Department of Anesthesia and Intensive Care, Singapore General Hospital, Singapore

Correspondence should be addressed to Harikrishnan Kothandan; harikrishnan.kothandan@singhealth.com.sg

Academic Editor: Latha Hebbar

The discordance between increased physiological demand during pregnancy and congenital cardiac pathology of a parturient is a perilous threat to the maternal-fetal well-being. Early involvement of a multidisciplinary team is essential in improving peripartum morbidity and mortality. Designing the most appropriate anesthetic care will require a concerted effort, with inputs from the obstetricians, obstetric and cardiac anesthesiologists, cardiologists, neonatologists, and cardiothoracic surgeons. We report the multidisciplinary peripartum care and anesthetic management for cesarean section (CS) of a 28-year-old primigravida who has partially corrected transposition of the great arteries, atrial and ventricular septal defect, dextrocardia, right ventricle hypoplasia, and tricuspid atresia.

1. Introduction

In Asia, congenital heart disease occurs in approximately 9.3 per 1000 live births [1]. Modern medicine has substantially improved the survival of patients with major congenital heart disease and extended their life expectancy beyond reproductive age. The complex nature of the cardiac anomaly coupled with the wide array of sophisticated temporizing or corrective procedures performed on these patients translates into a daunting task for the anesthesiologists. The physiological changes associated with pregnancy and delivery compound the problem further.

Written consent was obtained from the patient for publication with approval from local ethics committee. This manuscript adheres to the applicable EQUATOR guidelines.

2. Case Description

Our patient is a 28-year-old primigravida who presented with New York Heart Association (NYHA) class III symptoms at 17 weeks' gestation. She was diagnosed with complex congenital cyanotic heart disease at birth and her cardiac malformations included transposition of great arteries, large nonrestrictive ventricular septal defect (VSD) and atrial septal defect (ASD), dextrocardia with atrial and abdominal situs solitus, hypoplastic right ventricle, tricuspid atresia, and multiple aortopulmonary collaterals to the right lung. She had pulmonary artery banding at 6 weeks of age and bidirectional cavopulmonary connections (also known as Glenn's shunt) were performed at the age of 18 (see Figure 1.) Completion of Fontan's procedure was held off indefinitely because of an incidental finding of cerebral arteriovenous malformation (AVM). The AVM was deemed unsuitable for embolization due to its connection with a large venous pouch. She had been counselled against pregnancy by her cardiologist before conception. The patient's other comorbidities include mild scoliosis, prolapsed intervertebral disc between the fourth and fifth lumbar vertebrae, previous infective endocarditis complicated by a cerebrovascular accident (full neurological recovery from left-sided numbness), and compensatory polycythemia (hemoglobin concentration: 20–22 g/dL).

At 17 weeks' gestation, the patient was admitted by her cardiologist because of increasing cyanosis and dyspnea. Her oxygen saturation (SpO_2) on air decreased from 90% before pregnancy to 80% on admission. Obstetrical work-up revealed a healthy viable fetus. Serial transthoracic echocardiography showed an ejection fraction of 55% with bidirectional shunt across the VSD. Due to pulmonary artery

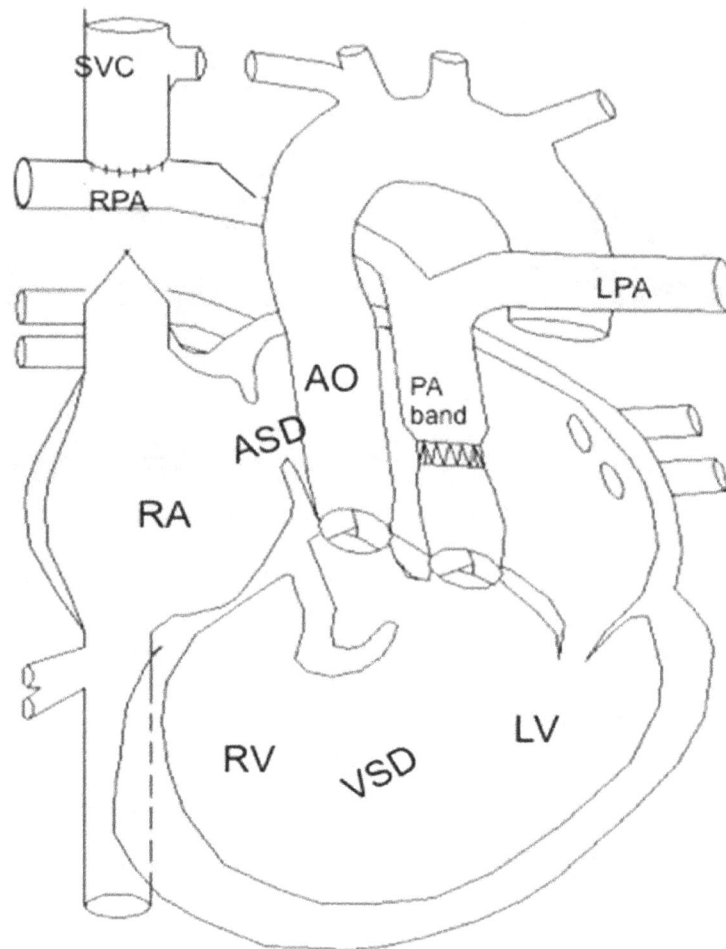

FIGURE 1: *Patient's abnormal cardiac anatomy (picture courtesy of cardiologist Dr. Tan Ju Le). (1) Transposition of great arteries*: the morphologic left ventricle is connected to the pulmonary artery (PA) and pulmonary circulation; the hypoplastic right ventricle is connected to the aorta and systemic circulation. *(2)* The *tight pulmonary artery band* limits blood flow from the left ventricle into the pulmonary circulation to prevent development of pulmonary hypertension and to direct oxygenated blood from left ventricle to right ventricle through the large nonrestrictive *ventricular septal defect (VSD)* and then from right ventricle to systemic circulation. *(3)* Systemic venous blood from the superior vena cava enters the pulmonary circulation for oxygenation via the *bidirectional cavopulmonary connection*. *(4)* Systemic venous blood from the inferior vena cava returns to the right atrium and enters left atrium via the large nonrestrictive *atrial septal defect (ASD)*, from left atrium to the morphologic left ventricle. Due to the congenital *tricuspid atresia*, there is no blood flow form right atrium to right ventricle. *(5)* Oxygenated blood from the lungs enters the pulmonary veins, flows to left atrium and left ventricle and then through the ventricular septal defect to right ventricle. Both the hypoplastic right ventricle and the left ventricle (via the ventricular septal defect) eject blood into the aorta. Bidirectional shunting occurs across the ventricular septal defect with mixing of oxygenated and deoxygenated blood.

banding, transpulmonary gradient was 41 mmHg. The obstetric anesthesiologist and obstetrician were alerted from the time of admission. The patient was again counselled extensively regarding the risks of further maternal decompensation and fetal anomaly. However, she remained keen to continue with the pregnancy. The patient stayed in the cardiology high dependency ward for bed rest, oxygen therapy, and monitoring by a cardiologist who was specialized in adult congenital heart disease from 17 weeks' gestation until the point of delivery.

A multidisciplinary team comprising cardiologists, obstetricians, obstetric and cardiothoracic anesthesiologists, cardiothoracic surgeons, and neonatologists was established from the time of admission. The discussions were led jointly by the obstetrician and the anesthesiologists. The team met regularly with the following agenda: (1) update on patient's condition, (2) update on fetal condition (after 24 weeks), (3) plans for an early elective delivery, and (4) formulation of an emergency plan in the event of acute maternal decompensation. The multidisciplinary team had consensus that maternal condition would deteriorate in the 3rd trimester, and cesarean section (CS) should happen before 28 weeks of gestation to avoid maternal decompensation. Nearing the end of 2nd trimester, the patient was demonstrating NYHA class IV symptoms and would desaturate during minimal efforts such as eating and speaking. Her highest SpO_2 value prior to delivery was 85% on a nonrebreathing mask with 15 L/min of oxygen. A decision was made for an elective

CS to be performed at 27 weeks of gestation in view of her worsening functional capacity. This was to allow the conduct of anesthesia and surgery under controlled conditions.

A general anesthetic technique was jointly agreed upon by the cardiac and obstetric anesthesiologists because of the potential for less hemodynamic instability. Members of the multidisciplinary team were present in the operating theatre on the day of surgery. The perfusionists were also on standby in preparation for the possible need for extracorporeal membrane oxygenation (ECMO).

Equipment necessary for both maternal and neonatal care and monitoring were available, including transesophageal echocardiography (TEE), nitric oxide for inhalation, and neonatal resuscitator (medical device). Intravenous cardiovascular drugs (nitroglycerine, norepinephrine, epinephrine, and milrinone) were prepared. Before the induction of anesthesia, the vascular access sites for emergency ECMO support were identified and marked. Standard monitors were attached, and the left radial artery and left internal jugular vein were cannulated for intra-arterial and central venous pressure lines. The left internal jugular vein was cannulated as the right internal jugular vein was noted to be small on ultrasound imaging. A pulmonary artery catheter was not considered in this patient as it would be technically difficult. This was because the superior vena cava was anastomosed to the right pulmonary artery. Typical pulmonary artery tracing would not be obtainable as the blood flow to the lung is passive in nature due to her altered anatomy.

The patient's airway was locally anesthetized with 5 mL of 1% nebulized lidocaine and cophenylcaine sprays to attenuate the sympathetic response to laryngoscopy and endotracheal intubation. Before induction of anesthesia, an antibiotic was prophylactically administered as per institutional protocol. The surgical site was cleansed with antiseptic solution, and surgical drapes were attached. Rapid sequence induction of anesthesia was performed with cricoid pressure. Induction drugs used include fentanyl 100 mcg, ketamine 25 mg, etomidate 10 mg, and rocuronium at 1 mg/kg (research papers have supported the use of 1 mg/kg for rapid sequence induction). The trachea was intubated with a 7.5 mm endotracheal tube.

Intraoperatively, the patient was hemodynamically stable with mean arterial pressure (MAP) remaining more than 70 mmHg throughout. The SpO_2 value remained within 10% of her baseline at 81–87%. Excessive airway pressure was avoided by setting a low tidal volume (350 mL) and a higher respiratory rate (15) for volume-controlled mechanical ventilation. Peak end expiratory pressure was set at zero. Peak airway pressure was consistently at or below 20 cm H_2O. The patient was closely monitored for hypercapnia and hypoxia. Hypothermia was prevented with the use of Bair hugger warming blanket and Hotline fluid warmer. Preload was optimized by trending the central venous pressure (CVP readings) and was guided by real-time TEE imaging. The CVP readings were, in fact, pulmonary artery pressure readings as the superior vena cava in this patient was anastomosed to the right pulmonary artery. The hemoglobin concentration was kept above 16 g/dL (patient's baseline was approximately 20–22 g/dL). Blood products were available on standby. Air bubbles in intravenous drip sets were carefully avoided in

view of the presence of VSD. Cardiac function was continuously monitored by TEE performed by the cardiologist in direct contact with the anesthesiologist.

Following the delivery of the baby, three intravenous boluses of oxytocin 1 U were administered, which achieved satisfactory uterine contraction. There were no noticeable changes in the vital signs during autotransfusion.

At the end of surgery and before tracheal extubation, bilateral transversus abdominis plane blocks were performed. The muscle relaxant was reversed with sugammadex 2 mg/kg. The hemodynamic stimulation during tracheal extubation was blunted by titrated boluses of esmolol.

After tracheal extubation, she was monitored in the intensive care unit for 1 day. She was subsequently transferred to a high dependency ward under the care of the cardiologist and had no episodes of acute desaturation during her stay. She was discharged home on postoperative day 10.

The baby was delivered weighing 870 g and was sent to neonatal intensive care unit. He was subsequently discharged well.

3. Discussion

In industrialized countries, maternal congenital heart disease is the most common cause of mortality in parturients with preexisting cardiovascular disease. Mortality risk of up to 30% is associated with poor NYHA class status, severe ventricular dysfunction, severe aortic stenosis, Marfan's syndrome with aortic valve lesion or aortic dilatation, or pulmonary hypertension [2].

A best evidence topic presented by Asfour et al. in 2013 deems vaginal delivery to be safer in patients who are NYHA classes I and II in labour, but an expedited instrument-assisted vaginal delivery in patients with poorer NYHA status is feasible with good analgesia. Right ventricular failure, pulmonary regurgitation, and pulmonary hypertension impart the greatest risk to both mother and baby [3]. Due to the poor maternal state of our patient antenatally and the prematurity of the fetus, the multidisciplinary team decided that CS under controlled conditions is the safest option.

After multidisciplinary discussions, we decided to perform the cesarean section under general anesthesia. We considered general anesthesia as the method of choice because of a possibly lower risk of hemodynamic instability compared to neuraxial anesthesia. Spinal and to a lesser extent epidural anesthesia will lead to profound sympathetic block. General anesthesia using carefully selected anesthetic agents known to produce less hemodynamic effects will offer more predictability and stability. In addition, general anesthesia will enable the use of TEE intraoperatively. The underlying lumbar scoliosis and disc prolapse might have complicated the administration of neuraxial anesthesia. Accidental or deliberate dural puncture occurring during attempted epidural or spinal anesthesia, respectively, might have caused rupture of the cerebral AVM secondary to a change in transmural pressure [4]. The patient was also too breathless to tolerate the supine position required for the surgery.

For patients with Glenn shunt in situ, the superior vena cava is anastomosed to the right pulmonary artery, such that blood bypasses the malformed chambers of the right heart and is shunted directly into the lungs for oxygenation. Anesthetic goals include (a) maintenance of adequate preload, (b) preservation of sinus rhythm and myocardial contractility, (c) maintenance of a low pulmonary and normal systemic vascular resistance, (d) avoidance of hypoxia, hypercarbia, acidosis, and hypothermia, which may increase right to left shunt, (e) avoidance of air bubbles in intravenous drip sets, (f) avoidance of excessive airway pressure by maintaining low tidal volume ventilation and avoiding the use of peak end expiratory pressure, and (g) maintenance of hemoglobin level above 16 g/dL. The stress response to intubation as well as surgery should be well blunted.

Central venous pressure (CVP) line was inserted in the left internal jugular vein. CVP in this patient denotes the pulmonary artery (PA) pressure as the superior vena cava is directly connected to the right PA. In addition, a central venous line is necessary for administration of inotropic drugs if required.

General anesthesia is not without its perils. A reduction in venous return due to vasodilation, myocardial depression due to anesthetic agents, and reduction in systemic vascular resistance will result in worsening of the right to left shunt in this patient [5]. Atelectasis following general anesthesia may also worsen the right to left shunt. Sympathetic discharge during laryngoscopy which is known to be more difficult in parturients [6] can lead to rupture of the AVM with devastating consequences.

Etomidate and ketamine were used as induction agents in view of their cardiovascular stability. Etomidate causes minimal changes in systemic and pulmonary vascular resistance and the cardiac output. Specifically, ketamine administration in patients with congenital heart disease has been shown to produce minimal changes in shunt direction or systemic oxygenation [7] and improve myocardial contractility [8]. Etomidate and ketamine are safe to use in obstetric anesthesia with minimal changes to uterine blood flow and no adverse neonatal outcomes [5].

After delivery of the baby, autotransfusion of blood from the uteroplacental bed back into the maternal circulation together with blood loss can increase or decrease preload causing unpredictable effects on right heart function and degree of right to left shunt. For this reason, glyceryl trinitrate, vasoconstrictors, and inotropes were made available intraoperatively to counteract these effects during surgery.

This complicated patient was under the care of the multidisciplinary team during her stay in the hospital. Without such conjoint effort, a desirable outcome would not have been possible in this complicated cardiac patient.

In conclusion, a multidisciplinary team involving obstetricians, adult congenital cardiologists, anesthesiologists, cardiothoracic surgeons, and neonatologists should be initiated at the earliest opportunity during pregnancy. Patients with partially or fully corrected congenital heart disease should also be managed in centres experienced in the care of these conditions. In the multidisciplinary team meetings, patient-specific concerns should be discussed. Detailed plans for delivery should be mapped out, and a contingency plan should be formulated in anticipation of maternal deterioration requiring emergency surgery.

The mode of anesthesia and delivery should be decided based on patient-specific factors, and the decision should be made in conjunction with the obstetrician, cardiologist, and neonatologist.

Authors' Contributions

Huili Lim, Chuen Jye Yeoh, and Jerry Tan contributed to literature review and drafting of the paper. Huili Lim, Chuen Jye Yeoh, Jerry Tan, May U. S. Mok, and Harikrishnan Kothandan contributed to revision of the paper. Huili Lim was responsible for submitting the paper.

Acknowledgments

The authors would like to thank Adjunct Assistant Professor Tan Ju Le (MBBS (UK), MRCP(UK), FAMS (Cardiology), FACC (USA), and FESC (France)) for allowing them to use her diagram of the patient's altered cardiac anatomy in this case report. Adjunct Assistant Professor Tan Ju Le is a senior consultant with the Department of Cardiology in National Heart Centre Singapore (NHCS); she is also the Director of the Adult Congenital Heart Disease Programme at NHCS.

References

[1] D. Van der Linde, E. E. M. Konings, M. A. Slager et al., "Birth prevalence of congenital heart disease worldwide: a systematic review and meta-analysis," *Journal of the American College of Cardiology*, vol. 58, no. 21, pp. 2241–2247, 2011.

[2] MBRRACE-UK, *Saving Lives, Improving Mothers' Care - Lessons Learned to Inform Future Maternity Care from the UK and Ireland Confidential Enquiries into Maternal Deaths and Morbidity 2009–1*, National Perinatal Epidemiology Unit, University of Oxford, Oxford, 2014.

[3] V. Asfour, M. O. Murphy, and R. Attia, "Is vaginal delivery or caesarean section the safer mode of delivery in patients with adult congenital heart disease?" *Interactive CardioVascular and Thoracic Surgery*, vol. 17, no. 1, pp. 144–150, 2013.

[4] C. A. Davie and P. O'Brien, "Stroke and pregnancy," *Journal of Neurology, Neurosurgery & Psychiatry*, vol. 79, no. 3, pp. 240–245, 2008.

[5] D. H. Chestnut, "Principles and practice of obstetric," in *Anesthesia*, pp. 703–733, Elsevier Mosby, Philadelphia, 3rd edition, 2004.

[6] B.-S. Kodali, S. Chandrasekhar, L. N. Bulich, G. P. Topulos, and S. Datta, "Airway changes during labor and delivery," *Anesthesiology*, vol. 108, no. 3, pp. 357–362, 2008.

[7] N. Dhawan, S. Chauhan, S. S. Kothari, U. Kiran, S. Das, and N. Makhija, "Hemodynamic responses to etomidate in pediatric patients with congenital cardiac shunt lesions," *Journal of Cardiothoracic and Vascular Anesthesia*, vol. 24, no. 5, pp. 802–807, 2010.

[8] J. Hanouz and E. Persehaye, "The inotropic and lusitropic effects of ketamine in isolated human atrial myocardium: the effect of adrenoceptor blockade," *Analgesia*, pp. 1689–1695, 2004.

35

Treatment of Digital Ischemia with Liposomal Bupivacaine

José Raul Soberón,[1] Scott F. Duncan,[2] and W. Charles Sternbergh[3]

[1] Department of Anesthesiology, Ochsner Clinic Foundation, 1514 Jefferson Highway, New Orleans, LA 70121, USA
[2] Department of Orthopedic Surgery, Ochsner Clinic Foundation, 1514 Jefferson Highway, New Orleans, LA 70121, USA
[3] Vascular and Endovascular Surgery, Ochsner Clinic Foundation, 1514 Jefferson Highway, New Orleans, LA 70121, USA

Correspondence should be addressed to José Raul Soberón; jsoberon@ochsner.org

Academic Editors: U. Deveci, A. Han, and J. Malek

Objective. This report describes a case in which the off-label use of liposomal bupivacaine (Exparel) in a peripheral nerve block resulted in marked improvement of a patient's vasoocclusive symptoms. The vasodilating and analgesic properties of liposomal bupivacaine in patients with ischemic symptoms are unknown, but our clinical experience suggests a role in the management of patients suffering from vasoocclusive disease. *Case Report.* A 45-year-old African American female was admitted to the hospital with severe digital ischemic pain. She was not a candidate for any vascular surgical or procedural interventions. Two continuous supraclavicular nerve blocks were placed with modest clinical improvement. These effects were also short-lived, with the benefits resolving after the discontinuation of the peripheral nerve blocks. She continued to report severe pain and was on multiple anticoagulant medications, so a decision was made to perform an axillary nerve block using liposomal bupivacaine (Exparel) given the compressibility of the site as well as the superficial nature of the target structures. *Conclusions.* This case report describes the successful off-label usage of liposomal bupivacaine (Exparel) in a patient with digital ischemia. Liposomal bupivacaine (Exparel) is currently FDA approved only for wound infiltration use at this time.

1. Introduction

Chemical sympathectomy from peripheral nerve blockade is well known and especially beneficial in vascular surgery [1]. Limited data are available regarding chemical sympathectomy in patients with digital ischemic pain and vasculopathy. Patients with these conditions, especially those with ischemic pain secondary to autoimmune disorders, benefit from chemical and surgical sympathectomy [2, 3]. The benefits of surgical sympathectomy often persist for years after the surgical procedure [3].

Exparel is a liposomal bupivacaine formulation that is currently FDA approved only for wound infiltration use. While this novel anesthetic is most commonly used during bunion and hemorrhoid surgery, it is also used in a number of other colorectal and orthopedic procedures and is gaining popularity in other surgical specialties [4, 5]. Its vasodilatory properties are unknown at this time.

2. Case Report

Written informed consent was obtained from the patient after a lengthy discussion of the known and potential risks and benefits of the block procedure, and all questions were answered. Witnessed verbal consent was obtained from the patient prior to the preparation of this case report. Additionally, the Ochsner Clinic Foundation Institutional Review Board was contacted and determined that IRB approval was not necessary for the submission of this case report.

A 45-year-old African American female presented with a two-week history of severe pain in the 4th and 5th digits of her right hand. Her past medical history was significant for poorly controlled type I diabetes, hypertension, peripheral vascular disease, and opiate dependence. Imaging studies of the extremity revealed diminished flow and occlusion of the distal ulnar artery. Her physical exam revealed cyanosis of the 4th and 5th digits with limited hand movement secondary to discomfort.

The vascular surgery team postulated that her ulnar artery was injured during attempts at intravascular catheter placement during a recent admission for diabetic ketoacidosis. After angiography, the vascular surgeons determined that she was not a candidate for direct revascularization with intra-arterial thrombolysis or operative intervention. The patient was not offered an amputation by the surgical team at this time because the ischemic regions of her hand had not fully demarcated and to allow the possibility of healing if nonsurgical interventions were successful. Additionally, she initially declined an amputation when the possibility of one was discussed during her hospitalization. A heparin infusion and oral aspirin were initiated for anticoagulation therapy. Anesthesiology was then contacted to place a nerve block to assist with pain control and provide a chemical sympathectomy. A supraclavicular nerve catheter was placed under Ultrasound guidance, and her pain and clinical symptoms modestly improved over the next two days. Her nerve catheter was removed and she was discharged home. Aspirin and clopidogrel were prescribed for outpatient use.

However, she was readmitted to the hospital two days later complaining of continued pain in her hand. Clinical examination showed that her condition had regressed to what it was during her initial presentation, with increased cyanosis when compared to prior to discharge. In addition to aspirin and clopidogrel, enoxaparin and coumadin were added to her anticoagulation regimen, and the anesthesia team was consulted to place a second nerve block.

A supraclavicular nerve catheter was placed but became dislodged less than 48 hours after its insertion. The patient was scheduled for a repeat block procedure with the expectation that she would be discharged home soon afterwards if her pain and symptoms improved. She was determined not to be a suitable candidate for an outpatient perineural catheter.

An ultrasound-guided Axillary block was performed using 1.3% liposomal bupivacaine (Exparel), with 3 mL injected incrementally around the musculocutaneous, radial, median, and ulnar nerves. A total of 12 mL of liposomal bupivacaine was used, corresponding to a total dose of 159.6 mg. A repeat supraclavicular catheter was not performed because of the patient's anticoagulated state and the possibility of hospital discharge if her symptoms improved. She was monitored in the block area 30 minutes after the procedure and placed on continuous telemetry monitoring for the remainder of her hospital stay.

She continued to report high pain scores in spite of appearing more comfortable following the procedure. The next day, the vascular surgeon noted an improvement in her physical examination, with normal color in the 5th digit and up to the dorsal aspect of the distal 1/3 and plantar to the proximal 1/3 of the 4th digit. She also had increased grip strength and hand movement.

These clinical improvements were markedly better than what she experienced with the previous supraclavicular blocks, and she was discharged home. She did not experience any signs or symptoms of local anesthetic toxicity at any point during her hospitalization, and she denied them on daily telephone followup for five days.

Photoplethysmography (PPG) flow studies provide a qualitative measure of digital arterial perfusion by measuring the digital artery pulsatility. Progressive reduction in digital arterial flow creates damping of the waveform. A "flatline" suggests very poor arterial flow. These PPG studies were performed during her hospital admissions, and the results are illustrated in Figure 1.

She demonstrated no pulsatility in the affected 4th and 5th digits prior to treatment, consistent with the clinical presentation. Although the patient's pain and clinical symptoms improved while receiving a perineural infusion of local anesthetics, these benefits did not persist after discontinuation of her peripheral nerve catheter, and no improvements in digital blood flow were seen in PPG studies. Moreover, increased flow in her 4th and 5th digits was observed on the PPG studies one week after the liposomal bupivacaine block.

Unfortunately, the patient's ischemic vasculopathy worsened over the subsequent six weeks, and her 4th finger became gangrenous. She was scheduled for a 4th digit amputation and surgical sympathectomy of the 4th and 5th digits as an outpatient. During her surgical procedure, however, it was found that her common digital arteries were clotted. A surgical sympathectomy was nonetheless performed even though the efficacy of doing this procedure in vessels that are already clotted is unknown. The patient underwent an amputation at the level of the proximal interphalangeal joint to remove the gangrenous digit. Her amputation site healed without complication, and she has had no other ischemic issues with the remaining digits. On followup, she reported better pain control and use of the hand compared to prior to surgery.

3. Discussion

Our decision to use an off-label medication was based on multiple factors, with patient safety being at the forefront. Our indication for a block in this scenario, unlike most of our routine cases, was not postoperative pain control, avoidance of a general anesthetic, or minimization of opioid-related side effects, but a last-effort attempt at preserving the patient's digits.

We believe that our clinical decisions, albeit controversial, were based on careful consideration of the benefits and risks, specifically improving blood flow in an attempt to salvage at least part of a limb against the possibility of nerve injury, local anesthetic toxicity, or other potential (currently unknown) risks associated with liposomal bupivacaine. Given her history of opioid dependence, her pain was difficult to control with oral and intravenous analgesics. At the time of the liposomal bupivacaine block, the patient was on multiple anticoagulant medications, each acting on a different facet of the coagulation process. An axillary block was deemed safer than a repeat supraclavicular block on an anticoagulated patient, because of ease of block performance and compressibility of the site should bleeding occur. Furthermore, the block was performed by a Fellowship trained regional anesthesiologist (J. R. Soberón) with extensive experience in Ultrasound-guided peripheral nerve blocks. A strict in-plane

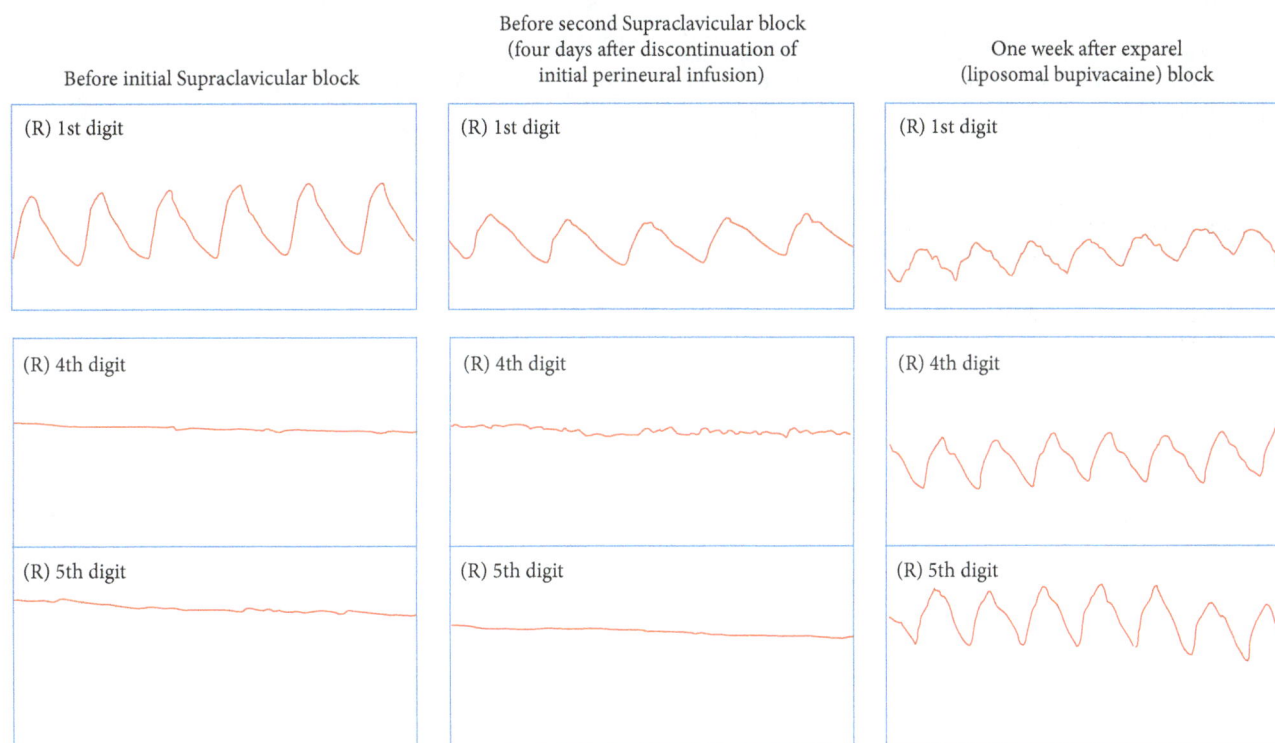

FIGURE 1: Results from photoplethysmography (PPG) studies obtained throughout the patient's hospitalizations. Of particular interest is the sustained blood flow seen in the 4th and 5th digits one week after her liposomal bupivacaine (Exparel) block. The 1st digit was nonischemic and included as a control.

technique was used to visualize the needle at all times to avoid vascular trespass or intraneural injection. Meticulous and frequent aspiration were negative for blood during the block procedure. Avoiding a block altogether would have likely led to worsening ischemia and the loss of the 5th digit, as well as a prolonged hospitalization for pain control purposes.

Exparel is a liposomal bupivacaine formulation that is currently FDA approved only for wound infiltration use, although FDA trials for perineural use approval are currently underway. Its vasodilatory properties are unknown at this time.

Patients with vaso-occlusive disorders benefit from peripheral nerve blocks because of their vasodilating and analgesic effects. In addition to chemical sympathectomy, surgical sympathectomy may be attempted to increase blood flow to the digits [2, 3]. The most common surgical approach involves identifying the common digital arteries and removing the adventitia from the vessels over a 1- to 2- centimeter segment. This removal of the adventitia disrupts the zone where the nerves lie, allowing for subsequent vasodilation and potentially increased blood flow.

It is unclear if improved control of the patient's medical issues, as well as increased adherence to therapy and medical recommendations, would have yielded a better outcome. Our patient was spared amputation of the 5th digit, which was also ischemic and cyanotic during her presentation. Our PPG results and clinical experience suggest that liposomal bupivacaine may increase blood flow and assist with pain control in patients with digital ischemia. Further research needs to be performed to determine the safety and potential role of liposomal bupivacaine in peripheral nerve block use, particularly with regards to analgesic and vasodilating effects in patients with ischemic symptoms.

Acknowledgments

The authors would like to thank Armin Schubert, M.D., and Bobby Nossaman, M.D., of the Ochsner Clinic Foundation Department of Anesthesiology as well as Kathleen McFadden, M.A., from Ochsner Clinic Foundation Publishing Services for proofreading and editing this paper. The authors are also grateful to Barbara Siede, M.S., from Ochsner Clinic Foundation Medical Illustration Services for her assistance in the labeling of their image.

References

[1] E. B. Malinzak and T. J. Gan, "Regional anesthesia for vascular access surgery," *Anesthesia and Analgesia*, vol. 109, no. 3, pp. 976–980, 2009.

[2] R. A. Greengrass, N. G. Feinglass, P. M. Murray, and S. D. Trigg, "Continuous regional anesthesia before surgical peripheral sympathectomy in a patient with severe digital necrosis associated with Raynaud's phenomenon and scleroderma," *Regional Anesthesia and Pain Medicine*, vol. 28, no. 4, pp. 354–358, 2003.

[3] K. Murata, S. Omokawa, Y. Kobata, Y. Tanaka, H. Yajima, and S. Tamai, "Long-term follow-up of periarterial sympathectomy for chronic digital ischaemia," *J Hand Surg Eur*, vol. 37, no. 8, pp. 788–793, 2012.

[4] K. Candiotti, "Liposomal bupivacaine: an innovative nonopioid local analgesic for the management of postsurgical pain," *Pharmacotherapy*, vol. 32, supplement 9, pp. 19S–26S, 2012.

[5] Pacira Pharmaceuticals Inc, *EXPAREL (Bupivacaine Liposome Injectable Suspension) Prescribing Information*, Pacira Pharmaceuticals Inc, Parsippany, NJ, USA, 2011.

36

Thoracic Anesthesia and Cross Field Ventilation for Tracheobronchial Injuries: A Challenge for Anesthesiologists

Sankalp Sehgal,[1] Joshua C. Chance,[1] and Matthew A. Steliga[2]

[1] Department of Anesthesiology and Pain Medicine, University of Arkansas for Medical Sciences, Little Rock, AR 72205, USA
[2] Department of Cardiothoracic Surgery, University of Arkansas for Medical Sciences, Little Rock, AR 72205, USA

Correspondence should be addressed to Sankalp Sehgal; sehgal_sankalp@yahoo.com

Academic Editors: J. Malek and D. A. Story

Tracheobronchial injuries are rare but life threatening sequel of blunt chest trauma. Due to the difficult nature of these injuries and the demanding attributes of the involved surgery, the anesthesiologist faces tough challenges while securing the airway, controlling oxygenation, undertaking one-lung ventilation, maintaining anesthesia during tracheal reconstruction, and gaining adequate postoperative pain control. Amongst the few techniques that can be used with tracheobronchial injuries, cross field ventilation is a remotely described and rarely used technique, especially in injuries around the carina. We effectively applied cross field ventilation in both our cases and the outcome was excellent.

1. Introduction

Tracheobronchial injuries (TBI) are life threatening complications encountered in blunt chest and neck trauma. Tracheal injuries should be suspected in all patients involved in high speed motor vehicle accidents. The first successful repair of a bronchial rupture caused by blunt chest trauma was reported in 1947 by Kinsella and Johnsrud [1]. They are found in 0.8% of blunt thoracic trauma victims presenting for emergency surgery [2]. Tragically, 30% to 80% of these patients die before reaching the hospital [3].

Surgical repair remains the treatment of choice for such injuries. Due to the difficult nature of these surgeries, the anesthesiologist faces tough challenges securing the airway, controlling oxygenation and ventilation, undertaking one-lung ventilation, maintaining anesthesia during tracheal reconstruction with loss of ventilation to the atmosphere, and gaining adequate postoperative pain control. For appropriate management of these injuries in the operating room, modified anesthetic techniques and effective communication with the thoracic surgeon are important. Key considerations are avoidance of excessive preoperative sedation, maintaining spontaneous ventilation during intubation, using bronchoscopy to visualize and secure the airway, avoiding blind instrumentation [4, 5], single-lumen tube endobronchial

intubation, cross field ventilation, and adequate postoperative pain control. Using these techniques, the outcome of our cases was excellent.

In the current case scenario, we shall discuss anesthetic management of two patients who presented to our level-1 trauma center, between years 2010 and 2012, with tracheobronchial injuries following severe blunt chest trauma in motor vehicle accidents.

2. Case Report Number 1

A 20-year-old male presented following a motor vehicle accident. His physical findings included a right-sided tension pneumothorax which was treated with a chest tube, subcutaneous emphysema, and left clavicle fracture. CT of the thoracic spine revealed a longitudinal defect in the posterior membranous wall of his trachea extending into the carina (Figure 1). With an impending respiratory failure and the possibility of mediastinitis and subsequent sepsis with nonoperative management, it was decided to operate upon the tracheal tear. His past medical history included reflux disease, smoking, and alcohol consumption but no major cardiopulmonary problems. His vital signs were stable so far. The airway was anesthetized in preparation for an awake oral fiberoptic bronchoscopy and a radial arterial line was placed

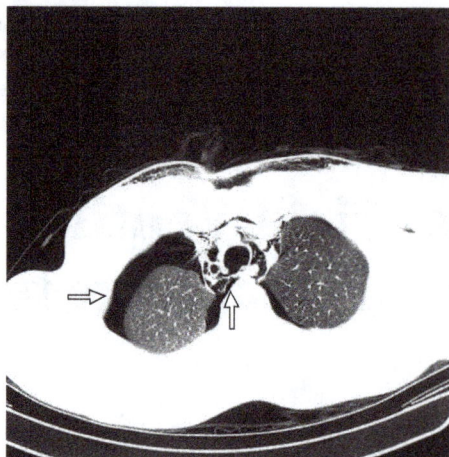

FIGURE 1: CT chest image depicting tear in the posterior part of the trachea with a right-sided pneumothorax.

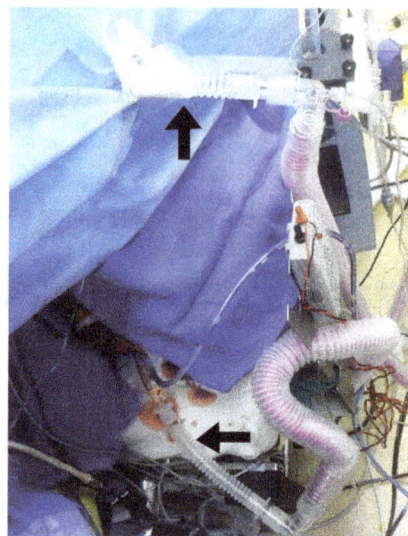

FIGURE 2: An oral endotracheal tube and a second cross field ventilation circuit that is passing through the drapes.

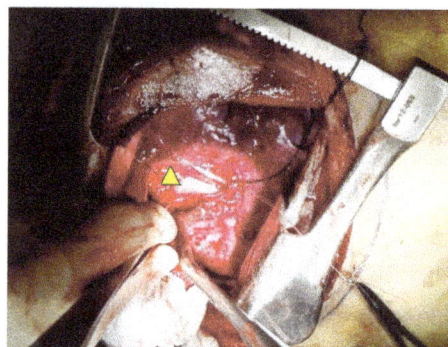

FIGURE 3: Cross field selective one-lung ventilation with a single-lumen endobronchial tube via the thoracotomy.

preoperatively. He was then transferred to the operating room and midazolam was titrated for sedation and anxiolysis. With the patient still awake, flexible bronchoscopy was performed to evaluate the posterior pharynx and arytenoids and to remove blood and debris from the airway. The bronchoscope was advanced into the left main-stem bronchus and a reinforced 7.5 size endotracheal tube was placed. The intubation was followed by induction using propofol, fentanyl, and cisatracurium and he was then placed on the ventilator thus ensuing one-lung ventilation via selective bronchial intubation. Due to the short length of the reinforced tube, it was replaced with a regular 7.5 size tube using a tube exchanger. He was then maintained under general anesthesia using sevoflurane with end-expiratory concentration of approximately 2%. Ventilator parameters included a tidal volume of 500 mL (approximately 7 mL/kg), a 12–14 cycles/min respiratory rate, and inspired oxygen fraction 0.55–0.7% and his oxygen saturation was maintained between 96 and 99%.

During the surgery, while briefly holding respirations, the endotracheal tube was withdrawn and a bronchoscope was used to visualize and assess the extent of the tear. A 9 to 10 cm long longitudinal tear was seen on the posterior membranous portion of the trachea. The tube was replaced into left main bronchus and selective left lung ventilation was undertaken. The patient was positioned in left lateral decubitus position. A right thoracotomy was done and the tracheal tear was noticed to extend from the right main-stem bronchus up to the apex of the chest. The cuff of the endotracheal tube was noted to be in the area requiring repair and hence cross field ventilation was planned. A size 6.0 sterile endotracheal tube was brought into the surgical field through the drapes, which was placed by the surgeon into the left main-stem bronchus via the thoracotomy. At the same time the oral endotracheal tube was withdrawn (Figure 2). Again selective left lung ventilation was undertaken. The endobronchial intubation via thoracotomy and cross field ventilation greatly facilitated the tracheal repair around the carina (Figure 3). A bronchoscopy using the fiberoptic scope was then performed through the oral tube and the tracheal repair was noted. Once

the carina was almost completely repaired and sutures around it were ready to be tied, the cross field tube was withdrawn and the oral endotracheal tube was reinserted into the left main-stem bronchus over the fiberoptic bronchoscope. Now the remaining part of the trachea was repaired and the repair was reinforced with an intercostal muscle flap. This was followed by closure of the chest. Two right-sided chest tubes were then placed by the surgeon. Hemodynamics and electrocardiogram remained stable. The patient's paralysis was fully reversed and he was extubated in the operating room and transferred to the intensive care unit.

He had an uneventful postoperative course and was discharged on tenth postoperative day.

3. Case Report Number 2

A 26-year-old male presented following a rollover motor vehicle accident. He was an unrestrained driver and was hemodynamically stable. He did not have any open injuries. He had a past medical history of asthma, drug and alcohol use, and smoking. Upon physical examination he had left-sided chest tenderness, bilateral breath sounds which were slightly decreased on the left side, subcutaneous emphysema in the neck, and normal heart sounds. He had a C-collar in place and hence poor mouth opening and difficult airway examination. Chest X-ray revealed bilateral pneumothoraces and left 1st and 3rd rib fractures. A CT of the thoracic spine confirmed bilateral pneumothoraces and showed left pulmonary contusion and extensive air tracking along soft tissue planes of the neck with a defect of posterior trachea at approximately T9 level; the latter finding was suspicious for tracheal injury. For the blunt tracheal rupture and bilateral pneumothoraces, a bronchoscopy, right thoracotomy, and tracheal repair with intercostal muscle flap was planned.

The patient was taken to the operating room. Due to the presence of a hemopneumothorax on the left, it was decided to operate on the right side. After induction with fentanyl, propofol, and succinylcholine, a fiberoptic bronchoscopy was performed to evaluate the airway and a several centimeters long longitudinal split was noted along the entire posterior wall of the trachea that extended to the carina. There was also a significant amount of blood in the airway which was suctioned and evacuated. A size 6.0 endotracheal tube was placed via the bronchoscope accomplishing a selective left main-stem intubation. A left-sided chest tube was placed by the surgeon for the hemopneumothorax. A radial arterial line was placed in addition to 2 large bore peripheral intravenous catheters. The patient was placed in left lateral decubitus position. General anesthesia was maintained using sevoflurane with an end tidal concentration of 2–2.5%. Blood pressure was maintained between systolic pressure of 90 and 120 mmHg. Selective left lung ventilation was undertaken. Ventilator parameters included pressure control ventilation with tidal volume 400–500 mL, a respiratory rate between 12 and 16 cycles/min, peak end-expiratory pressure of 5 cm H_2O, and inspired O_2 100% which maintained an oxygen saturation of 94–99%. A nasogastric tube was passed and esophageal injury was ruled out after no leak was detected upon injecting methylene blue through the nasogastric tube.

The tracheal tear was repaired along its length, except at the carina where the endotracheal tube cuff was present. To accomplish this repair, the oral endotracheal tube was withdrawn and the left main-stem bronchus was intubated via the open-chest thoracotomy site with a size 6.0 sterile endotracheal tube; a sterile anesthesia circuit was used to provide cross field ventilation. The carina was then repaired. After all the sutures were in place (Figure 4) and the trachea was repaired along its full length, the cross field tube was removed and the oral endotracheal tube was advanced from the oral cavity and secured in place to ventilate both the lungs. A positive pressure breath was held to help detect any air leaks in the sutured trachea. Repeat fiberoptic bronchoscopy was performed and the airway was cleared of blood, mucus, and secretions, indicating that the back wall of the trachea appeared intact.

After the surgeons finished closing the thoracotomy, with the patient in left lateral decubitus position, a thoracic epidural was placed and dosed with 100 mcg fentanyl for postoperative pain control. Paralysis reversal was achieved using

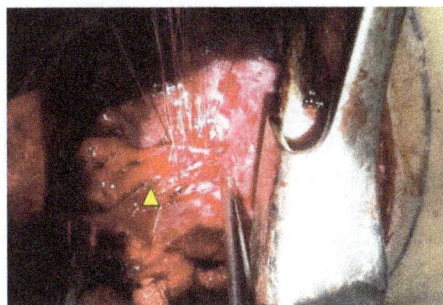

FIGURE 4: Tracheal repair with sutures along its length while the cross field endobronchial tube is in place.

glycopyrrolate and neostigmine. The patient was then extubated while deeply anesthetized to prevent coughing. Once in recovery with the patient awake and no evident neurological deficit, an epidural test dose was given to rule out intravascular or intrathecal placement. The epidural was then bolused with 0.25% bupivacaine to achieve an appropriate level of anesthesia and patient controlled epidural analgesia (PCEA) was initiated. Postoperative recovery was uneventful. The patient was discharged home on fourth postoperative day.

4. Discussion

4.1. Etiology of Tracheal Injuries. Injury to the trachea can be extra- or intrathoracic with complete or partial disruption. Etiology of tracheal injuries includes iatrogenic causes (e.g., traumatic endotracheal intubation, the use of tube exchange catheters, percutaneous dilatational tracheostomy, and cricothyroidotomy), blunt trauma which frequently involves injuries of the trachea within 2 cm of the carina, penetrating trauma, usually to the cervical trachea, and mucosal tears, which are usually self-limiting.

4.2. Mechanism of Tracheal Injury in Blunt Chest Trauma. Blunt trauma usually involves the membranous portion of the intrathoracic trachea. In motor vehicle accidents, it may occur due to impact of the steering wheel or dashboard on the chest [6]. Three patters of injuries have been described [7]. In the first, rapid compression of the anteroposterior diameter of the thorax with a simultaneous widening of the transverse diameter of the chest produces lateral motion, causing traction on the trachea at the carina. Secondly, rapid deceleration causes shearing forces at cricoid cartilage and carina along the trachea, leading to their disruption. And thirdly a sudden increase in the airway pressure with a closed glottis at the time of rapid deceleration shears the bronchus from its points of fixation near the cricoids and carina. In blunt chest trauma, tracheobronchial injuries occur within 2.5 cm of the carina in 40–80% of the times [8–10] and the most common injury associated with penetrating tracheal injuries is esophageal perforation [11, 12].

4.3. Clinical Presentation of Tracheobronchial Injuries. If the patient is hemodynamically unstable, it is important to stabilize the airway prior to diagnosis [6]. Such injuries may also present in a subtle way. The most common presentations are dyspnea and subcutaneous emphysema [13, 14]. Other symptoms may include hoarseness, signs of external trauma, stridor, pneumothorax, pneumomediastinum or pneumopericardium, oxygen desaturation, cyanosis, and hemoptysis [15]. Extra-anatomic air is present in approximately 90% at the time of chest radiography [6]. Suspicion should be high when pneumomediastinum and pneumothorax are refractory to adequate pleural drainage [16]. In a stable patient with a chest radiograph suggestive of TBI, prompt bronchoscopy should be performed in the anticipation of surgical exploration and to confirm the location and extent of injury [13]. Computed tomographic scans may also provide additional information regarding the severity of the injury [17], such as in the cases described here.

4.4. Airway and Ventilation.

4.4. Airway and Ventilation. These patients require careful airway management. A partially disrupted trachea may become completely disrupted by the passage of an endotracheal tube. There are several possible ways of airway management in these cases: (1) induction using short acting neuromuscular blocker followed by direct laryngoscopy and intubation with a double-lumen tube, (2) using short acting neuromuscular blocker followed by fiberoptic endobronchial intubation using a single-lumen tube, (3) awake fiberoptic endobronchial intubation using a single-lumen tube, (4) using a jet ventilator, and (5) cardiopulmonary bypass (CPB).

The mainstay of intraoperative management, as described in our cases, remained a single-lumen endotracheal tube [18]. An endobronchial tube may be chosen instead of a standard double-lumen tube because the double-lumen tube is usually too bulky to permit tracheal surgery [19]. Cricoid pressure can dislocate a fractured cricoid or thyroid cartilage and should thus be avoided [19]. The safest course is to maintain spontaneous ventilation, either with deep inhalation agents or topical anesthesia followed by fiberoptic intubation [19]. Tracheostomy cannot be performed in these cases due to injury in the distal airway.

After securing the airway, ventilation can be challenging due to one-lung ventilation and loss of ventilation to the atmosphere from the tracheal defect. Cross field ventilation may be set up (as described in the next section).

Other methods of ventilation such as with low-frequency or high-frequency jet ventilation and CPB have been reported earlier [20–22].

4.5. Cross Field Ventilation. For ventilation during tracheal reconstruction around the carina, cross field ventilation may be required, especially if the defect involves the carina. This technique has also been described in the surgical literature as being used in complex tracheal surgeries in which a part of the trachea has to be resected due to tumor or malignancy. It involves retracting the oral endobronchial tube and intubating the bronchus across the operative field (Figure 5). A sterile anesthesia circuit attached to an endotracheal tube at its end is passed through/around the drapes across the surgical field to be placed and secured into the main bronchus for ventilating the dependent lung. Usually a small sized tube like size 6.0 or 6.5 is used. Withdrawing the existing oral endotracheal tube proximally allows the cross field tube to

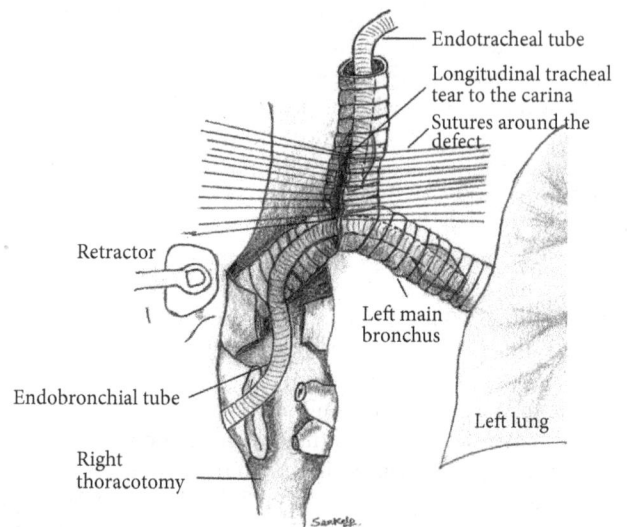

FIGURE 5: A sketch depicting a tracheal defect involving carina, the two main-stem bronchi, a retracted oral endotracheal tube, and an endobronchial tube placed via the open-chest thoracotomy to ventilate the left lung.

ventilate. This setup allows ventilation while facilitating the process for the surgeon to repair the defect around the carina. Once the anastamotic sutures are in place to repair the tracheal defect at the carina, the oral tube is advanced back into the bronchus while withdrawing the cross field endotracheal tube and the repair is then completed by tying the sutures.

4.6. Monitoring during Anesthesia for Tracheal Injuries. Monitoring required for tracheal surgeries, besides standard ASA monitors, includes invasive blood pressure and arterial blood gases monitoring. Oxygenation is confirmed by pulse oximetry and blood gases. An arterial catheter is also helpful in the postoperative period. It is possible to surgically compress the innominate artery that crosses the trachea at the sternal notch which may impair blood flow to the right arm and right carotid vessels. Either an arterial line or pulse oximeter on the right arm provides warning as to its occurrence [19]. A central venous catheter may be indicated for administering fluids or blood products rapidly or vasopressors and inotropes.

There are several reasons to prefer extubation after repair of such injuries. Leaving the endotracheal tube in place will irritate the tracheal anastamosis, especially if the end of the tube or cuff is at the suture line of the repaired defect. In addition, continuing positive pressure ventilation will place additional strain on the suture line that will tend to push air into the tissues [19]. Extubating the patient while deeply anesthetized may prevent disruption of the fresh repair from coughing. Constant communication between the anesthesiologist and the thoracic surgeon is imperative.

4.7. Postoperative Pain Control. For pain control in such injuries, while systemic narcotics remain the most prevalent modality, compared to epidural such patients retain more CO_2, have lower PaO_2, do not improve maximum inspiratory pressure or tidal volume, and have more respiratory and cough suppression and increased sedation. Intrapleural anesthesia, either via indwelling thoracostomy tube or placement of dedicated intrapleural catheter, provides unilateral pain control and risks pneumothorax, and compared to epidural analgesia it provides less pain relief and more narcotic use. Intercostal nerve blocks, although effective, carry high risk of pneumothorax and local anesthetic toxicity. Paravertebral blocks are unilateral, are simple to perform, improve pain, blood gases with less hypotension and urinary retention than epidural analgesia. Epidural carries procedure related complications but improves lung function and may decrease risk of pneumonia and shorten the duration of ICU stay. Postoperative pain control is improved and there is a likely decreased length of hospital stay with epidural [23] as seen in our second case.

References

[1] T. J. Kinsella and L. W. Johnsrud, "Traumatic rupture of the bronchus," *The Journal of Thoracic Surgery*, vol. 16, pp. 571–583, 1947.

[2] J. H. Devitt, R. F. McLean, and J.-P. Koch, "Anaesthetic management of acute blunt thoracic trauma," *Canadian Journal of Anaesthesia*, vol. 38, no. 4, pp. 506–510, 1991.

[3] J. F. Burke, "Early diagnosis of traumatic rupture of the bronchus," *The Journal of the American Medical Association*, vol. 181, pp. 682–686, 1962.

[4] M. M. Kirsh, M. B. Orringer, D. M. Behrendt, and H. Sloan, "Management of tracheobronchial disruption secondary to nonpenetrating trauma," *Annals of Thoracic Surgery*, vol. 22, no. 1, pp. 93–101, 1976.

[5] F. J. Baumgartner, B. Ayres, and C. Theuer, "Danger of false intubation after traumatic tracheal transection," *Annals of Thoracic Surgery*, vol. 63, no. 1, pp. 227–228, 1997.

[6] W. C. Wilson, *Trauma: Emergency Resuscitation, Perioperative Anesthesia, Surgical Management*, vol. 1, Google eBooks: Informa Healthcare, 2007.

[7] J. M. Unger, G. G. Schuchmann, J. E. Grossman, and J. R. Pellett, "Tears of the trachea and main bronchi caused by blunt trauma: radiologic findings," *American Journal of Roentgenology*, vol. 153, no. 6, pp. 1175–1180, 1989.

[8] A. C. Kiser, S. M. O'Brien, and F. C. Detterbeck, "Blunt tracheobronchial injuries: treatment and outcomes," *Annals of Thoracic Surgery*, vol. 71, no. 6, pp. 2059–2065, 2001.

[9] M. M. Rossbach, S. B. Johnson, M. A. Gomez, E. Y. Sako, O. LaWayne Miller, and J. H. Calhoon, "Management of major tracheobronchial injuries: a 28-year experience," *Annals of Thoracic Surgery*, vol. 65, no. 1, pp. 182–186, 1998.

[10] R. B. Lynn and K. Iyengar, "Traumatic rupture of the bronchus," *Chest*, vol. 61, no. 1, pp. 81–83, 1972.

[11] P. N. Symbas, C. R. Hatcher Jr., and G. A. W. Boehm, "Acute penetrating tracheal trauma," *Annals of Thoracic Surgery*, vol. 22, no. 5, pp. 473–477, 1976.

[12] R. R. Ecker, R. V. Libertini, W. J. Rea, W. L. Sugg, and W. R. Webb, "Injuries of the trachea and bronchi," *Annals of Thoracic Surgery*, vol. 11, no. 4, pp. 289–298, 1971.

[13] D. C. Cassada, M. P. Munyikwa, M. P. Moniz, R. A. Dieter Jr., G. F. Schuchmann, and B. L. Enderson, "Acute injuries of the trachea and major bronchi: importance of early diagnosis," *Annals of Thoracic Surgery*, vol. 69, no. 5, pp. 1563–1567, 2000.

[14] J. H. Devitt and B. R. Boulanger, "Lower airway injuries and anaesthesia," *Canadian Journal of Anaesthesia*, vol. 43, no. 2, pp. 148–159, 1996.

[15] S. Sengupta, A. Saikia, S. Ramasubban et al., "Anaesthetic management of a patient with complete tracheal rupture following blunt chest trauma," *Annals of Cardiac Anaesthesia*, vol. 11, no. 2, pp. 123–126, 2008.

[16] W. J. Grant, R. L. Meyers, R. L. Jaffe, and D. G. Johnson, "Tracheobronchial injuries after blunt chest trauma in children with hidden pathology," *Journal of Pediatric Surgery*, vol. 33, no. 11, pp. 1707–1711, 1998.

[17] H. Porte, M. Langlois, C. H. Maquette, J. Dupont, J. M. Anselin, and A. Wurtz, "Successful esophageal tracheobronchoplasty for combined tracheal and bronchial traumatic rupture," *Journal of Thoracic and Cardiovascular Surgery*, vol. 115, no. 5, pp. 1216–1218, 1998.

[18] R. Karmy-Jones and D. E. Wood, "Traumatic injury to the trachea and bronchus," *Thoracic Surgery Clinics*, vol. 17, no. 1, pp. 35–46, 2007.

[19] H. C. Grillo, *Anesthesia for Tracheal Injuries. Surgery of the Trachea and Bronchi*, B.C. Decker, 1st edition, 2001.

[20] R. C. DeWitt and C. H. Hallman, "Use of cardiopulmonary bypass for tracheal resection: a case report," *Texas Heart Institute Journal*, vol. 31, no. 2, pp. 188–190, 2004.

[21] T. Misao, T. Yoshikawa, M. Aoe et al., "Bronchial and cardiac ruptures due to blunt trauma," *General Thoracic and Cardiovascular Surgery*, vol. 59, no. 3, pp. 216–219, 2011.

[22] P. N. Symbas, A. G. Justicz, and R. R. Ricketts, "Rupture of the airways from blunt trauma: treatment of complex injuries," *Annals of Thoracic Surgery*, vol. 54, no. 1, pp. 177–183, 1992.

[23] R. C. Mackersie, S. R. Shackford, D. B. Hoyt, and T. G. Karagianes, "Continuous epidural fentanyl analgesia: ventilatory function improvement with routine use in treatment of blunt chest injury," *Journal of Trauma*, vol. 27, no. 11, pp. 1207–1212, 1987.

37

Spinal Anaesthesia for Cesarean Section in a Patient with Vascular Type Ehlers-Danlos Syndrome

Jeffrey M. Carness ⓘ[1] **and Mark J. Lenart**[2]

[1]*Department of Anesthesiology, United States Naval Hospital Yokosuka, Yokosuka, Japan*
[2]*Department of Anesthesiology, Naval Medical Center Portsmouth, Portsmouth, VA, USA*

Correspondence should be addressed to Jeffrey M. Carness; jeffrey.m.carness.mil@mail.mil

Academic Editor: Alparslan Apan

We report the administration of spinal anaesthesia for cesarean delivery in a parturient with vascular Ehlers-Danlos syndrome. Parturients who genetically inherit this disorder are at risk for significant morbidity and mortality. Risks during pregnancy include premature labor, uterine prolapse, and uterine rupture. Additionally, such laboring parturients are at increased risk of hemodynamic volatility, vascular stress, and severe postpartum hemorrhage. Instrumented delivery and cesarean delivery bring additional risks. Nonpregnancy-related complications include excessive bleeding, intestinal rupture, cardiac valvular dysfunction, and arterial dissection. Despite the complexity of this condition, literature focusing on specific intraoperative anaesthetic management is sparse.

1. Introduction

Ehlers-Danlos syndromes (EDS) comprise connective tissue disorders affecting multiple organ systems to include the integumentary, musculoskeletal, pulmonary, digestive, and cardiovascular systems. These disorders are classified according to the Villefranche Nosology which was originally adopted in 1997 [1]. To date, six underlying types of disease have been identified and are categorised as follows: classical (formerly type I/II), hypermobility (formerly type III), vascular (formerly type IV), kyphoscoliosis (formerly type VI), arthrochalasia (formerly type VIIA/VIIB), and dermatosparaxis (formerly type VIIC) [1]. Each type possesses unique clinical manifestations and anaesthetic implications. Peripartum complications associated with vascular EDS include preterm premature rupture of membranes, arterial dissection/rupture (e.g., aorta, iliac, splenic, and coronary), uterine rupture, uterine incision dehiscence, 3rd-/4th-degree lacerations, and postpartum hemorrhage [2]. Peripartum mortality rates are highly variable and range from 4.3% to 25% [2]. Case reports in the literature specifically focusing on the intraoperative anaesthetic management of these patients are sparse [3, 4]. Here, we report the perioperative anaesthetic management of a parturient with vascular EDS. The patient provided written permission for publication of the report.

2. Case Description

The patient was a 23-year-old female (Gravida 1, Para 0) presenting for obstetric care at eight weeks gestational age with genetic documentation of a *COL3A1* mutation confirming vascular type EDS. She reported emergency room visits for significant hematomas in addition to current treatment with losartan for a history of cerebral aneurysm. First trimester brain MRI revealed full resolution of the aneurysm. Her second trimester transthoracic echocardiogram was unremarkable. A complete blood count, comprehensive electrolyte panel, and electrocardiogram were also unremarkable. Hemoglobin and hematocrit concentrations were 9.2 g·dl^{-1} and 28.9%. Prothrombin time, partial thromboplastin time, and platelet function analysis were within normal limits. We planned for surgical delivery at 34 + 0 weeks of gestational age. This gestational age represented a balance of fetal risk due to premature delivery and maternal risk due to increasing fetal size and an active second stage of labor. We elected for an ultrasound-guided arterial catheter, central venous catheter, and spinal anaesthetic.

A multidisciplinary team including physicians from the blood bank, cardiologists, cardiothoracic and vascular surgeons, neonatologists, and obstetric anaesthesiologists was assembled. On the day of surgery, the patient presented to the labor and delivery ward with normal vital signs and a reassuring airway. Two 18-gauge peripheral IV catheters were placed. The surgical procedure was performed in the cardiothoracic/vascular operating suite, where infusions of 1 g tranexamic acid and 0.3 μg·kg^{-1} deamino-D-arginine vasopressin (DDAVP) were initiated upon patient arrival. While in the supine position, a 20-gauge catheter was introduced into the right radial artery under ultrasound guidance. The patient was then placed in a sitting position for placement of the spinal anaesthetic where 2+ pitting edema was noted. A curvilinear low-frequency ultrasound probe was obtained and the lumbar anatomy visualised. After sterile preparation and draping, a 25-gauge 3.5″ Pencan® Spinal Needle was advanced at the L3/L4 interspace. Following subarachnoid puncture, 13.5 mg of 0.75% bupivacaine, 100 μg of epinephrine, 30 μg of clonidine, and 100 μg of morphine were injected. She was then placed in the supine position and the femoral region prepared and draped aseptically. The femoral vein was cannulated with a triple lumen catheter under ultrasound guidance. Spinal level was verified at T6 prior to bladder catheterization and subsequent uncomplicated cesarean section. Blood loss was 700 ml and the patient's postoperative hemoglobin and hematocrit concentrations were 7.2 g·dl^{-1} and 22.9%. Twenty units oxytocin in 1-liter normal saline was given via IV infusion. Following the procedure, the patient was transferred to the intensive care unit to utilise the combined resources of obstetric and critical care nursing. Hourly neurologic checks were performed to monitor for symptoms of a neuraxial hematoma. Maternal postoperative pain management was dictated by the surgeon and included the use of a patient-controlled analgesic device. Maternal complications were limited to an ileus requiring nasogastric tube placement and a brief extension of her hospital stay. The ileus resolved without complication permitting discharge to home within one week of surgery. During phone follow-up two weeks later, the patient reported satisfaction with her anaesthetic and denied any complaints or concerns.

3. Discussion

Vascular EDS is a single subtype of a heterogeneous collection of connective tissue disorders associated with mutations in the genes that code for the production of collagen. Vascular EDS is associated with mutations in type III procollagen (COL3A1: OMIM #120180). The diagnosis, which carries a significant risk of peripartum morbidity, requires both genetic identification and the presence of at least two of the following major clinical criteria: "(1) arterial, gastrointestinal or uterine fragility or rupture, (2) thin, translucent skin without hyper-elasticity, (3) extensive bruising, or (4) characteristic facial appearance (thin lips and nose, hollow cheeks, large eyes, small chin)" [1]. Vascular EDS represents less than 10%

of all EDS patients and carries a relatively low prevalence of 1 : 100,000–1 : 200,000 patients [5]. As such, few case reports have addressed the anaesthetic management of parturients with vascular EDS [3, 4]. Our preoperative deliberations focused on options for vascular access (peripheral versus central; standard peripheral IV versus rapid infusion catheter; multilumen central venous access versus large-bore introducer), blood pressure monitoring (noninvasive versus intra-arterial; radial versus femoral arterial), anaesthetic approach (general versus spinal versus epidural anaesthesia), neuraxial anaesthetic technique (single injection versus continuous administration of local anaesthetic), blood management (type of blood products; intraoperative cell salvage), and coagulation (antifibrinolysis).

In this context, we reviewed a publication which reported the management of a vascular EDS patient undergoing elective cesarean section at 36 weeks of gestational age [4]. Coagulation studies, complete blood count, and transthoracic echocardiogram were obtained preoperatively. Vascular access included two large-bore IV catheters, a radial arterial catheter, and an antecubital central venous catheter. Volume preloading consisted of 1-liter crystalloid and 0.5-liter colloid solutions. Tuohy needle-guided spinal anaesthesia was established by subarachnoid injection of 2.8 ml of 0.5% bupivacaine via a 25-gauge Whitacre spinal needle. An epidural catheter was inserted for postoperative analgesia.

Another report described successful continuous epidural anaesthesia with ropivacaine and fentanyl administered via a 20-gauge polyurethane catheter for labor and forceps delivery in a patient with vascular EDS [3]. In the absence of further case reports specific to the anaesthetic management of vascular type EDS parturients, we referenced an algorithm by Wiesmann et al. suggesting a preoperative approach to the EDS patient [6]. Specifically, we confirmed the genetic subtype, discussed prior EDS complications, and confirmed we had prolonged postoperative care facilities available. We focused extra care on patient positioning, cross-matched the patient for blood products, and administered desmopressin intraoperatively due to the patient's history of recurrent hematomas. We pursued a multidisciplinary approach and were influenced by these preoperative recommendations. We further obtained a first trimester brain MRI to evaluate for cerebral aneurysm and a second trimester transthoracic echocardiogram to evaluate for aortic root widening, aortic aneurysm, or valvular pathology. We noted several factors in considering the intraoperative approach to her cesarean delivery. Risks of general anaesthesia include the difficulties of tracheal intubation and the potential complications encountered in vascular EDS patients (i.e., arterial dissection/cerebral hemorrhage during hypertensive response to intubation, possible pneumothorax from positive pressure ventilation, and unstable cervical spine with potential for atlantoaxial subluxation) [3, 7, 8]. Alternatively, neuraxial anaesthesia is potentially less consistently reliable and may increase the risk of epidural hematoma [7]. Though the majority of vascular EDS patients have normal coagulation, there is a tendency toward prolonged bleeding and platelet dysfunction [9]. Furthermore, the vascular fragility combined with the tendency for platelet dysfunction, and in this patient the additional history of recurrent hematomas, raised our concern for an increased risk of epidural hematoma. After counseling, however, the patient chose a spinal anaesthetic, desired her spouse to be in the operating room at delivery, and requested to be awake at delivery. No cases of neuraxial hematoma in a parturient with vascular EDS were noted during literature review. Explanations for a negative literature review likely include the extremely low incidences of both vascular EDS and neuraxial hematoma. Due to the risk of platelet dysfunction, postpartum hemorrhage, difficult uterine closure, and vascular fragility and in the setting of relatively benign side effect profiles, we elected to administer tranexamic acid and DDAVP [10, 11]. Historically, both medications have been used to mitigate the potential for postpartum hemorrhage. We considered the risk and benefit of administering these medications with the risk and benefit of the patient receiving an autologous blood transfusion. Ultimately, we selected a single spinal injection and a small 25-gauge spinal needle to minimise tissue trauma. We added epinephrine and clonidine to the local anaesthetic solution to lengthen the duration of the nerve block. We used invasive arterial monitoring with central venous access to allow for the potential use of vasoactive agents and/or blood product administration, should the loss of peripheral IV access occur. Due to the patient's history of hematoma formation, we chose femoral vascular access. The literature does not support an optimal site for central venous access in this patient population. Though a peripherally inserted central catheter (PICC line) provides continuous IV access, it is unreliable for resuscitation. In the event of significant vascular trauma with bleeding, the subclavian is noncompressible and the internal jugular's juxtaposition to the airway is undesirable. The femoral site is, however, recognizably not visible to the anaesthetist during the procedure. Of note, urgent interventional radiology, if necessary, remains possible using the contralateral vasculature. Abiding by National Institute for Clinical Excellence (NICE) guidelines, and in line with recommendations from Wiesmann et al., we employed ultrasound-guided techniques for all of our invasive procedures in effort to reduce the risk of vascular injury and neuraxial hematoma.

In conclusion, we have presented the safe and uneventful delivery of a 34-week gestational aged parturient with documented vascular EDS who underwent primary elective cesarean section under spinal anaesthesia. In this rare case, which had significant anaesthetic implications, the potential for morbidity was great. However, our patient had none of the complications documented in the literature, suggesting that this patient may have done well with any number of anaesthetic alternatives.

Disclosure

The study was carried out at Department of Anesthesiology, Naval Medical Center Portsmouth. The views expressed in the manuscript are those of the authors and do not reflect the official policy or position of the Department of the Navy, Department of Defense, or the Unites States Government.

This manuscript was screened for plagiarism and cryptomnesia using Grammarly. LCDR Carness and CAPT Lenart are military service members. This work was prepared as part of their official duties. Title 17 USC 105 provides that "copyright protection under this title is not available for any work of the United States Government." Title 17 USC 101 defines a United States Government work as a work prepared by a military service member or employee of the United States Government as part of that person's official duties.

Authors' Contributions

Jeffrey M. Carness and Mark J. Lenart conducted the manuscript compilation and dissemination.

Acknowledgments

The authors would like to thank Dr. Aaron T. Poole, MD, FACOG, LCDR MC USN (Obstetrician/Gynecologist, Maternal Fetal Medicine, Naval Medical Center Portsmouth, Portsmouth, Virginia, USA), and Dr. Timothy E. Sayles, MD, FACOG, CAPT MC USN (Obstetrician/Gynecologist, Naval Medical Center Portsmouth, Portsmouth, Virginia, USA), for their consultation and assistance. They would also like to express appreciation to the patient for providing her input, revisions, and ultimate consent for the publication of this manuscript.

References

[1] P. Beighton, A. De Paepe, B. Steinmann, P. Tsipouras, and R. J. Wenstrup, "Ehlers-danlos syndromes: revised nosology, Villefranche, 1997," *American Journal of Medical Genetics*, vol. 77, no. 1, pp. 31–37, 1998.

[2] M. L. Murray, M. Pepin, S. Peterson, and P. H. Byers, "Pregnancy-related deaths and complications in women with vascular Ehlers-Danlos syndrome," *Genetics in Medicine*, vol. 16, no. 12, pp. 874–880, 2014.

[3] N. Campbell and O. P. Rosaeg, "Anesthetic management of a parturient with Ehlers Danlos syndrome type IV," *Canadian Journal of Anesthesia*, vol. 49, no. 5, pp. 493–496, 2002.

[4] D. Brighouse and B. Guard, "Anaesthesia for caesarean section in a patient with ehlers-danlos syndrome type IV," *British Journal of Anaesthesia*, vol. 69, no. 5, pp. 517–519, 1992.

[5] N. Volkov, V. Nisenblat, G. Ohel, and R. Gonen, "Ehlers-Danlos syndrome: Insights on obstetric aspects," *Obstetrical & Gynecological Survey*, vol. 62, no. 1, pp. 51–57, 2007.

[6] T. Wiesmann, M. Castori, F. Malfait, and H. Wulf, "Recommendations for anesthesia and perioperative management in patients with Ehlers-Danlos syndrome(s)," *Orphanet Journal of Rare Diseases*, vol. 9, article 109, 2014.

[7] V. Sood, D. A. Robinson, and I. Suri, "Difficult intubation during rapid sequence induction in a parturient with Ehlers-Danlos syndrome, hypermobility type," *International Journal of Obstetric Anesthesia*, vol. 18, no. 4, pp. 408–412, 2009.

[8] G. J. Halko, R. Cobb, and M. Abeles, "Patients with type IV Ehlers-Danlos syndrome may be predisposed to atlantoaxial subluxation," *The Journal of Rheumatology*, vol. 22, no. 11, pp. 2152–2155, 1995.

[9] A. Anstey, K. Mayne, M. Winter, J. Van de pette, and F. M. Pope, "Platelet and coagulation studies in Ehlers-Danlos syndrome," *British Journal of Dermatology*, vol. 125, no. 2, pp. 155–163, 1991.

[10] D. E. Trigg, I. Stergiotou, P. Peitsidis, and R. A. Kadir, "A Systematic Review: The use of desmopressin for treatment and prophylaxis of bleeding disorders in pregnancy," *Haemophilia*, vol. 18, no. 1, pp. 25–33, 2012.

[11] N. Novikova and G. J. Hofmeyr, "Tranexamic acid for preventing postpartum haemorrhage," *Cochrane Database of Systematic Reviews (Online)*, vol. 7, 2010.

38

Anaesthetic Management of Parturient with Acute Atrial Fibrillation for Emergency Caesarean Section

Madhu Gupta, Shalini Subramanian, and Preeti Adlakha

Department of Anaesthesiology, ESI-PGIMSR, Basaidara Pur, New Delhi, India

Correspondence should be addressed to Madhu Gupta; madhugupta2602@gmail.com

Academic Editors: M. Dauri, M. Kodaka, and D. Lee

A 31-year-antenatal lady with critical mitral stenosis presented for emergency caesarean section with fetal distress. She had acute onset atrial fibrillation. She was given a combined spinal epidural (CSE) anaesthesia and her arrhythmia was successfully managed after delivery of the baby with intravenous calcium channel blocker. Mitral stenosis is the most common valvular heart disease complicating pregnancy in developing countries. The physiological changes during pregnancy may exacerbate their cardiac symptoms. They may present with complications like congestive cardiac failure, atrial fibrillation, or pulmonary thromboembolism during the antenatal, intrapartum, or postpartum period. Here we discuss the management of parturient woman with high maternal and fetal risk presenting for emergency caesarean. The merits of regional anaesthesia and the importance of invasive monitoring are also discussed.

1. Introduction

A 31-year-old lady presented to the antenatal clinic at 34 weeks of gestation with increasing shortness of breath. She was a known case of rheumatic heart disease with mitral stenosis and had undergone balloon mitral valvotomy 12 years ago and closed mitral commissurotomy 7 years ago. She was gravida 8, para 2 with 5 spontaneous abortions and had undergone caesarean section twice since the commissurotomy but had only one living issue who was 3 years old. The other had died a neonatal death. She was on oral Digoxin 0.25 mg od and penicillin prophylaxis since the past seven years. During the present pregnancy, her dyspnea had progressed from NYHA class II to class III. She was put on bed rest and started on diuretics. As part of her workup for elective caesarean section for obstetric reasons, she presented for preanaesthesia evaluation. On auscultation of the heart, she had a mid-diastolic murmur in the mitral area and loud P2. She had no signs of congestive cardiac failure. Her electrocardiogram showed a normal sinus rhythm with a heart rate of 80/min. She had a normal coagulation profile with prothrombin time 13/13, activated partial thromboplastin time 29/31, and platelet count 210×10^9/litre. Her haemoglobin was 11.7 g%. She was advised a fresh echocardiograph and the

risk of anaesthesia was explained to her. The next day she presented for emergency CS with onset of preterm labour and a nonreassuring fetal heart rate. She was immediately taken to the operating room. On examination, the patient was dyspneic at rest and unable to lie supine. She had pedal edema and her jugular venous pulse was raised. A 2D echocardiography done only that morning revealed critical mitral stenosis with mitral valve area of 0.7 cm^2, severe tricuspid regurgitation, mild aortic regurgitation, and pulmonary artery hypertension. Her ejection fraction was 60%. She was propped up with 2 pillows and given O_2 by face mask at 12 L/min. An intravenous access was secured with an 18G cannula, Ringer lactate was started, and a defibrillator was kept ready. ECG, NIBP, and SpO$_2$ monitors were attached. Her pulse was irregularly irregular and the ECG showed atrial fibrillation with a ventricular rate of 142/min. Her blood pressure (BP) was 106/60 mmHg. Her respiratory rate was 32/min but her chest was clear and saturation was 100% with oxygen therapy. A 20G arterial cannula was inserted in the radial artery for invasive blood pressure monitoring. The arterial blood gas analysis showed pH 7.5, PO$_2$ 98 mmHg, PCO$_2$ 30 mmHg, HCO$_3$ 20 mmol/L, Na$^+$ 134 mmol/L, and K$^+$ 3.8 mmol/L. Combined spinal epidural (CSE) anesthesia was planned for the surgery. An 18G CSE was inserted in the first attempt at L3/4 intervertebral space using loss of resistance to air in the sitting position. In the subarachnoid block, 6 mg (1.2 mL) of 0.5% Bupivacaine with 25 μg fentanyl was injected through a 27G needle after CSF aspiration. The epidural catheter was inserted 5 cm into the epidural space and fixed. The patient was made to lie over 2 pillows as she could not tolerate a supine position. A wedge was also placed below her right hip to allow left uterine displacement to prevent aortocaval compression. Her BP dropped to 72/50 mmHg which increased to 92/54 mmHg with 6 mg ephedrine. The sensory level achieved was T10 and epidural top up of 3 mL of 2% Xylocaine with adrenaline was given in aliquots of 1 mL to achieve a level of T6 when the surgery commenced. She required one more dose of 6 mg Ephedrine to maintain her systolic BP above 90 mmHg. Her ventricular rate rose to 172/min during this period. The baby was delivered within 5 minutes of abdominal incision. The 2.2 kg male baby had aspirated thick meconium and required endotracheal intubation, tracheobronchial suctioning, and mechanical ventilation. After delivery of the baby, 10 units of oxytocin was added to the mother's drip. Her BP was 92/60 mmHg and keeping all preparations ready for emergency cardioversion, she was given 15 mg of Diltiazem injection in 5 mg boluses to obtain a ventricular rate of 90/min. Her ECG reverted to sinus rhythm. Her systolic BP rose to 110 mmHg and she did not require any further vasopressors. A peripherally inserted central venous catheter was inserted to measure the central venous pressure. The rest of the surgery was uneventful. She received 500 mL of RL including 10 units of oxytocin and her urine output was 50 mL. She was shifted to the ICU for postoperative observation and monitoring. In the ICU, she received oxygen therapy, diuretics, epidural analgesia, and intravenous fluids guided by central venous pressure. Invasive BP monitoring was continued for 24 hours. An infusion of amiodarone was used to maintain sinus rhythm and rate. Postoperatively, continuous hemodynamic monitoring was done with invasive monitors, intra-arterial blood pressure, and central venous pressure monitoring. She remained hemodynamically stable and had no episode of tachyarrhythmia, pulmonary edema, or thromboembolism during her stay. The next day, she was started on oral diltiazem and subcutaneous low molecular weight heparin and shifted to the ward on the postoperative day 2 from where she was discharged 7 days later. The neonate developed meconium aspiration pneumonia and died on day 3 of life.

2. Discussion

Rheumatic mitral stenosis is not uncommon in developing countries and can complicate up to 88% of pregnant patients with heart disease [1]. As in our case, many of them present for the first time in the third trimester when cardiac symptoms worsen because of the physiological changes of increased cardiac output, heart rate, oxygen consumption, and hemodilution [2]. The preferred mode of delivery in these patients is the vaginal route with labor analgesia to alleviate the increased demand on the heart. Caesarean section is reserved for obstetric indications. The maternal complications that may occur are pulmonary edema, tachyarrhythmia, stroke, cardiac arrest, or death [3–5].

Here, we discuss the case of a 34, week antenatal lady with critical mitral stenosis who presented for emergency Caesarean section with acute atrial fibrillation (AF). The acute onset (<48 hours) of her arrhythmia was evident as her preanaesthetic evaluation done the day earlier showed her to be in sinus rhythm. As her BP was 100/60 with severe fetal distress and no symptoms of angina or acute heart failure [6], we decided to urgently deliver the baby and then manage the tachyarrhythmia. Administering general anaesthesia to this patient involved the risk of hemodynamic instability with the use intravenous induction agents. Etomidate [7] has been used but was not available in our hospital. Using high dose opioids was not also an option in view of the parturient being full stomach. Secondly, the stress of laryngoscopy and intubation might precipitate pulmonary edema. Thirdly, cardiovascular collapse or arrest during induction would necessitate urgent hysterotomy and delivery of the baby to facilitate maternal resuscitation [8]. This would increase the maternal and fetal morbidity manifold. Positive pressure ventilation would further reduce the preload. Considering the above risks, the absence of coagulopathy, and the option of providing postoperative epidural analgesia, a regional anaesthesia technique was decided upon.

The CSE anaesthesia has been used for CS successfully in several cardiac patients [9]. A CSE was given as using spinal anaesthesia alone would cause sudden severe hypotension. The CSE offered the combined advantage of immediate dense blockade, with a low dose spinal, to start the urgent surgical procedure, and the gradual increase in the height of the block with epidural if necessary. The height achieved with the subarachnoid block was only T10. The reason may be small dose of local anaesthetic used and the head up position that the patient had to assume because of her dyspnea. Epidural top up was required to achieve a level of T6. The hypotension after spinal was successfully managed with Ephedrine injection.

Once the baby was delivered, the increased venous return enabled us to achieve rate control with Diltiazem. As rate control is not inferior to rhythm control [6] in prevention of death or morbidity, we used calcium channel blocker to achieve rate control. The same drug also provided rhythm control in our patient though this is unusual [6]. Amiodarone infusion was started in the ICU to maintain the sinus rhythm and heart rate <110/min [10]. She required no further vasopressor therapy during the surgery or in the postoperative period. Thromboprophylaxis was started once the risk of surgical bleeding was absent [10]. Our patient had high maternal and fetal risk [5]. The factors predicting primary cardiac events in our patient were NYHA class >II at presentation and left heart obstruction (mitral valve area < 2 cm^2) [11]. The causes for the poor neonatal outcome [4, 11] were prematurity, meconium aspiration, uterine hypoperfusion, and preexisting intrauterine factors as suggested by her bad obstetric history. In retrospect, our decision to deliver the baby first in the face of maternal tachyarrhythmia was justified as fetal distress due to meconium aspiration would not have responded to merely maternal stabilization and consequent improvement in uterine perfusion. There have been reports in the literature of patients with uncontrolled atrial fibrillation who have been managed and then had an uncomplicated vaginal delivery at a later date [12, 13], but none with acute atrial fibrillation for caesarean section. Acute atrial fibrillation in valvular heart disease has a high risk of heart failure, stroke, and death [6]. The factors that abetted a favourable maternal outcome in our case were good left ventricular ejection fraction (>40%), hemodynamic stability in the face of acute atrial fibrillation, and the use of regional anaesthesia to aid urgent delivery of the gravid uterus, which improved preload and facilitated rhythm control.

References

[1] N. Bhatla, S. Lal, G. Behera et al., "Cardiac disease in pregnancy," *International Journal of Gynecology and Obstetrics*, vol. 82, no. 2, pp. 153–159, 2003.

[2] M. Kannan and G. Vijayanand, "Mitral stenosis and pregnancy: current concepts in anaesthetic practice," *Indian Journal of Anaesthesia*, vol. 54, no. 5, pp. 439–444, 2010.

[3] U. Elkayam and F. Bitar, "Valvular heart disease and pregnancy part I: native valves," *Journal of the American College of Cardiology*, vol. 46, no. 2, pp. 223–230, 2005.

[4] S. C. Siu, J. M. Colman, S. Sorensen et al., "Adverse neonatal and cardiac outcomes are more common in pregnant women with cardiac disease," *Circulation*, vol. 105, no. 18, pp. 2179–2184, 2002.

[5] S. C. Reimold and J. D. Rutherford, "Valvular heart disease in pregnancy," *The New England Journal of Medicine*, vol. 349, no. 1, pp. 52–59, 2003.

[6] V. Fuster, L. E. Rydén, D. S. Cannom et al., "ACC/AHA/ESC 2006 Guidelines for the Management of Patients With Atrial Fibrillation. A Report of the American College of Cardiology/American Heart Association Task Force on Practice Guidelines and the European Society of Cardiology Committee for Practice Guidelines (Writing Committee to Revise the 2001 Guidelines for the Management of Patients With Atrial Fibrillation)," *Journal of the American College of Cardiology*, vol. 48, no. 4, pp. e149–e246, 2006.

[7] R. M. L. E. Orme, C. S. Grange, Q. P. Ainsworth, and C. R. Grebenik, "General anaesthesia using remifentanil for caesarean section in parturients with critical aortic stenosis: a series of four cases," *International Journal of Obstetric Anaesthesia*, vol. 13, no. 3, pp. 183–187, 2004.

[8] "Cardiac arrest associated with pregnancy," *Circulation*, vol. 112, pp. IV-150–IIV153, 2005.

[9] E. Langesæter, M. Dragsund, and L. A. Rosseland, "Regional anaesthesia for a Caesarean section in women with cardiac disease: a prospective study," *Acta Anaesthesiologica Scandinavica*, vol. 54, no. 1, pp. 46–54, 2010.

[10] L. S. Wann, A. B. Curtis, C. T. January, K. A. Ellenbogen, and J. E. Lowe, "Estes NAM 3rdet al writing on behalf of the 2006 ACC/AHA/ESC Guidelines for the Management of Patients With Atrial Fibrillation Writing Committee. 2011 ACCF/AHA/HRS focused update on the management of patients with atrial fibrillation (updating the 2006 guideline): a report of the American College of Cardiology Foundation/American Heart Association Task Force on Practice Guidelines," *Journal of the American College of Cardiology*, vol. 57, pp. 223–242, 2011.

[11] S. C. Siu, M. Sermer, J. M. Colman et al., "Prospective multicenter study of pregnancy outcomes in women with heart disease," *Circulation*, vol. 104, no. 5, pp. 515–521, 2001.

[12] S. K. Sharma, D. R. Gambling, N. M. Gajraj, C. Truong, and E. J. Sidawi, "Anesthetic management of a parturient with mixed mitral valve disease and uncontrolled atrial fibrillation," *International Journal of Obstetric Anesthesia*, vol. 3, no. 3, pp. 157–162, 1994.

[13] D. K. Desai, M. Adanlawo, D. P. Naidoo, J. Moodley, and I. Kleinschmidt, "Mitral stenosis in pregnancy: a four-year experience at King Edward VIII hospital, Durban, South Africa," *British Journal of Obstetrics and Gynaecology*, vol. 107, no. 8, pp. 953–958, 2000.

39

A Rare Central Venous Catheter Malposition in a 10-Year-Old Girl

Ali Movafegh, Alireza Saliminia, Reza Atef-Yekta, and Omid Azimaraghi (iD)

Department of Anesthesiology and Critical Care, Dr. Ali Shariati Hospital, Tehran University of Medical Sciences, Tehran, Iran

Correspondence should be addressed to Omid Azimaraghi; o.azimaraghi@gmail.com

Academic Editor: Kuang-I Cheng

Central venous catheters (CVCs) are placed in operating rooms worldwide via different approaches. Like any other medical procedure, CVC placement can cause a variety of complications. We report the case of an unexpected malposition of a catheter in the right internal jugular vein, where it looped back on itself during placement and went upward into the right internal jugular vein. CVC line placement should always be viewed as a procedure that could become complicated, even in the hands of the most experienced operators.

1. Introduction

Central venous catheterization plays an important role in modern medical practice.

It is estimated that approximately 8% of hospitalized patients require central venous access during the course of their hospital stay, and it has been estimated that more than five million CVCs are inserted in patients in the United States each year [1, 2]. Indications for CVC placement are diverse. Some of the more common indications include invasive hemodynamic monitoring, parenteral nutrition support, dialysis, chemotherapy, fluid resuscitation, drug administration, and renal replacement therapy.

Although CV catheterization is a simple and relatively safe procedure, many complications have been reported during or after the procedure. Malposition is one of the complications observed.

In this report, we describe a rare case of malposition in a 10-year-old girl.

2. Case Presentation

The patient was a 10-year-old girl, recently diagnosed with leukemia and hospitalized for treatment. She required central venous (CV) line placement for chemotherapy. Other than her diagnosed leukemia, she had no other significant medical history.

After the procedure was explained thoroughly to the patient and her parents, a consent form was completed by her parents, and she was transferred to the CV line room. The patient was very alert and cooperative. Based on the local protocols, all patients requiring CV line placement are transferred to a room dedicated for CV line placement (the intravenous access room), which is located in the operating room. Standard monitoring including an electrocardiogram (ECG), noninvasive blood pressure, and pulse-oximetry were initiated. A 20-gauge cannula was inserted into the vein on the dorsum of the patient's left hand.

The right internal jugular vein was selected for CV cannulation.

Propofol was used for sedation, and after adequate sedation, a single-lumen 14-gauge catheter was inserted in the right internal jugular vein using ultrasound sonography under sterile conditions by an experienced anesthesiologist. No problem was encountered during the procedure, and after blood was aspirated, the catheter was fixed at 13 cm. Normal saline infusion was initiated through the CV. Central venous waveforms were not used for catheter position confirmation.

A chest radiograph was immediately arranged to confirm the catheter position.

On chest radiograph, the catheter could be seen looping back and going upward at the junction of the right internal jugular vein and the right subclavian vein (Figure 1). The team decided to use ultrasonography to verify that the catheter was

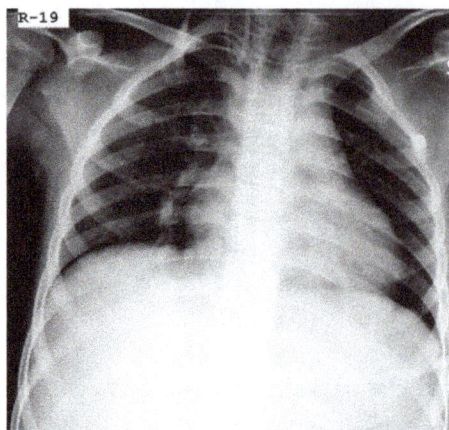

FIGURE 1: The catheter can be seen looping back and going upward at the junction of the right internal jugular vein and the right subclavian vein.

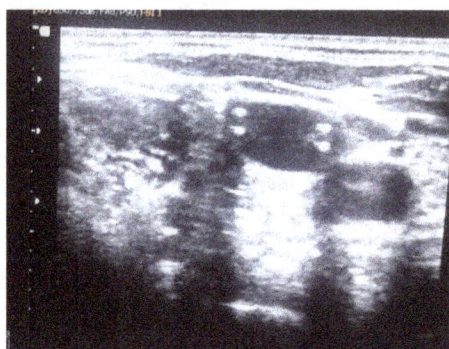

FIGURE 2: The right internal jugular vein is clearly evident on ultrasonography. Two lumens of the catheter can also be seen.

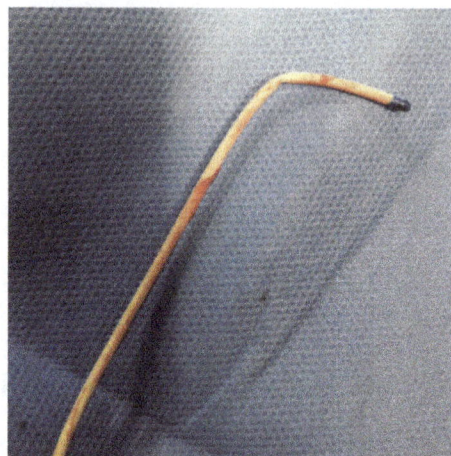

FIGURE 3: The bended catheter.

in the jugular vein and had not punctured the dorsal wall of the vein. During scanning of the right internal jugular vein, only a single lumen of the catheter could be seen until we scanned the bottom third of the jugular vein (Figure 2).

We decided to pull back the catheter under the guidance of ultrasonography until only one lumen could be visualized and then pass a guidewire over the catheter to reposition the catheter. While doing so and after only one lumen was visualized following extraction of the central venous line under the guidance of ultrasonography, passage of the guidewire was attempted, but resistance was encountered. Therefore, we decided to completely remove the catheter and reinsert another catheter.

When the catheter was removed, it was observed that the catheter had bent at the distal end (Figure 3).

Subsequently, we placed another CVC through the internal jugular vein without any complications. The position of the CVC was confirmed by radiograph.

3. Discussion

CV catheterization is being performed every day in medical centers around the world. The internal jugular vein is one of the most common sites that anesthesiologists use, and this site is chosen because CVC can be securely inserted in this location.

It is difficult to estimate the rate of early and late complications that occur during insertion of CV lines. Many of the complications may go unseen, and many are unreported. Some complications may be life threatening or may cause morbidity, and some may not be recognized as a complication at all [3]. The incidence and occurrence of complications depend on various factors, such as the experience of the operator, the site of insertion, and the placement technique [4].

At our center, Shariati Hospital, we insert over 2000 CV lines every year. The Hematology-Oncology Research Center and Stem Cell Transplantation (HORCSCT) Center, which is affiliated to Tehran University of Medical Sciences (TUMS), is based in Shariati Hospital, and over two-thirds of our patients are individuals who have hematological cancer and require CV line placement for chemotherapy.

The low price of CV lines compared to other options for CV access has favored their use at our center. However, using CV lines for chemotherapy has its own hazards, especially in the pediatric population.

We use single-lumen 14-gauge CV lines for all our patients (aged 2 months and above), and the main route of insertion and technique of insertion for adults at our center is the subclavian vein via the landmark technique. Regarding the route and technique of insertion, we have found that patients are much more satisfied and can handle their daily tasks much easier when the catheter is fixed at a level below the clavicle.

In the pediatric patients, we usually use an ultrasound-guided approach to the right internal jugular vein, as we are inserting a very large catheter and the risk of complications is much higher via the subclavian vein approach.

In the case described here, the procedure went smoothly with no resistance, and the blood was successfully aspirated at the end of the first attempt at placement, which led us to refrain from scanning the catheter placement with ultrasound. This example shows that although insufficient blood flow from the catheter during aspiration is a possible warning sign of misplacement of the CV line, adequate blood aspiration cannot be totally relied on as a sign of successful placement.

Ultrasonography has aided in the placement of CVCs in many ways, especially in pediatric patients. However, as can be seen in this case, relying on ultrasound only for finding the vein and guiding the needle is not enough and did not prevent the malposition of the catheter. Based on this report, it is advised to scan along the vein to localize the catheter, even after a seemingly uneventful catheter placement. This is especially important when placing catheters via the subclavian vein, which is a site where a catheter risks going upward into the internal jugular vein.

Chest radiographs have always helped us determine early and late complications. The immediate chest radiograph that was taken in this patient proved to be vital in showing the complication.

Although we have had different types of malposition of catheters, this is the first time that we encounter a catheter looping back on itself. A probable mechanism could have been the angle of the internal jugular vein and subclavian vein, facilitating the malposition and pushing the j-shaped tip of the guidewire upward and back on itself. The right-sided bevel of the needle at the time of internal jugular vein puncture and guidewire insertion may also have contributed to the looping back of the guidewire and, consequently, the catheter.

Another issue that needs to be highlighted is the need for a specific facility for intravenous access procedures. Due to the large number of CVCs placed at our center, a few years ago we decided to dedicate a room with trained personnel for CV placement. Having a dedicated room for this purpose has not only decreased the time spent during each procedure but also decreased the rate of complications and increased patient satisfaction.

A variety of rare complications such as perforation of the left brachiocephalic vein and massive hemothorax, chylothorax, internal mammary artery malposition of catheter, and inadvertent placement of a CVC in the left pericardiophrenic vein have been reported previously [5–8].

It should be noted that a bending catheter has the risk of occlusion or perforation of the vein which fortunately did not occur in the described report above.

Many practical techniques such as using surface landmarks for estimating the length of catheter insertion, ultrasound-guided localization of the vein and guidance of the needle, echocardiography, electrocardiographic guided catheter tip placement using $NaHCO3$-filled catheters, and immediate postprocedure X-rays have been proposed for aiding a safe placement of CVC [9, 10].

We believe that to decrease the rate of complications associated with CVC placement, a multimodal approach is required. An appropriate setting with trained personnel, in combination with ultrasound guidance during and after the procedure, is helpful but not enough. Making sure the operator is focused throughout the procedure with attention to any atypical events such as resistance during any of the stages of catheter placement may help to decrease complications.

CV line placement should always be looked on as a procedure that could become complicated, even in the hands of the most experienced operators.

Therefore, it should be remembered that follow-up and checking of the correct function and placement of the CVC are as important as the procedure itself.

References

[1] S. Ruesch, B. Walder, and M. R. Tramèr, "Complications of central venous catheters: Internal jugular versus subclavian access - a systematic review," *Critical Care Medicine*, vol. 30, no. 2, pp. 454–460, 2002.

[2] D. C. McGee and M. K. Gould, "Preventing complications of central venous catheterization," *The New England Journal of Medicine*, vol. 348, no. 12, pp. 1123–1133, 2003.

[3] C.-C. Chen, P.-N. Tsao, and K.-I. Tsou Yau, "Paraplegia: complication of percutaneous central venous line malposition," *Pediatric Neurology*, vol. 24, no. 1, pp. 65–68, 2001.

[4] W. Schummer, C. Schummer, N. Rose, W.-D. Niesen, and S. G. Sakka, "Mechanical complications and malpositions of central venous cannulations by experienced operators: a prospective study of 1794 catheterizations in critically ill patients," *Intensive Care Medicine*, vol. 33, no. 6, pp. 1055–1059, 2007.

[5] L. R. Wetzel, P. R. Patel, and N. L. Pesa, "Central venous catheter placement in the left internal jugular vein complicated by perforation of the left brachiocephalic vein and massive hemothorax: a case report," *A&A Case Reports*, vol. 9, no. 1, pp. 16–19, 2017.

[6] U. S. D. Kumar, S. Shivananda, and M. Wali, "Malpositioned central venous catheters: a diagnostic dilemma," *Journal of the Association for Vascular Access*, vol. 21, no. 1, pp. 35–38, 2016.

[7] K. Kumada, N. Murakami, H. Okada et al., "Rare central venous catheter malposition - an ultrasound-guided approach would be helpful: a case report," *Journal of Medical Case Reports*, vol. 10, article 248, 2016.

[8] M. H. Trujillo and K. Arai, "Hydrothorax after inadvertent placement of a central venous catheter in the left pericardiophrenic vein," *Journal of Intensive Care Medicine*, vol. 9, no. 5, pp. 257–260, 1994.

[9] K.-S. Chu, J.-H. Hsu, S.-S. Wang et al., "Accurate central venous port-a catheter placement: intravenous electrocardiography and surface landmark techniques compared by using transesophageal echocardiography," *Anesthesia & Analgesia*, vol. 98, no. 4, pp. 910–914, 2004.

[10] J.-H. Hsu, C.-K. Wang, K.-S. Chu et al., "Comparison of radiographic landmarks and the echocardiographic SVC/RA junction in the positioning of long-term central venous catheters," *Acta Anaesthesiologica Scandinavica*, vol. 50, no. 6, pp. 731–735, 2006.

40

Anesthesiological Management of a Patient with Williams Syndrome Undergoing Spine Surgery

Federico Boncagni,[1] Luca Pecora,[2] Vasco Durazzi,[3] and Francesco Ventrella[4]

[1]*Clinica di Rianimazione Generale, Respiratoria e del Trauma Maggiore,*
 Azienda Ospedaliero-Universitaria "Ospedali Riuniti Umberto I-G. M. Lancisi-G. Salesi", 60126 Ancona, Italy
[2]*Anestesia e Rianimazione dei Trapianti e della Chirurgia Maggiore,*
 Azienda Ospedaliero-Universitaria "Ospedali Riuniti Umberto I-G. M. Lancisi-G. Salesi", 60126 Ancona, Italy
[3]*Clinica di Neurologia, Azienda Ospedaliero-Universitaria "Ospedali Riuniti Umberto I-G. M. Lancisi-G. Salesi", 60126 Ancona, Italy*
[4]*Anestesia e Rianimazione Pediatrica, Azienda Ospedaliero-Universitaria "Ospedali Riuniti Umberto I-G. M. Lancisi-G. Salesi",*
 60126 Ancona, Italy

Correspondence should be addressed to Federico Boncagni; fede.boncagni@gmail.com

Academic Editor: Maria Jose C. Carmona

Williams Syndrome (WS) is a complex neurodevelopmental disorder associated with a mutation on chromosome 7. Patients with WS usually display dysmorphic facial and musculoskeletal features, congenital heart diseases, metabolic disturbances and cognitive impairment. Structural cardiovascular abnormalities are present in the majority of the children and may provide a substrate for perioperative Sudden Cardiac Death, as presented by several reports, something that creates a great challenge to the anesthetic conduct. We present the case of a 12-year old girl who required anesthetic care for surgical correction of an acquired kyphoscoliosis. Potential anesthesiological implications of WS are subsequently reviewed.

1. Introduction

Williams-Beuren Syndrome (WBS) is a genetic autosomal dominant disorder associated with *de novo* deletion in the long arm of chromosome 7 (7q11.23), occurring 1 : 10.000 live births [1–3]. Patients with WBS show mild to moderate mental retardation and musculoskeletal and craniofacial abnormalities, such as hypertelorism, flat nasal bridge, long philtrum, and wide mouth with a hypoplastic or short mandible [1, 3]. Considering the association with congenital heart defects, Supravalvular Aortic Stenosis (SVAS) and Pulmonary Artery Stenosis (PAS) are reported in up to 80% of pediatric patients [2], clinical conditions that create enormous difficulty in the anesthetic approach, something that can be translated by the high probability of refractory intraoperative cardiac arrest [4–8]. Given to the multiorgan involvement of the syndrome and to the anecdotal nature of case descriptions, anesthesiological management of affected patients is often challenging and it implies special considerations to cardiovascular, metabolic, and technical aspects of anesthesia delivering. In this case report, we describe the anesthetic management of a 12-year-old girl undergoing anesthesia for surgical correction of an acquired kyphoscoliosis and we subsequently discuss perioperative implications of WBS.

Written informed consent from patient's relatives was obtained before case report publication and it is available on editors' request.

2. Case Presentation

A 12-year-old girl with WBS was referred to our centre for definitive correction of a developmental, thoracic kyphoscoliosis. She already underwent the provisional placement of a posterior extensible distractor three years ago. The diagnosis of WBS, based on *stellata iris* pattern of the eyes, umbilical hernia, interatrial septal defect, and failure to thrive, was presumed at 7 months by her paediatrician and further

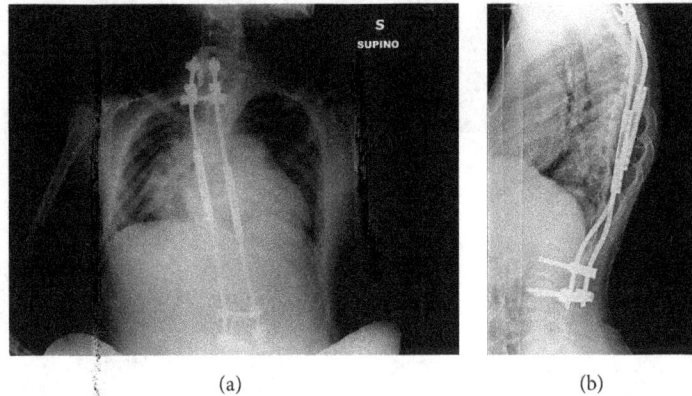

FIGURE 1: Anteroposterior (a) and lateral (b) chest X-ray showing patient's pronounced spinal curvature and dorsal hump. A provisional extensible distractor is in place.

confirmed by genetic analysis (FISH hybridization) which showed the typical hemizygosity at 7q11.23.

During the follow-up, a spontaneous closure of cardiac septal defect, hypercalcemia, controlled by dietary interventions, repeated episodes of fever of unknown origin by one year, and occurrence of Schönlein-Henoch purpura by two months, both, before admission to surgery were found.

Physical examination showed the characteristic appearance of WBS patients with broad forehead, flat nasal bridge, wide mouth with a prominent lower lip, dental malocclusion, and a short mandible. Spinal curvature was more than 80° in the coronal plane with an associated dorsal hump (Figure 1). She weighed 35 Kg and her vital signs were within the limits, with blood pressure (BP) of 130/90 mmHg. Baseline ECG showed sinus rhythm at 88 beats/min with a normal QRS and no ST-T alterations. Cardiopulmonary physical examination only showed slight 2/6 systodiastolic murmur at the precordium. Preoperative laboratory exams included TSH, thyroid hormones, and calcium, which were within normal range. A transthoracic echocardiogram, performed to rule out previously unrecognized cardiac abnormalities, showed a nonsignificant interventricular septal defect, absence of SVAS, or interatrial septal defect. Color-Doppler examination of supra-aortic trunks showed no thickening of the carotids. Given that the patient was asymptomatic under the cardiovascular point of view and doing well with everyday activities, we chose not to perform a coronary angiography.

A 4.5-French central venous catheter was placed in the right internal jugular vein under light sedation and local anesthesia, in the day before the surgical procedure. The child was kept quiet for eight hours and transported to the operating room the day of the surgery. Atropine 0.4 mg was given intravenously soon before anesthesia induction with fentanyl 100 mcg and propofol 120 mg. No neuromuscular blocking agent was used. Prior to intubation, the glottis was irrigated under direct laryngoscopy with 10 mL of 2% lidocaine via a Optispray® syringe, revealing grade I Cormack-Lehane visualization of vocal cords. Tracheal intubation was achieved at first attempt after local anesthesia with a 6.5 mm ID cuffed tube. After intubation, left radial artery was cannulated and a urinary catheter was placed. Finally, the patient was prone

positioned. The maintenance of the anesthesia consisted of 2% sevoflurane in O_2/air mixture and remifentanil continuous infusion. Intraoperative monitoring included pulse oximetry, continuous ECG tracing, invasive blood pressure, and hemodynamic monitoring via a FloTrac/Vigileo® device, end tidal carbon dioxide, and bladder temperature. Neurophysiological monitoring was provided by continuous EEG and somatosensory evoked potentials (SSEPs) to detect spinal lesions occurring during surgery. We attempted to maintain blood pressure of 90/50 mmHg throughout the whole procedure, with an average cardiac index (CI) around 4.5 L/min/m². Minimum bladder temperature at the end of the surgery was 35°C. No alteration of SSEPs propagation compared to baseline was noted (Figure 2). Total surgical time was 7 h 16 min, with an estimated blood loss of 500 mL. In turn, during the surgery, it was observed that the correction of the original kyphoscoliosis was impossible, due to excessive rigidity of the spine. Therefore, only definitive spinal fusion was performed. After supine repositioning, the maintenance of anesthesia was stopped and the patient extubated, without complications. Clinical observation continued for about 30 min in the operating theatre, and then the child was moved to the department of orthopaedics. Analgesia was provided by means of continuous infusion of morphine 20 mg, ketorolac 30 mg, and ketamine 100 mg, over the following 24 hours. The postoperative course was uneventful and the child was discharged home on day 8.

3. Discussion

Williams-Beuren Syndrome (WBS), originally first described by Williams et al. in 1961 [9], is a congenital disease that occurs due to deletion in the long arm of chromosome 7. Typically, the deletion involves a region spanning 1.5 to 1.8 Mb that encodes for several genes, including the elastin (ELN) gene, and it occurs during meiotic crossover as a result of chromosome misalignment [1, 10]. Either the maternally or the paternally inherited chromosome 7 may be involved, the phenomenon being sporadic in the majority of the cases. Elastin deficiency and defective expression of contiguous genes have been regarded, as possible explanations of the

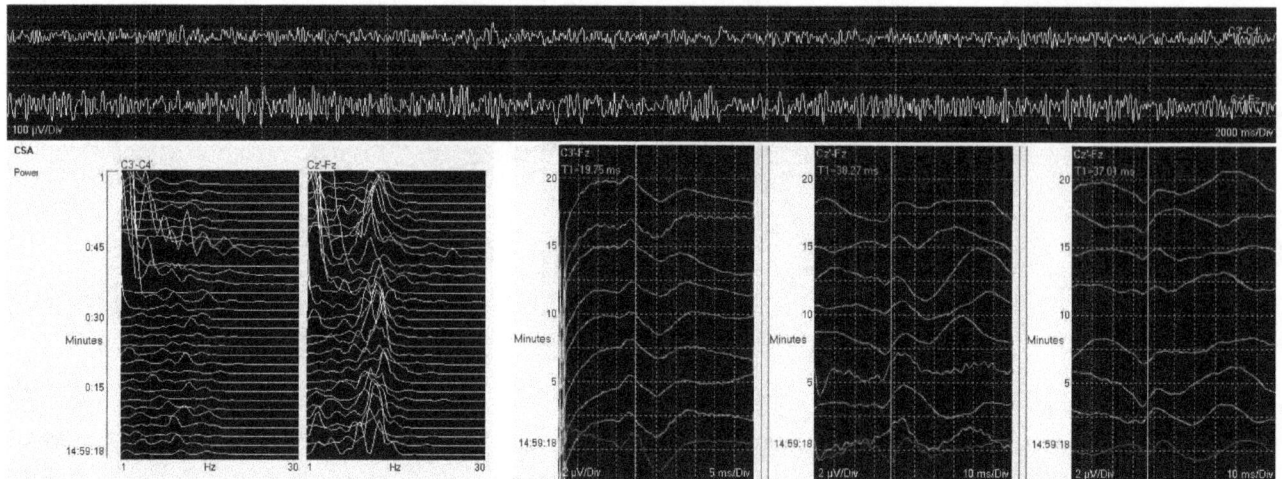

FIGURE 2: Screenshot of continuous EEG, spectral EEG analysis, and SSEPs (somatosensory evoked potentials) at the end of the procedure. EEG monitoring under general anesthesia shows persistence of α-like activity (top) with a peak frequency around 9-10 Hz (left). Right corner of the image: SSEPs monitoring is shown. Physiological neuraxial propagation of peripheral stimuli (darker line) with no time delay is seen (from left to right: the first column is right upper limb channel, and then the right lower limb and the left lower limb channels are shown, second and third column, resp.).

multiorgan involvement of the disease [1, 10, 11]. Typically, affected individuals display a variable degree of mental retardation (mean IQ range 41–80), a friendly and hypersocial personality with characteristic facial stigmata, such as epicanthal folds, wide-set eyes, flat nasal bridge, a prominent lower lip, and puffy cheeks ("elfin face"). The mandible is often short or hypoplastic. Blue-eyed patients may have a "stellate" pattern of their irides (stellata iris) [12].

Pediatric patients may turn to anesthesiologists early in their lives, for surgical repair of cardiovascular defects, multiple hernias of the abdominal wall, and ENT procedures [8, 12, 13]. Anesthesiological management is often challenging and implies in careful preoperative evaluation, aiming to exclude potential comorbidities.

Supravalvular Aortic Stenosis (SVAS) is the most common congenital cardiac defect encountered in children with WBS. It may appear as hourglass narrowing, at the sinotubular junction, or as diffuse stenosis of the ascending aorta, involving the brachiocephalic vessels [3, 9, 14], with frequently stenotic and tortuous coronary arteries [15]. Cardiac arrest under general anesthesia has been reported in several case series, likely as a result of a perfusion mismatch in the presence of a severe left ventricular outflow tract (LVOT) obstruction [4–8]. Since WBS clinical presentation is variable, less severe forms of cardiac defects are possible, as in our case. A detailed review of previous medical history and a preoperative work-up, including at least 4-limb blood pressure measurement, ECG, and a transthoracic echocardiogram screening, will help the identification of high-risk of adverse events, which serve as reference for the care to be adopted by the teams. Although questionable, a coronary angiography has been recommended by some authors for any WBS patient requiring anesthetic care [5]. Besides congenital heart diseases, elastin gene knockout leads to diffuse arteriopathy: specific lesions imply a thickening of

supra-aortic trunks [16] and renovascular involvement [17, 18]. Actually, early-onset hypertension is a common finding among affected patients [19–21].

The presence of a difficult airway may be a reason for concern, too. Despite the fact that clinical reports are substantially lacking, distinct anatomic features of WBS patients are predictors of both difficult intubation and bag-mask ventilation, especially mandible hypoplasia, dental abnormalities, and flattened maxillary profile [13, 22]. It is not clearly established whether WBS patients are at higher risk for airway obstruction. Nonetheless, it has been inferred that elastin deficiency may affect vocal cords function, thereby providing an explanation for WBS individuals' hoarse voice. There are at least two descriptions of laryngeal stridor; one of these is occurring in the postoperative setting and successfully managed with inhaled epinephrine [13, 23]. Joint laxity and muscle weakness are commonly reported in WBS, and a variable degree of myopathy has been demonstrated. Caution has been advocated in the use of neuromuscular blocking agents (NMBAs), since the risk of a prolonged response could not be excluded [13, 24].

Endocrine anomalies are commonly represented by hypercalcemia and hypothyroidism. Infantile hypercalcemia has been reported in up to 15% of pediatric patients and usually resolves in the first years of life. It is generally mild and rarely accompanied by nephrocalcinosis. However, calcium imbalances may be recurrent during puberty and preoperative screening is recommended [12, 25]. Subclinical hypothyroidism has been described in 15 to 30% of WBS screened patients. Although overt hypothyroidism is a rare finding, clinical implications on cardiac function, blood volume, perioperative anemia, and temperature homeostasis prompt preoperative thyroid function evaluation [26, 27].

In summary, anesthetic care of WBS patients demands particular attention. The identification of cardiovascular comorbidities is the most challenging task and meticulous preoperative evaluation of heart defects should be warranted. However, anesthesiologists should be aware of the fact that the management of these patients should address all the multisystemic aspects of this complex syndrome.

References

[1] B. R. Pober, "Williams-Beuren syndrome," *The New England Journal of Medicine*, vol. 362, no. 3, pp. 239–252, 2010.

[2] C. P. Hornik, R. T. Collins II, R. D. Jaquiss et al., "Adverse cardiac events in children with Williams syndrome undergoing cardiovascular surgery: an analysis of the Society of Thoracic Surgeons Congenital Heart Surgery Database," *The Journal of Thoracic and Cardiovascular Surgery*, vol. 149, no. 6, pp. 1516–1522, 2015.

[3] R. T. Collins II, "Cardiovascular disease in Williams syndrome," *Circulation*, vol. 127, no. 21, pp. 2125–2134, 2013.

[4] L. M. Bird, G. F. Billman, R. V. Lacro et al., "Sudden death in Williams syndrome: report of 10 cases," *Journal of Pediatrics*, vol. 129, no. 6, pp. 926–931, 1996.

[5] P. E. Horowitz, S. Akhtar, J. A. Wulff, F. Al Fadley, and Z. Al Halees, "Coronary artery disease and anesthesia-related death in children with Williams syndrome," *Journal of Cardiothoracic and Vascular Anesthesia*, vol. 16, no. 6, pp. 739–741, 2002.

[6] P. Gupta, J. D. Tobias, S. Goyal et al., "Sudden cardiac death under anesthesia in pediatric patient with Williams syndrome: a case report and review of literature," *Annals of Cardiac Anaesthesia*, vol. 13, no. 1, pp. 44–48, 2010.

[7] K. Bragg, G. M. Fedel, and A. DiProsperis, "Cardiac arrest under anesthesia in a pediatric patient with Williams syndrome: a case report," *AANA Journal*, vol. 73, no. 4, pp. 287–293, 2005.

[8] A. Monfared and A. Messner, "Death following tonsillectomy in a child with Williams syndrome," *International Journal of Pediatric Otorhinolaryngology*, vol. 70, no. 6, pp. 1133–1135, 2006.

[9] J. C. Williams, B. G. Barratt-Boyes, and J. B. Lowe, "Supravalvular aortic stenosis," *Circulation*, vol. 24, pp. 1311–1318, 1961.

[10] A. K. Ewart, C. A. Morris, D. Atkinson et al., "Hemizygosity at the elastin locus in a developmental disorder, Williams syndrome," *Nature Genetics*, vol. 5, no. 1, pp. 11–16, 1993.

[11] D. Kotzot, F. Bernasconi, L. Brecevic et al., "Phenotype of the Williams-Beuren syndrome associated with hemizygosity at the elastin locus," *European Journal of Pediatrics*, vol. 154, no. 6, pp. 477–482, 1995.

[12] Committee on Genetics, "American Academy of Pediatrics: health care supervision for children with Williams syndrome," *Pediatrics*, vol. 107, no. 5, pp. 1192–1204, 2001.

[13] J. Medley, P. Russo, and J. D. Tobias, "Perioperative care of the patient with Williams syndrome," *Paediatric Anaesthesia*, vol. 15, no. 3, pp. 243–247, 2005.

[14] M. P. Suárez-Mier and B. Morentin, "Supravalvular aortic stenosis, Williams syndrome and sudden death. A case report," *Forensic Science International*, vol. 106, no. 1, pp. 45–53, 1999.

[15] D. Bonnet, V. Cormier, E. Villain, P. Bonhoeffer, and J. Kachaner, "Progressive left main coronary artery obstruction leading to myocardial infarction in a child with Williams syndrome," *European Journal of Pediatrics*, vol. 156, no. 10, pp. 751–753, 1997.

[16] Y. Aggoun, D. Sidi, B. I. Levy, S. Lyonnet, J. Kachaner, and D. Bonnet, "Mechanical properties of the common carotid artery in Williams syndrome," *Heart*, vol. 84, no. 3, pp. 290–293, 2000.

[17] C. Rose, A. Wessel, R. Pankau, C.-J. Partsch, and J. Bürsch, "Anomalies of the abdominal aorta in Williams-Beuren syndrome—another cause arterial hypertension," *European Journal of Pediatrics*, vol. 160, no. 11, pp. 655–658, 2001.

[18] J. R. Ingelfinger and J. W. Newburger, "Spectrum of renal anomalies in patients with Williams syndrome," *Journal of Pediatrics*, vol. 119, no. 5, pp. 771–773, 1991.

[19] S. R. Daniels, J. M. H. Loggie, D. C. Schwartz, J. L. Strife, and S. Kaplan, "Systemic hypertension secondary to peripheral vascular anomalies in patients with Williams syndrome," *The Journal of Pediatrics*, vol. 106, no. 2, pp. 249–251, 1985.

[20] K. Broder, E. Reinhardt, J. Ahern, R. Lifton, W. Tamborlane, and B. Pober, "Elevated ambulatory blood pressure in 20 subjects with Williams syndrome," *American Journal of Medical Genetics*, vol. 83, no. 5, pp. 356–360, 1999.

[21] G. B. Ferrero, E. Biamino, L. Sorasio et al., "Presenting phenotype and clinical evaluation in a cohort of 22 Williams-Beuren syndrome patients," *European Journal of Medical Genetics*, vol. 50, no. 5, pp. 327–337, 2007.

[22] M. G. Butler, B. G. Hayes, M. M. Hathaway, and M. L. Begleiter, "Specific genetic diseases at risk for sedation/anesthesia complications," *Anesthesia and Analgesia*, vol. 91, no. 4, pp. 837–855, 2000.

[23] K. K. Vaux, H. Wojtczak, K. Benirschke, and K. L. Jones, "Vocal cord abnormalities in Williams syndrome: a further manifestation of elastin deficiency," *American Journal of Medical Genetics*, vol. 119, no. 3, pp. 302–304, 2003.

[24] T. Voit, H. Kramer, C. Thomas, W. Wechsler, H. Reichmann, and H. G. Lenard, "Myopathy in Williams-Beuren syndrome," *European Journal of Pediatrics*, vol. 150, no. 7, pp. 521–526, 1991.

[25] A. P. Cagle, S. G. Waguespack, B. A. Buckingham, R. Ravi Shankar, and L. A. Dimeglio, "Severe infantile hypercalcemia associated with williams syndrome successfully treated with intravenously administered pamidronate," *Pediatrics*, vol. 114, no. 4, pp. 1091–1095, 2004.

[26] V. Cammareri, G. Vignati, G. Nocera, P. Beck-Peccoz, and L. Persani, "Thyroid hemiagenesis and elevated thyrotropin levels in a child with Williams syndrome," *American Journal of Medical Genetics*, vol. 85, no. 5, pp. 491–494, 1999.

[27] S. Stagi, G. Bindi, A. S. Neri et al., "Thyroid function and morphology in patients affected by Williams syndrome," *Clinical Endocrinology*, vol. 63, no. 4, pp. 456–460, 2005.

A Rare Case of C2 Sensory Blockade with Preserved Phrenic Nerve Function in an Obstetric Patient

John C. Coffman, Kasey Fiorini, Meghan Cook, and Robert H. Small

Department of Anesthesiology, The Ohio State University Wexner Medical Center, Columbus, OH 43210, USA

Correspondence should be addressed to John C. Coffman; john.coffman@osumc.edu

Academic Editor: Latha Hebbar

High neuraxial blockade is a serious complication in obstetric patients and requires prompt recognition and management in order to optimize patient outcomes. In cases of high neuroblockade, patients may present with significant hypotension, dyspnea, agitation, difficulty speaking or inability to speak, or even loss of consciousness. We report the unusual presentation of an obstetric patient that remained hemodynamically stable and had the preserved ability to initiate breaths despite sensory blockade up to C2. The presence of differential motor and sensory block documented in this case helped enable the patient to be managed with noninvasive ventilatory support until the high blockade regressed and we are not aware of any other similar reports in literature.

1. Introduction

High neuroblockade is an important cause of anesthesia-related maternal morbidity and mortality [1–3] and has been reported as the most common among serious complications in obstetric patients with an incidence of 1 in 4,336 neuraxial anesthetics [2]. We present an uncommon case of rapid epidural dosing for emergent cesarean delivery that led to sensory blockade up to the C2 dermatomal level, which remarkably did not result in hypotension, altered mentation, or loss of consciousness. The patient also retained at least partial diaphragmatic motor function despite the C2 sensory blockade, and this differential block along with her hemodynamic stability allowed her to be managed with mask-assisted respirations.

2. Case Presentation

A healthy 33-year-old nulliparous patient (weight = 94 kg, body mass index = 33.6 kg/m^2) of 40 weeks' gestation presented in active labor and had uncomplicated epidural catheter placement at L3-4. Epidural catheter aspiration and test dose with 1.5% lidocaine with 1 : 200,000 epinephrine 3 mL were negative for signs or symptoms of intravascular or intrathecal catheter placement. Labor analgesia was initiated with 0.125%

bupivacaine 10 mL and fentanyl 20 mcg, given in divided doses over five minutes, and this resulted in effective pain relief with a T10 sensory blockade to pinprick stimuli and partial motor blockade (Bromage score = 1). For the next three hours, she had good labor analgesia with a continuous epidural infusion of 0.0625% bupivacaine + 2 mcg/mL fentanyl at 12 mL/hr with patient-controlled epidural analgesia (6 mL bolus, 15 minute lockout). At this time, recurrent late fetal heart rate (FHR) decelerations became apparent, including a prolonged FHR deceleration to the 60–70 bpm range that resolved after a minute. The nonreassuring FHR pattern persisted despite placing the patient on supplemental oxygen and attempts at repositioning her in order to optimize uteroplacental perfusion, and at this point the obstetrician communicated the need for emergent cesarean delivery. The patient received oral sodium citrate 15 mL and was rapidly transitioned to the operating room. A T12 sensory block to pinprick stimuli and Bromage score of 0 were noted prior to epidural dosing with fentanyl 50 mcg and 2% lidocaine with 1 : 200,000 epinephrine 20 mL, given in 5 mL increments over five minutes' time. As the epidural was being dosed, a sterile surgical field was prepared and she was placed on nasal cannula oxygen 3 L/min given the nonreassuring fetal status. She was also given intravenous (IV) ephedrine 10 mg and glycopyrrolate 0.2 mg during this interval. The overnight anesthesia provider commonly administers these IV medications when dosing labor epidurals for cesarean delivery in order to minimize incidence of hypotension due to neuraxial blockade, though this is not the regular practice of other providers at our institution. Three minutes after epidural dosing, she was noted to have a T9-10 block to pinprick stimuli and almost complete motor block (Bromage score = 2). Epidural 3% 2-chloroprocaine 5 mL was administered to try and achieve a higher level for surgical anesthesia, and after one minute a T6-7 sensory level was noted immediately before skin incision.

The anesthesia staff began transitioning to the daytime shift as surgery was beginning. Delivery of a healthy female infant occurred two minutes after skin incision, and neonatal Apgar scores were 8 at one minute and 9 at five minutes. No intraoperative cause for the nonreassuring FHR tracing was identified. Just prior to delivery, the patient reported difficulty breathing and was immediately transitioned to hand-assisted ventilation through the anesthesia circuit and facemask. On further examination, she was completely unable to move her upper extremities or turn her head. However, she was able to speak quietly, initiate breaths, cough, blink her eyes, protrude her tongue, and move her facial muscles. She had sensory blockade at the C2 dermatome level, as she was unable to feel pinprick stimuli on her arms, neck, and posterior scalp areas. Her facial sensation remained intact. Repeat epidural catheter aspiration appeared negative for cerebrospinal fluid (CSF).

She did not display any hypotension, bradycardia, or loss of consciousness with the development of high neuroblockade. Her blood pressure ranged within 105–125/50–65 mm Hg and heart rate was 103–112 beats/min during the operative course, and she did not require additional vasopressor or inotropic or chronotropic support. She maintained a respiratory rate of 20–24 breaths/min and pulse oximetry 99-100% on mask-assisted ventilation with fraction of inspired oxygen of 50% and peak inspiratory pressure kept at 10–12 cm H_2O using the adjustable pressure limiting valve. The mask-assisted ventilation, supplemental oxygen, and potentially the initial doses of IV ephedrine and glycopyrrolate allowed her to remain stable and comfortable. She did not desire intubation despite counseling regarding the potential risks of respiratory compromise due to muscle weakness and aspiration, though it was agreed that intubation would be performed if her clinical condition worsened. The willingness of the anesthesia providers and patient to continue with noninvasive ventilatory support was impacted by the patient's hemodynamic stability, normal mentation, ease of mask-assisted ventilation, preserved laryngeal motor function, and at least partially preserved diaphragmatic function. Additionally, she had not had oral food intake for more than twelve hours and no clear liquid intake for more than three hours. IV metoclopramide 10 mg was administered to increase gastric emptying. The patient remained remarkably calm despite the high neuroblockade that occurred, though she eventually began to have mild anxiety and received IV midazolam 2 mg for anxiolysis, given in divided doses five minutes apart. The midazolam was given incrementally to minimize the risk of oversedation and hypoventilation in this patient requiring mask-assisted respirations. Epidural morphine 2 mg is usually given for postcesarean analgesia at our institution, but in this case it was decided to withhold epidural morphine given the complication of high neuroblockade and the fact that an intrathecal catheter could not be completely ruled out.

Forty-five minutes after the 3% 2-chloroprocaine dose, the sensory blockade to pinprick had regressed to the C3-4 level. Respirations were assisted for a total of one hour, at which point testing revealed a C5-6 sensory level. She was then able to resume unassisted ventilation with supplemental oxygen administered by simple facemask at 5 L/min. After another hour, she had a T2-3 sensory level, demonstrated full grip strength, and was breathing comfortably on nasal cannula at 2 L/min. She was transferred to the recovery area in stable condition. After two hours in recovery, her sensory blockade had regressed to the L1 level and motor function was returning in her lower extremities. The remainder of her hospital stay was uncomplicated and she was discharged along with her baby on postpartum day three.

3. Discussion

The incidence of high neuraxial block requiring intubation or conversion to general anesthesia was recently reported to be 1 of 4,336 neuraxial anesthetics in obstetric patients [2]. High neuroblockade has been associated with unrecognized intrathecal administration of local anesthetic [2, 3] and with spinal anesthesia after failed epidural block [2, 4, 5] but can also occur with epidural catheter dosing [2, 3]. While an unrecognized intrathecal catheter cannot be completely ruled out in this case, it is very unlikely given the patient had a continuous epidural infusion for three hours without developing high neuroblockade and catheter aspiration remained negative for CSF. In addition, the volume of local anesthetic dosed for cesarean delivery likely would have resulted in a total spinal blockade if it were an intrathecal catheter. Rapid dosing of epidural medications under emergent circumstances most likely led to the high blockade observed. Epidural 2% lidocaine with 1 : 200,000 epinephrine has been observed to take ten minutes to achieve a surgical blockade for cesarean delivery [6, 7], and thus the onset of neuraxial blockade from the initial dosing had not fully taken effect prior to the epidural administration of 3% 2-chloroprocaine. Anesthesia providers may be pressed to rapidly provide extension of epidural blockade for cesarean anesthesia in emergent or urgent circumstances, but this case serves as an important example that epidural dosing should be performed gradually and incrementally in order to optimize patient safety [8].

IV ephedrine and glycopyrrolate administration during epidural dosing may have aided in preventing the onset of hypotension, bradycardia, or loss of consciousness that can occur with high neuroblockade of this magnitude. It should be noted that there is not good evidence to support routine administration of IV ephedrine and glycopyrrolate to prevent onset of hypotension or bradycardia induced by neuraxial blockade. Phenylephrine is considered the first-line vasopressor for routine management of spinal or epidural-induced hypotension in obstetric patients at our institution and many others given that it is more effective at preventing hypotension and is associated with less fetal acidosis compared to ephedrine [9]. When given prior to spinal anesthesia for cesarean delivery, glycopyrrolate has been shown to increase heart rate and cardiac output while lowering vasopressor dosing requirements, though it has not been shown to improve maternal or neonatal outcomes and is not routinely administered in many practices [10]. In cases of high neuroblockade accompanied by significant hypotension or bradycardia, IV epinephrine is likely a more appropriate vasopressor selection given its rapid onset and the direct adrenergic agonist can effectively manage bradycardia due to blockade of cardioaccelerator fibers or from diminished venous return [11].

The phrenic nerve arises from C3–5 before providing motor innervation to the diaphragm [12], and despite demonstrating a C2 sensory blockade our patient retained at least partial diaphragmatic function exhibited by the ability to initiate breaths. Differential nerve block in which sensory blockade is several levels higher than motor blockade may occur with both spinal and epidural anesthesia [13, 14]. Differential motor and sensory blockade can be observed in routine clinical practice if lower extremity motor function and sensory levels are closely evaluated during initiation of spinal or epidural anesthesia, though we are unaware of any previous reports of preserved phrenic nerve function despite C2 sensory blockade. The differential blockade observed in this case contributed to the patient's ability to remain stable with hand-assisted ventilation for approximately 60 minutes, and this approach avoided the need for intubation and general anesthesia.

Obstetric patients undergoing cesarean delivery are considered to be at elevated risk for pulmonary aspiration of gastric contents, and aspiration risk was an important consideration in the management of our patient. Aspiration accounted for 23% of anesthesia-related maternal deaths in the United States from 1979 to 1990, though a more recent report did not list aspiration as a cause of anesthesia-related mortality from 1990 to 2002 [1, 15]. A recent report of serious complications in obstetric anesthesia did not document any cases of aspiration in more than 257,000 anesthetics, including more than 5000 general anesthetics [2]. The decreasing incidence of significant aspiration events may be due to increased use of neuraxial anesthesia for cesarean delivery, adherence to *nil per os* standards for parturients, and use of aspiration prophylaxis medications. Based on these reports, it is apparent that maternal aspiration is rare in current practice, though it is difficult to counsel patients on the exact incidence of aspiration in obstetric patients. The patient in this case had not had recent oral intake and also received aspiration prophylaxis in the form of sodium citrate and metoclopramide in an attempt to reduce the likelihood or severity of a potential aspiration event. Importantly, she maintained the ability to cough and protect her airway from aspiration, which was expected even in the setting of sensory blockade up to C2 given that laryngeal innervation is through the recurrent laryngeal and superior laryngeal nerve branches of the vagus nerve [16]. Endotracheal intubation at the time high neuraxial blockade became apparent was considered as an option, but the anesthesia providers and patient felt comfortable

continuing with mask-assisted ventilation in the setting of hemodynamic stability, normal mentation, preserved vocal cord function, no recent oral intake, and relative ease of mask-assisted breathing. Changes in any of these factors would likely have prompted endotracheal intubation, and thus it was important to have IV induction medications and intubating equipment immediately available.

Competing Interests

The authors declare that there is no conflict of interests in regard to the publication of this paper.

References

[1] J. L. Hawkins, J. Chang, S. K. Palmer, C. P. Gibbs, and W. M. Callaghan, "Anesthesia-related maternal mortality in the United States: 1979–2002," *Obstetrics and Gynecology*, vol. 117, no. 1, pp. 69–74, 2011.

[2] R. D'Angelo, R. M. Smiley, E. T. Riley, and S. Segal, "Serious complications related to obstetric anesthesia: the serious complication repository project of the society for obstetric Anesthesia and Perinatology," *Anesthesiology*, vol. 120, no. 6, pp. 1505–1512, 2014.

[3] J. M. Davies, K. L. Posner, L. A. Lee, F. W. Cheney, and K. B. Domino, "Liability associated with obstetric anesthesia: a closed claims analysis," *Anesthesiology*, vol. 110, no. 1, pp. 131–139, 2009.

[4] S. R. Furst and L. S. Reisner, "Risk of high spinal anesthesia following failed epidural block for cesarean delivery," *Journal of Clinical Anesthesia*, vol. 7, no. 1, pp. 71–74, 1995.

[5] G. M. Stocks, "When using spinal anaesthesia for caesarean section after the epidural has failed, the normal dose of spinal anaesthetic should be used," *International Journal of Obstetric Anesthesia*, vol. 14, no. 1, pp. 55–57, 2005.

[6] D. T. C. Lam, W. D. Ngan Kee, and K. S. Khaw, "Extension of epidural blockade in labour for emergency Caesarean section using 2% lidocaine with epinephrine and fentanyl, with or without alkalinisation," *Anaesthesia*, vol. 56, no. 8, pp. 790–794, 2001.

[7] D. N. Lucas, G. K. Ciccone, and S. M. Yentis, "Extending low-dose epidural analgesia for emergency Caesarean section. A comparison of three solutions," *Anaesthesia*, vol. 54, no. 12, pp. 1173–1177, 1999.

[8] D. Wlody, "Complications of regional anesthesia in obstetrics," *Clinical Obstetrics and Gynecology*, vol. 46, no. 3, pp. 667–678, 2003.

[9] W. D. Ngan Kee, A. Lee, K. S. Khaw, F. F. Ng, M. K. Karmakar, and T. Gin, "A randomized double-blinded comparison of phenylephrine and ephedrine infusion combinations to maintain blood pressure during spinal anesthesia for cesarean delivery: the effects on fetal acid-base status and hemodynamic control," *Anesthesia & Analgesia*, vol. 107, pp. 1295–1302, 2008.

[10] W. D. Ngan Kee, S. W. Y. Lee, K. S. Khaw, and F. F. Ng, "Haemodynamic effects of glycopyrrolate pre-treatment before phenylephrine infusion during spinal anaesthesia for caesarean

delivery," *International Journal of Obstetric Anesthesia*, vol. 22, no. 3, pp. 179–187, 2013.

[11] J. B. Pollard, "Cardiac arrest during spinal anesthesia: common mechanisms and strategies for prevention," *Anesthesia and Analgesia*, vol. 92, no. 1, pp. 252–256, 2001.

[12] T. Hamada, A. Usami, A. Kishi, H. Kon, and S. Takada, "Anatomical study of phrenic nerve course in relation to neck dissection," *Surgical and Radiologic Anatomy*, vol. 37, no. 3, pp. 255–258, 2016.

[13] B. R. Fink, "Mechanisms of differential axial blockade in epidural and subarachnoid anesthesia," *Anesthesiology*, vol. 70, no. 5, pp. 851–858, 1989.

[14] D. P. Chamberlain and R. D. Crawford, "Integrated electromyographic measurement of abdominal motor blockade during bupivacaine epidural anesthesia for lower abdominal and pelvic surgery," *Anesthesia & Analgesia*, vol. 66, no. 1, pp. 57–63, 1987.

[15] J. L. Hawkins, L. M. Koonin, S. K. Palmer, and C. P. Gibbs, "Anesthesia-related deaths during obstetric delivery in the United States, 1979–1990," *Anesthesiology*, vol. 86, no. 2, pp. 277–284, 1997.

[16] J. W. Dankbaar and F. A. Pameijer, "Vocal cord paralysis: anatomy, imaging and pathology," *Insights into Imaging*, vol. 5, no. 6, pp. 743–751, 2014.

42

Anesthetic Management for Laser Excision of Ball-Valving Laryngeal Masses

Benjamin B. Bruins,[1] Natasha Mirza,[2] Ernest Gomez,[3] and Joshua H. Atkins[4]

[1]Department of Anesthesiology & Critical Care, Hospital of the University of Pennsylvania, Philadelphia, PA 19104, USA
[2]Department of Otorhinolaryngology, Head and Neck Surgery, Perelman School of Medicine, The University of Pennsylvania, Philadelphia, PA 19104, USA
[3]Department of Otorhinolaryngology, Head and Neck Surgery, Hospital of the University of Pennsylvania, Philadelphia, PA 19104, USA
[4]Department of Anesthesiology & Critical Care, Department of Otorhinolaryngology, Head and Neck Surgery, Perelman School of Medicine, The University of Pennsylvania, PA 19104, USA

Correspondence should be addressed to Joshua H. Atkins; atkinsj@uphs.upenn.edu

Academic Editor: Pavel Michalek

A 47-year-old obese woman with GERD and COPD presents for CO_2-laser excision of bilateral vocal fold masses. She had a history of progressive hoarseness and difficulty in breathing. Nasopharyngeal laryngoscopy revealed large, mobile, bilateral vocal cord polyps that demonstrated dynamic occlusion of the glottis. We describe the airway and anesthetic management of this patient with a topicalized C-MAC video laryngoscopic intubation using a 4.5 mm Xomed Laser Shield II endotracheal tube. We examine the challenges of anesthetic management unique to the combined circumstances of a ball-valve lesion and the need for a narrow-bore laser compatible endotracheal tube.

1. Introduction

Airway management of the patient with a glottic lesion producing dynamic total airway occlusion (ball-valve effect) requires a specialized management plan [1]. Induction of general anesthesia, loss of hypopharyngeal tone, abolition of spontaneous ventilation, and initiation of positive pressure ventilation can result in the inability to ventilate and/or intubate. For these reasons, airway management in patients with large or periglottic airway masses is often accomplished with awake or minimally sedated fiberoptic bronchoscopic endotracheal tube placement [2, 3]. The added requirement for laser surgery at the glottis around a narrow-bore (<6 mm) endotracheal tube limits this approach. We describe successful topicalized-sedated intubation with Storz C-MAC (Karl Storz, Tuttlingen, Germany) videolaryngoscopy and characterize technical limitations associated with blind techniques and laser tubes.

The patient gave written consent for publication of the details of the case.

2. Case Description

A 47-year-old, obese (BMI 33) woman with GERD, COPD, and 60-pack year smoking history presented to the operative theater for CO_2-laser excision of bilateral vocal fold polyps. Home medications included a proton pump inhibitor and inhaled beta-2 agonist. Preoperative nasopharyngeal laryngoscopy demonstrated a left highly mobile polyp that herniated from a supraglottic position during expiration to a subglottic position during inspiration and a smaller right polyp. Airway occlusion was estimated at 70–80% by the surgical team as depicted in video 1 in Supplementary Material available online at http://dx.doi.org/10.1155/2015/875053. The patient declined tracheostomy and was scheduled for an elective resection of the polyps in the operating room. Physical examination revealed full neck mobility, the ability to sublux her mandible, intact dentition, 3 cm mentohyoid distance, 4 cm interincisor distance, and Mallampati score of 1. History was significant for hoarseness and an exaggerated gag reflex. The surgical plan was mass excision employing the CO_2-laser and a 4.5 mm laser-resistant endotracheal tube was requested to facilitate exposure.

Nebulized lidocaine (2%, 8 mL, 8 L/min) was administered in the holding area over 15 minutes. The patient was brought to the operating room, positioned 40 degrees head-up on the operating room table, ASA standard monitors were applied, and ondansetron (4 mg) was administered. Nasal cannula oxygen (4 L/min) with end-tidal CO_2 sampling was placed. A bolus of intravenous dexmedetomidine (1 mcg/kg) was administered over 10 minutes during which a remifentanil infusion was started (0.05 mcg/kg/min). An Ovassapian intubating oral airway with a dollop of 5% lidocaine ointment on the tip was placed and allowed to sit for 5 minutes. A first attempt at laryngoscopy with a C-MAC D-Blade produced gagging, so additional lidocaine 2% (4 mL) was administered to the posterior oropharynx with a MADgic atomizer (Teleflex Medical, Research Triangle Park, NC) and a 0.2 mcg/kg bolus of remifentanil delivered. The CMAC D-Blade was reintroduced with minimal coughing to reveal a grade I view of the glottis and the lesions. A 4.5 mm ID Xomed Laser Shield II endotracheal tube (Medtronic Xomed, Jacksonville, FL) with stylet was passed through the cords under indirect visualization. The endotracheal tube cuff was inflated to a minimal occlusion volume with methylene blue tinted normal saline. General anesthesia was induced with propofol and remifentanil and maintained with those agents and a background dexmedetomidine infusion (0.3 mcg/kg/h). Empiric dexamethasone (10 mg) was administered to limit airway edema. Additional measures to minimize risk of airway fire included reduction of FiO_2 to 40% and the use of moist gauze in and around the airway.

Suspension laryngoscopy and CO_2-laser excision commenced. During the repositioning of the surgical laryngoscope for resection of the second lesion the patient developed two episodes of profound bradycardia that evolved to transient asystole. This was effectively treated with immediate removal of the laryngoscope, sixty seconds of CPR, intravenous atropine (0.5 mg), and cessation of dexmedetomidine infusion. Suspension laryngoscopy was repeated and the second lesion was resected without further event. The patient emerged smoothly from anesthesia, evidenced no postoperative respiratory distress, and required no additional medications (e.g., racemic epinephrine and albuterol) for airway maintenance. The patient was wide-awake 30 minutes after surgery and expressed a strong preference for the same-day discharge and signed out against medical advice.

3. Discussion

Airway management of the patient with a glottic lesion producing dynamic, airway occlusion (ball-valve effect) requires a specialized management plan [1]. Induction of general anesthesia, loss of hypopharyngeal tone, abolition of spontaneous

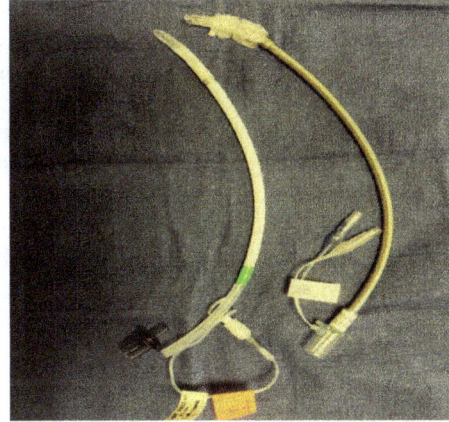

FIGURE 1: 4.5 mm ID Xomed Laser Shield II (left) and laser-safe (right) endotracheal tubes.

ventilation, and initiation of positive pressure ventilation can promote total airway obstruction and result in the inability to ventilate and/or intubate. Traditional airway rescue techniques of cricothyrotomy or LMA will be limited in the event of an obstructing into the glottis. Awake tracheostomy may be considered in this setting, but the patient refused this option and the surgeon was confident that a near total resection was feasible without the associated morbidity of a tracheostomy. While we have previously described the technique of subglottic HFJV [4], in light of the complexity of the resection, the anticipated duration, and the pulmonary comorbidities of the patient, the team elected endotracheal intubation.

Airway management of the "difficult airway" is often accomplished with awake or minimally sedated fiberoptic bronchoscopic intubation. The added requirement for laser surgery at the glottis around a narrow-bore (<6 mm) endotracheal tube with a mobile glottic lesion limits the appeal of this approach. The "blind" translation of an endotracheal tube over a gum-elastic bougie, tube exchange catheter (e.g., if downsizing to a smaller tube), or fiberoptic scope is commonly associated with tube impingement on the arytenoid or vocal folds [5]. Such an approach also risks obstruction or bleeding into the airway should the tube encounter the airway lesions during passage.

Selection of the appropriate laser-resistant endotracheal tube is of utmost importance. The Xomed Laser Shield Tube II (Medtronic, Minneapolis, MN) is made of silicone rubber wrapped with aluminum and Teflon (see Figure 1) and offers several advantages. In contrast with the Laser Flex endotracheal tube (Mallinckrodt, St. Louis, MO), the connector is removable and the pilot balloon connectors are external to the lumen allowing a 2.9 mm fiberoptic bronchoscope to tightly translate through even the smallest 4.5 mm ID tube. Additionally, the Xomed Laser Shield Tube II is more pliable which facilitates manipulation and may limit tube related trauma to friable lesions.

Sustained airway obstruction is unlikely in the spontaneously ventilating patient under minimal sedation. Surgical direct laryngoscopy (MDL) with introduction of a cannula across the lesion for oxygen delivery would be one rescue option. Rigid bronchoscopy and formal awake tracheostomy should be considered as alternative strategies. Awake videolaryngoscopy (VL) offers a safe and practical approach to intubation, preserving the ability to visualize the glottis, the lesion, and movements of the endotracheal tube during intubation. The entire surgical and anesthesia team can follow the intubation in an effort to maximize safety and facilitate immediate expert input should intubation prove challenging. A growing body of evidence supports awake VL or combined awake VL and fiberoptic guidance for complex airway management [6–9]. Each respective VL technique offers unique advantages. For a glottic lesion it is important to visualize the tip of the blade as it transits towards the larynx. The GlideScope (Verathon Medical, Bothell, WA) does not allow for continuous distal tip visualization [10]. Stylet options are also important. The traditional rigid GlideScope stylet, recommended for most intubations, cannot pass through a 4.5 ID laser tube. Some devices such as the PENTAX Airway Scope (AWS, Ambu A/S, Ballerup, Denmark) offer an intubating channel that eliminates the need for a stylet altogether but are recommended to use with a straight blade approach that might not be suitable for all lesions. Similarly when using some devices it can be challenging to reliably introduce suction directly to the area of the glottis to clear bleeding or secretions during laryngoscopy. We selected the Storz CMAC VL for the ability to continuously visualize the tip of the blade, reliably deliver surgical suction to the glottis if bleeding should occur, and use a narrow, malleable stylet if needed.

Various approaches to patient sedation and airway preparation for awake laryngoscopy have been described and largely parallel those adopted for fiberoptic intubation. Dexmedetomidine is a useful sedative in this setting as respiratory depression is minimal and patients retain the ability to follow commands, including deep inspiration and expiration that promote opening of the airway. Dexmedetomidine decreases sympathetic circulating norepinephrine levels and is associated with bradycardia [11]. Remifentanil is also associated with bradycardia and laryngoscopy exerts a profound stimulus of vagal activity. We believe that the drug combination along with the self-reported history of a profound gag reflex and the receding effects of topical lidocaine 60 minutes into the procedure contributed to the asystole. Pretreatment with an anticholinergic agent should be considered when the combination of dexmedetomidine and remifentanil is used for suspension laryngoscopy.

Acknowledgment

The authors acknowledge the helpful suggestions of Jeff E. Mandel, M.D., M.S., in preparation of the paper.

References

[1] R. E. Dalmeida, J. F. Mayhew, B. Driscoll, and R. McLaughlin, "Total airway obstruction by papillomas during induction of general anesthesia," *Anesthesia and Analgesia*, vol. 83, no. 6, pp. 1332–1334, 1996.

[2] C. V. Rosenstock, B. Thøgersen, A. Afshari, A.-L. Christensen, C. Eriksen, and M. R. Gätke, "Awake fiberoptic or awake video laryngoscopic tracheal intubation in patients with anticipated difficult airway management: a randomized clinical trial," *Anesthesiology*, vol. 116, no. 6, pp. 1210–1216, 2012.

[3] W. H. Rosenblatt, P. J. Wagner, A. Ovassapian, and Z. N. Kain, "Practice patterns in managing the difficult airway by anesthesiologists in the United States," *Anesthesia and Analgesia*, vol. 87, no. 1, pp. 153–157, 1998.

[4] J. E. Mandel, G. E. R. Weller, S. K. Chennupati, and N. Mirza, "Transglottic high frequency jet ventilation for management of laryngeal fracture associated with air bag deployment injury," *Journal of Clinical Anesthesia*, vol. 20, no. 5, pp. 369–371, 2008.

[5] D. M. Johnson, A. M. From, R. B. Smith, R. P. From, and M. A. Maktabi, "Endoscopic study of mechanisms of failure of endotracheal tube advancement into the trachea during awake fiberoptic orotracheal intubation," *Anesthesiology*, vol. 102, no. 5, pp. 910–914, 2005.

[6] V. K. Dimitriou, I. D. Zogogiannis, and D. G. Liotiri, "Awake tracheal intubation using the Airtraq laryngoscope: a case series," *Acta Anaesthesiologica Scandinavica*, vol. 53, no. 7, pp. 964–967, 2009.

[7] J. Jeyadoss, N. Nanjappa, and D. Nemeth, "Awake intubation using Pentax AWS video-laryngoscope after failed fibreoptic intubation in a morbidly obese patient with a massive thyroid tumour and tracheal compression," *Anaesthesia and Intensive Care*, vol. 39, no. 2, pp. 311–312, 2011.

[8] A. A. Abdellatif and M. A. Ali, "Glidescopespi videolaryngoscope versus flexible fiberoptic bronchoscope for awake intubation of morbidly obese patient with predicted difficult intubation," *Middle East Journal of Anesthesiology*, vol. 22, no. 4, pp. 385–392, 2014.

[9] S.-Q. Li, J.-L. Chen, H.-B. Fu, J. Xu, and L.-H. Chen, "Airway management in pediatric patients undergoing suspension laryngoscopic surgery for severe laryngeal obstruction caused by papillomatosis," *Paediatric Anaesthesia*, vol. 20, no. 12, pp. 1084–1091, 2010.

[10] P. B. Richardson and I. Hodzovic, "Awake tracheal intubation using videolaryngoscopy: importance of blade design," *Anaesthesia*, vol. 67, no. 7, pp. 798–799, 2012.

[11] C. Liu, Y. Zhang, S. She, L. Xu, and X. Ruan, "A randomised controlled trial of dexmedetomidine for suspension laryngoscopy," *Anaesthesia*, vol. 68, no. 1, pp. 60–66, 2013.

43

Is It Possible to Maintain Consciousness and Spontaneous Ventilation with Chest Compression in the Early Phase of Cardiac Arrest?

Menekse Oksar and Selim Turhanoglu

Department of Anesthesiology and Reanimation, Mustafa Kemal University Faculty of Medicine, 31100 Hatay, Turkey

Correspondence should be addressed to Menekse Oksar; menekseoksar@gmail.com

Academic Editor: Pavel Michalek

Chest compression is important in cardiopulmonary resuscitation. However, life support algorithms do not specify when chest compression should be initiated in patients with persistent spontaneous normal breathing in the early phase after cardiac arrest. Here we describe the case of a 69-year-old man who underwent femoral bypass surgery and was extubated at the end of the procedure. After extubation, the patient's breathing pattern and respiratory rate were normal. The patient subsequently developed ventricular fibrillation, evident on two monitors. Because defibrillation was ineffective, chest compression was initiated even though the patient had spontaneous normal breathing and defensive motor reflexes, which were continued throughout resuscitation. He regained consciousness and underwent tracheal extubation without neurological sequelae on postoperative day 1. This case highlights the necessity of chest compression in the early phase of cardiac arrest.

1. Introduction

The 2010 American Heart Association recommendations and European Resuscitation Council guidelines for cardiopulmonary resuscitation (CPR) focus on the requirement of immediately initiating chest compression and ventilation to maintain cerebral blood flow and adequate gas exchange, respectively [1]. Maintaining cerebral perfusion prevents neurological damage. Some studies have shown that conscious, spontaneous breathing may continue for a short time after cerebral perfusion stops; for example, repeated rhythmic coughs every 1–3 s maintained consciousness for up to 39 s in three patients who developed ventricular fibrillation during coronary arteriography [2]. Cardiac arrest survivors recall memories of awareness, fear, and persecution after CPR [3]. Early diagnosis of cardiac arrest may prolong spontaneous breathing and consciousness by maintaining cerebral perfusion through effective chest compression. We present a 69-year-old man with uninterrupted spontaneous normal breathing during CPR.

2. Case Report

A 69-year-old man (American Society of Anesthesiologists class 2; weight 70 kg; height 1.72 m) with peripheral arterial disease and diabetes mellitus underwent femoral bypass surgery. Anesthesia was induced using 2 mg midazolam, 100 μg fentanyl, and 2 mg/kg propofol. Endotracheal intubation was achieved with 40 mg rocuronium, anesthesia was maintained by 2% sevoflurane with N_2O and 50% O_2, and diuretic and insulin infusions were administered as required. The patient showed normal blood gas levels (pH, 7.36; $PaCO_2$, 43 mmHg; PaO_2, 92 mmHg; lactate, 3.5 mmol/L; and base excess, 1.2 mmol/L). His blood glucose level was 220 mg/dL, O_2 saturation level was 99% on 50% O_2, heart rate (HR) was 88 beats/min, and mean arterial pressure (MAP) was 70 mmHg. Neuromuscular blockade was reversed using 200 mg sugammadex, and the patient was extubated. Thereafter, his breathing pattern was regular, with a respiratory rate of 17 breaths/min and a tidal volume of 600 mL. Oxyhemoglobin saturation determined using pulse oximetry was 99%, invasive arterial blood pressure was 140/90 mmHg (MAP, 106 mmHg), and HR was 100 beats/min. Further, a transport monitor was connected.

The patient subsequently developed ventricular fibrillation (VF), evident on 2 monitors. A biphasic 150-J shock was administered immediately, and ventilation was initiated with a facemask supplying O_2 at 6 L/min before his trachea was reintubated without a neuromuscular blocking agent. Ventilatory support was manually administered because he was breathing spontaneously. After the first shock, external cardiac massage was applied for 2 min. However, the patient remained in VF; therefore, a second shock was administered, followed by further chest compression. The patient became asystolic and received 1 mg intravenous epinephrine. Although spontaneous breathing persisted, CPR was continued. Shocks and chest compression continued for 1 h, with epinephrine administered every 3–5 min with short breaks to assess cardiac rhythm. The chest compression evoked defensive motor reflexes, such as flexion of the neck, trunk, and arms, and arterial traces were determined to originate from external cardiac massage during resuscitation.

During resuscitation, arterial blood gas recordings showed acidosis with an abnormally low pH, high lactate, and low base excess. $PaCO_2$ was normal during VF and resuscitation, but it increased by the end of resuscitation. Although assisted breathing was provided throughout resuscitation, the rate of spontaneous breathing was 16-17 breaths/min with a tidal volume of 600 mL/min. During resuscitation, end-tidal CO_2 was 19–22 mmHg. The potassium level was normal intraoperatively (3.6 mmol/L), reduced during resuscitation (2.0 mmol/L), and increased with potassium replacement therapy by the end of resuscitation (3.2 mmol/L). The patient remained asystolic until circulation resumed spontaneously. After resuscitation, the HR was recorded at 51 beats/min with ST depression observed on electrocardiography (ECG) (Table 1). Measurements recorded at baseline, preoperatively, during CPR, and after CPR are shown in Table 1. Spontaneous breathing continued without interruption throughout the entire CPR period. Following tracheal intubation, ventilation was manually assisted with the balloon of a breathing circuit throughout the entire CPR period and an Ambu bag during patient transfer following resuscitation. The actual measured duration of asystole was 50 min. VF lasted for approximately 10 minutes. During cardiac arrest, defibrillation attempts were made and chest compression was initiated in order to maintain adequate blood pressure. CPR was continued until potential underlying correctable causes of VF (such as the hypokalemia and low arterial pH levels in the present case) were determined and corrective interventions could be performed. Approximately 1 hour after correction of the metabolic causes of VF, during which spontaneous breathing and continued motor responses to chest compression without QRS complexes on electrocardiography were observed, the patient was reviewed by a cardiologist and was subsequently transferred to coronary angiography for further investigations. ECG and ventilatory data at the end of CPR were given as supplementary material (Figure S1 in Supplementary Material available online at http://dx.doi.org/10.1155/2016/3158015).

During angiography, the patient again developed asystole requiring further chest compression but responded to CPR and was transferred to the cardiovascular surgery intensive care unit. Coronary angiography was reported as normal. The patient regained consciousness on postoperative day 1, was extubated, and showed no evidence of neurological sequelae. Written consent for the publication of this report was obtained from the patient postoperatively.

3. Discussion

A significantly increased incidence of ventricular tachycardia (VT) and VF has been reported after reperfusion therapy for patients with myocardial infarction and systemic acidosis [4]. There is evidence that systemic metabolic acidosis is a strong predictor of VT/VF after reperfusion of ST-elevation myocardial infarction associated with inflammation [5]. However, the causal relationship between systemic acidosis secondary to myocardial ischemia and VT/VF is complex, and the trigger is not always obvious. In this case, the lactic acidosis after surgical clamping coupled with the final low HCO_3^- may have created a high-anion-gap metabolic acidosis that caused VF. Another possibility is that using insulin or diuretics caused hypokalemia, which induced VF.

Although VF is the most frequent cause of cardiac arrest and death, it is reversible if treated early. Failure to commence CPR between cardiac arrest and the cessation of spontaneous breathing may cause irreversible brain injury. Therefore, current guidelines recommend immediate chest compression for unresponsive patients who are breathing abnormally [6]. For spontaneously breathing patients who are unresponsive or unconscious, guidelines recommended they should be placed in the recovery position because spontaneous breathing is considered a reliable sign of effective cardiac activity [1]. However, a few reports have demonstrated that normal spontaneous breathing, and even consciousness, continues for a short time after a cardiac arrest.

In one study of 8 patients, breathing pattern, frequency, and tidal volume were found to be unchanged in the first 12–15 s of VF [7]. These findings were confirmed in adult sheep, where breathing patterns were unchanged for 15 s and minute ventilation increased for 55 ± 44 s before stopping abruptly. Agonal breathing efforts have been reported to begin 37 ± 38 s into the apneic period, whereas there is evidence that normal breathing ceases after 12–60 s and that agonal breathing can persist for up to 6 min [8]. Agonal breathing was reported in 40% of 445 out-of-hospital cardiac arrests, where it was more frequent in patients with VF and was associated with increased survival [9]. Our patient continued to breathe spontaneously throughout CPR, perhaps because of the early and uninterrupted breathing support, and we did not detect agonal breathing.

As mentioned previously, rhythmic coughs have been shown to prolong consciousness in VF [2], whereas survivors of cardiac arrest have reported a broad range of cognitive experiences. Furthermore, 2% (2 of 101 patients) have reported retaining full awareness [3]. Although it is unclear whether the experiences during cardiac arrest refer to actual events or hallucinations, the finding that conscious

TABLE 1: Perioperative arterial blood gas, peak end-tidal partial CO$_2$ pressure, and concomitant hemodynamic parameter measurements (*bold column, time of VF initiation; italic columns, cardiac arrest period*).

Measurement number	T1	T2	**T3**	*T4*	*T5*	*T6*	*T7*	T8	T9	T10
pH	7.45	7.36	**7.01**	*No result*	*7.19*	*7.26*	*7.05*	7.12	7.39	7.40
PaCO$_2$ (mmHg)	40	43	**39**	*No result*	*47*	*61*	*78*	56	34	68
ETCO$_2$ (mmHg)	25	25	**Not monitored ETCO$_2$**	*Not monitored ETCO$_2$*	*19*	*19*	*21*	22	Not monitored	Not monitored
Base excess	3.5	−1.2	**−21**	*No result*	*−9.9*	*−0.2*	*−9.3*	−10.7	−3.7	−3.1
PaO$_2$ (mmHg)	126	220	**126**	*No result*				92	93	68
Lactate (mMol/L)	2.0	3.5	**7.5**	*7.5*	*8.0*	*8.0*	*8.5*	11.7	6.0	3.5
Glucose (mg/dL)	126	220	**205**					256		
Potassium (mMol/L)	3.5	3.6	**2.0**	*2.2*	*2.8*	*3.0*	*3.2*	4.0	3.6	3.2
FiO$_2$ (%)	50	50	**Room air**	*100*	*100*	*100*	*100*	100	100	Room air
Cardiac rhythm	Sinus	Sinus	**VF**	*Asystole*	*Asystole*	*Asystole*	*Asystole*	Bradycardia	Sinus	Sinus
HR (beat/minute)	67	70	**Not applicable**	*0*	*100*	*100*	*100*	51	80	88
MAP (mmHg)	60	60	**No pressure**	*No pressure*	*60*	*65*	*65*	60	68	85
SpO$_2$ (%)	99	99	**Unreadable**	*Unreadable*	*Unreadable*	*Unreadable*	*Unreadable*	Unreadable	97	95

CPR, cardiopulmonary resuscitation; ETCO$_2$, peak end-tidal partial pressure of CO$_2$; FiO$_2$, fractional inspired O$_2$ concentration; HR, heart rate; MAP, mean arterial pressure; PaCO$_2$, arterial partial pressure of CO$_2$; PaO$_2$, arterial partial pressure of O$_2$; SpO$_2$, O$_2$ saturation; VF, ventricular fibrillation.
T1, baseline; T2, intraoperative period; T3, postoperative VF and defibrillation; T4, after 2 min of CPR after defibrillation attempts; T5, resuscitation 1; T6, resuscitation 2; T7, resuscitation 3; T8, resuscitation 4; T9, postoperative day 1; T10, after tracheal extubation on postoperative day 1.

awareness can remain during cardiac arrest is intriguing and supports other recent studies indicating that consciousness may be present despite clinically undetectable consciousness. Another report has suggested that functional neuroimaging techniques can assist with the prognosis and diagnosis of patients with disorders of consciousness [10]. Notably, our patient displayed defensive motor reflexes in response to painful stimuli (chest compression) but denied any recollection.

In conclusion, because respiratory neurons can maintain respiration immediately after cardiac arrest, it can be misleading to assume that any normal breathing movements preclude a diagnosis of cardiac arrest. Therefore, the first 10–15 s of a witnessed cardiac arrest are crucial to save patients' lives and prevent neurological sequelae. Although intervention during this time is critical, it will be difficult to implement appropriate interventions with unmonitored patients.

References

[1] J. P. Nolan, J. Soar, D. A. Zideman et al., "European resuscitation council guidelines for resuscitation 2010 section 1. Executive summary," *Resuscitation*, vol. 81, no. 10, pp. 1219–1276, 2010.

[2] J. M. Criley, A. H. Blaufuss, and G. L. Kissel, "Self administered cardiopulmonary resuscitation by cough induced cardiac compression," *Transactions of the American Clinical and Climatological Association*, vol. 87, pp. 138–146, 1976.

[3] S. Parnia, K. Spearpoint, G. de Vos et al., "AWARE-AWAreness during REsuscitation—a prospective study," *Resuscitation*, vol. 85, no. 12, pp. 1799–1805, 2014.

[4] T. Nagai, T. Anzai, H. Kaneko et al., "Impact of systemic acidosis on the development of malignant ventricular arrhythmias after reperfusion therapy for ST-elevation myocardial infarction," *Circulation Journal*, vol. 74, no. 9, pp. 1808–1814, 2010.

[5] S. Niwano and T. Tojo, "Systemic acidosis in acute myocardial ischemia—cause or result of life-threatening ventricular arrhythmia?" *Circulation Journal*, vol. 74, no. 9, pp. 1794–1795, 2010.

[6] R. A. Berg, R. Hemphill, B. S. Abella et al., "Part 5: adult basic life support: 2010 American Heart Association Guidelines for Cardiopulmonary Resuscitation and Emergency Cardiovascular Care," *Circulation*, vol. 122, no. 3, pp. S685–S705, 2010.

[7] P. Haouzi, N. Ahmadpour, H. J. Bell et al., "Breathing patterns during cardiac arrest," *Journal of Applied Physiology*, vol. 109, no. 2, pp. 405–411, 2010.

[8] M. W. Kroll, D. R. Lakkireddy, J. R. Stone, and R. M. Luceri, "TASER electronic control devices and cardiac arrests: coincidental or causal?" *Circulation*, vol. 129, no. 1, pp. 93–100, 2014.

[9] J. J. Clark, M. P. Larsen, L. L. Culley, J. R. Graves, and M. S. Eisenberg, "Incidence of agonal respirations in sudden cardiac arrest," *Annals of Emergency Medicine*, vol. 21, no. 12, pp. 1464–1467, 1992.

[10] D. Cruse and A. M. Owen, "Consciousness revealed: new insights into the vegetative and minimally conscious states," *Current Opinion in Neurology*, vol. 23, no. 6, pp. 656–660, 2010.

44

Ultrasound-Guided Multiple Peripheral Nerve Blocks in a Superobese Patient

Alper Kilicaslan,[1] **Ahmet Topal,**[1] **Atilla Erol,**[1] **Hale Borazan,**[1]
Onur Bilge,[2] **and Seref Otelcioglu**[1]

[1] Department of Anaesthesiology, Meram Medical Faculty, Necmettin Erbakan University, 42080 Konya, Turkey
[2] Department of Orthopaedic Surgery, Meram Medical Faculty, Necmettin Erbakan University, 42080 Konya, Turkey

Correspondence should be addressed to Alper Kilicaslan; dralperkilicaslan@gmail.com

Academic Editors: P. Michalek, C. Seefelder, D. A. Story, and E. A. Vandermeersch

The number of obese patients has increased dramatically worldwide. Morbid obesity is associated with an increased incidence of medical comorbidities and restricts the application choices in anesthesiology. We report a successfully performed combined ultrasound-guided blockade of the femoral, tibial, and common peroneal nerve in a superobese patient. We present a case report of a 31-year-old, ASA-PS II, super obese man (190 kg, 180 cm, BMI: 58 kg/m^2) admitted to the emergency department with a type II segmental tibia shaft fracture and ankle dislocation after a vehicle accident. After two failed spinal anesthesia attempts, we decided to apply a femoral block combined with a sciatic block. Femoral blocks were successfully performed with US guided in-plane technique. Separate blocks of the tibial and common peroneal nerves were planned after the sciatic nerve could not be located due to the thick subcutaneous tissue. We performed a tibial nerve block at 2 cm above the popliteal crease and common peroneal nerve at the level of the fibular head with US guided in-plane technique. The blocks were successful and no block-related complications were noted. Ultrasound guidance allows new approaches for multiple peripheral nerve blocks with low local anesthetic doses in obese patients.

1. Introduction

The number of obese patients is gradually increasing worldwide. The World Health Organization estimates that, by 2015, there will be 2.3 billion overweight (BMI 25–30 kg/m^2) and 700 million obese (BMI $>$ 30 kg/m^2) adults worldwide [1]. Anatomic and physiological alterations occur in association with obesity, particularly in the airway and in the cardiovascular, respiratory, gastrointestinal, and neurological organ systems. These changes increase the incidence of comorbidities and cause limitations and problems in anesthesiology procedures [2].

For obese patients, regional anesthesia provides many advantages compared to general anesthesia, such as avoiding airway manipulation and systemic effects of anesthetic agents, and provides better postoperative pain control [3]. However, the failure rate increases in regional anesthesia procedures performed in obese patients due to the increased depth of nerve structures, the disappearance of landmarks, and difficulties in positioning [4].

On the other hand, the increase in the use of ultrasonography in recent years eliminates many limitations. Ultrasonography enables direct visualization of nerve structures, reduction in complications, and identification of new peripheral nerve block approaches [5].

In this study, we aimed to present the anesthesia management of a superobese patient who underwent ultrasound-guided multiple peripheral nerve blocks (the femoral, tibial, and common peroneal nerves) following the failure of spinal anesthesia.

2. Case Report

A 31-year-old, ASA II, superobese male patient (190 kg, 180 cm, BMI: 58 kg/m^2) was admitted to the emergency department with a segmental Gustilo-Anderson type IIIA

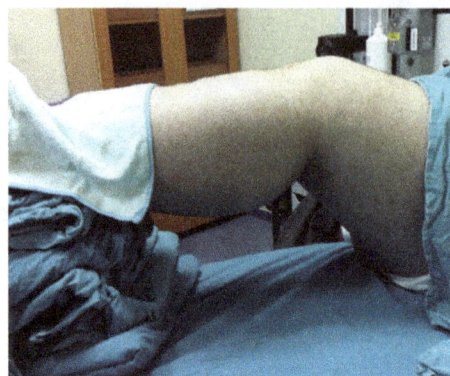

(a)

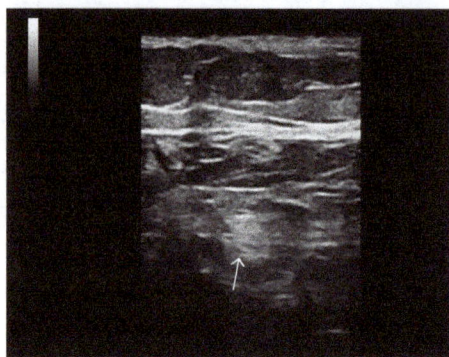

(b)

FIGURE 1: (a) Positioning for popliteal approach to the tibial nerve block. (b) Transverse sonogram in the popliteal region showing the tibial nerve as a hyperechoic nodule (arrow).

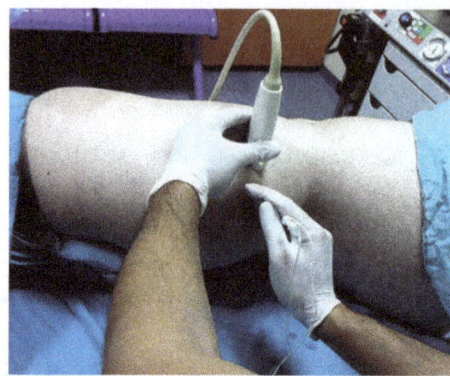

(a)

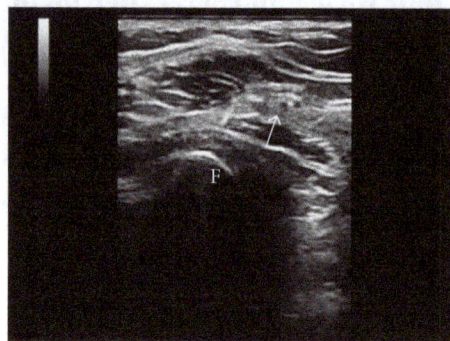

(b)

FIGURE 2: (a) Ultrasound probe placement for common peroneal nerve block at the head of the fibula. (b) Sonogram of the common peroneal nerve at the head of the fibula (arrow). F: fibula.

open tibial fracture and ankle dislocation following an in-vehicle traffic accident. The initial proper management of open fracture and joint dislocation was performed by orthopaedic and traumatology surgeons in the emergency department. The patient had no history of additional diseases. The preoperative airway examination revealed a class 3 Mallampati airway and, in light of the difficulty of intubation, an intrathecal block with a 150 mm needle was planned. After the written consent was obtained, 2 mg IV midazolam and 50 μg fentanyl were administered for sedation. The vertebral anatomical structures were barely distinguishable despite ultrasound guidance. After two unsuccessful attempts, we decided not to use spinal anesthesia and planned to perform a combined sciatic and femoral nerve block. As a tourniquet was not required above the knee, the blockade of these two nerves would be adequate for surgical anesthesia.

Before the femoral nerve block, the pannus was taped cephalad as the fatty tissue hanging from the abdomen made it difficult to access the inguinal region. The femoral nerve was identified at a depth of 5 cm with a linear US probe (Esaote, 10–18 MHz, Florence, Italy). Fifteen mL (8 mL of 0.5% levobupivacaine and 7 mL of 2% lidocaine) of local anesthetic mixture was administered around the femoral nerve using the in-plane approach. Due to the difficulties in situating the patient in the prone position, the distal extremities of the patient were elevated with folded blankets

in the supine position (Figure 1(a)). The sciatic nerve could not be visualized despite several attempts using both linear and convex probes; therefore separate blocks of the tibial and common peroneal nerves were planned. The tibial nerve was identified in the popliteal fold, posterior to the popliteal artery at a depth of 3 cm (Figure 1(b)). Visualization of the tibial nerve was highly difficult in areas more proximal than the point 2 cm above the popliteal fossa. The common peroneal nerve (CPN) and the bifurcation of the sciatic nerve could not be visualized despite several attempts using both linear and convex probes. Therefore, 10 mL (7 mL of 0.5% levobupivacaine and 3 mL of 2% lidocaine) of local anesthetic mixture was administered around the tibial nerve 2 cm above the popliteal fold by using a linear probe. Screening was performed in the distal direction over the lateral side of the patient's leg with the linear probe placed transversely on the edge of the patella to identify the CPN (Figure 2(a)). The nerve was visualized posteriorly and laterally to the fibular head, 4 cm distally to the edge of the patella at a depth of 2 cm (Figure 2(b)). At this level, 10 mL (7 mL of 0.5% levobupivacaine and 3 mL of 2% lidocaine) of local anesthetic mixture was administered around the nerve with the in-plane technique using a linear probe. A 100 mm 21-G echogenic needle (Pajunk, Geisingen, Germany) was used for all blocks. A nerve stimulator was not used for any blocks since the patient had extremity pain associated with trauma. Surgical anesthesia was established within 30 minutes after anesthetic administration and no complications occurred in association with the blocks. Emergent reduction and fixation with an external fixator were performed for the ankle dislocation and fracture of the tibia. Additional local anesthetic injection or additional sedation was not required during the operation. The operation lasted for approximately 1.5 hours and was completed without problems. The patient's consent was obtained for the publication of this case report.

3. Discussion

The likelihood of the presence of medical comorbidities such as hypertension, cardiopulmonary disease, type 2 diabetes, obstructive sleep apnea and venous thromboembolism increases in superobese (BMI ≥ 50) patients [6]. Obesity is associated with increased perioperative risks of difficult airway, cardiopulmonary dysfunction, acid aspiration, and mortality. The use of regional anesthesia instead of general anesthesia in obese patients decreases these risks and additionally it provides safe and effective postoperative analgesia [7, 8]. Unfortunately, our attempt at spinal anesthesia failed in this case despite ultrasound guidance. In the application of neuraxial blockade on obese patients, palpation of bony landmarks and the identification of the midline are more difficult, and the presence of fat packets may cause false-positive loss of resistance during the advancement of the needle. The identification of the intervertebral structures using ultrasonography is even more difficult in these patients [3]. Cases with failure and complications were reported even with the use of ultrasonography during epidural anesthesia [9]. Additionally, the decrease in the epidural space volume in obese patients leads to an unpredictable spread of local anesthetics and variable block levels. The risk of cardiopulmonary collapse and respiratory problems associated with increased block levels is higher in obese patients [7].

Despite the technical difficulties, peripheral nerve blocks may help to reduce these problems. Peripheral nerves are under dense adipose tissues and located more deeply in obese patients. During the use of ultrasonography, the needles should be positioned at a more vertical angle since the target tissue is more deeply located and thus the visualization of the needle tip is more difficult. Therefore, more experience and expertise is required for the use of ultrasonography in obese patients [10]. The increase in adipose tissue leads to alteration of the sonoanatomy learnt for normal-weight individuals and makes it more difficult to identify the target structures; therefore we may need to try new approaches by changing our perspectives.

The CPN block is uncommon in clinical practice. The CPN passes around the fibular head laterally after passing through the popliteal fossa. The block of the CPN in this region was described by Ting et al. [11]. This level is ideal for visualization with US, since the nerve is superficially located and the fibular head can be used as a sonoanatomical landmark. The absence of major vasculature at this level is another advantage, since the popliteal artery passes medially below the knee. On the other hand, the proximity of the CPN

to the fibular head in this region increases the risk of injury associated with compression [12]. Since there is inadequate data on the safety of this uncommon approach, the local anesthetic was limited to a volume of 10 mL in order to minimize the risk of nerve compression; no complications were observed following the block.

The curvilinear probe might be an appropriate option for obese patients because it uses lower frequencies and has improved penetration [13]. However, we do not have curvilinear probes in our department so we generally use linear probe for peripheral nerve blocks.

In conclusion, in the case of this superobese patient with difficult airway revealed by the preoperative examination, ultrasound-guided multiple peripheral nerve blocks were successfully performed following unsuccessful attempts for spinal block. Ultrasonography enables direct visualization of the nerves and reduction in the required local anesthetic doses and thus allows for multiple nerve blockade. In addition, ultrasound guidance enables the use of new peripheral nerve block approaches in obese patients. Due to these reasons, ultrasound-guided peripheral nerve blocks may be a good alternative to general anesthesia and central blocks for extremity surgeries in obese patients despite their technical difficulties. Based on our experience, the identification of more distal and superficial block points by individualized scanning instead of using common regions may be useful in the identification of physiological changes induced by obesity. Further studies are needed for the optimization of nerve block techniques and local anesthetic doses in obese patients.

References

[1] World Health Organization, "Obesity," 2008, http://www.who.int/topics/obesity/en/.

[2] Y. Leykin, T. Pellis, E. Del Mestro, B. Marzano, G. Fanti, and J. B. Brodsky, "Anesthetic management of morbidly obese and super-morbidly obese patients undergoing bariatric operations: hospital course and outcomes," *Obesity Surgery*, vol. 16, no. 12, pp. 1563–1569, 2006.

[3] J. Ingrande, J. B. Brodsky, and H. J. M. Lemmens, "Regional anesthesia and obesity," *Current Opinion in Anaesthesiology*, vol. 22, no. 5, pp. 683–686, 2009.

[4] M. C. Parra and R. W. Loftus, "Obesity and regional anesthesia," *International Anesthesiology Clinics*, vol. 51, pp. 90–112, 2013.

[5] Z. J. Koscielniak-Nielsen, "Ultrasound-guided peripheral nerve blocks: what are the benefits?" *Acta Anaesthesiologica Scandinavica*, vol. 52, no. 6, pp. 727–737, 2008.

[6] R. J. Garrison and W. P. Castelli, "Weight and thirty-year mortality of men in the Framingham Study," *Annals of Internal Medicine*, vol. 103, no. 6, pp. 1006–1009, 1985.

[7] J. P. Adams and P. G. Murphy, "Obesity in anaesthesia and intensive care," *British Journal of Anaesthesia*, vol. 85, no. 1, pp. 91–108, 2000.

[8] Z. Shenkman, Y. Shir, and J. B. Brodsky, "Perioperative management of the obese patient," *British Journal of Anaesthesia*, vol. 70, no. 3, pp. 349–359, 1993.

[9] R. J. Whitty, C. V. Maxwell, and J. C. A. Carvalho, "Complications of neuraxial anesthesia in an extreme morbidly obese patient for cesarean section," *International Journal of Obstetric Anesthesia*, vol. 16, no. 2, pp. 139–144, 2007.

[10] K. J. Chin, A. Perlas, V. W. S. Chan, and R. Brull, "Needle visualization in ultrasound-guided regional anesthesia: challenges and solutions," *Regional Anesthesia and Pain Medicine*, vol. 33, no. 6, pp. 532–544, 2008.

[11] P. H. Ting, J. G. Antonakakis, and D. C. Scalzo, "Ultrasound-guided common peroneal nerve block at the level of the fibular head," *Journal of Clinical Anesthesia*, vol. 24, no. 2, pp. 145–147, 2012.

[12] W. Ryan, N. Mahony, M. Delaney, M. O'Brien, and P. Murray, "Relationship of the common peroneal nerve and its branches to the head and neck of the fibula," *Clinical Anatomy*, vol. 16, no. 6, pp. 501–505, 2003.

[13] S. Carty and B. Nicholls, "Ultrasound-guided regional anaesthesia," *Continuing Education in Anaesthesia, Critical Care and Pain*, vol. 7, no. 1, pp. 20–24, 2007.

45

Successful Perioperative Management of a Patient with the Left Ventricular Assist Device for Brain Tumor Resection

Rashmi Vandse and Thomas J. Papadimos

Department of Anesthesiology, Wexner Medical Center, Ohio State University, Columbus, OH 43210, USA

Correspondence should be addressed to Rashmi Vandse; rashmi.vandse@osumc.edu

Academic Editor: Jian-jun Yang

Heart failure is the leading cause of death in the United States. Our increasingly aged population will contribute to an increased incidence and prevalence of heart failure, thereby augmenting the need for mechanical circulatory devices. Here we present the first successful resection of a brain tumor in a left ventricular device- (LVAD-) dependent patient with increased intracranial pressure and address pertinent perioperative anesthetic considerations and management.

1. Background

Heart failure continues to be the leading cause of death in United States. It is estimated to affect >5 million Americans and 550,000 new cases are diagnosed annually [1]. Although cardiac transplantation carries an excellent result for the treatment of end-stage heart failure, this option is severely limited by the number of available donor hearts. Ventricular assist devices (LAD; left (L) and (R) right) were initially developed to temporarily support the failing heart as a bridge to transplantation. Following the landmark Randomized Evaluation of Mechanical Assistance in the Treatment of Congestive Heart Failure (REMATCH) trial, which proved LVAD to be superior to any known medical therapy, LVAD is more frequently being used now as a destination therapy in patients with advanced heart failure ineligible for transplantation [2–5].

As the number of patients with long term LVAD therapy is increasing, the anesthesiologists are faced with the task of providing care to these patients for various noncardiac surgical procedures. Anesthetic considerations and perioperative management of patients with LVAD undergoing various types of noncardiac surgery have been discussed in the literature [6–12]. With this case report, we address the key anesthetic implications and issues in an LVAD supported patient undergoing elective craniotomy for resection of a brain tumor associated with increased intracranial pressure (ICP).

2. Case Presentation

Patient was a 60-year-old female who had an implantation of a Heart Mate II LVAD for ischemic cardiomyopathy about 2 years ago. She presented with a history of persistent severe headaches associated with confusion and balance problems. Brain imaging demonstrated four different ring-enhancing lesions within the brain. The largest one was located within the right temporal lobe measuring 4.4×5.3 cm. There was significant mass effect and edema in the right cerebral hemisphere including uncal herniation and 8 mm of right-to-left midline shift. Her past medical history was significant for chronic obstructive pulmonary disease (COPD), myocardial infarction, arrhythmia, congestive heart failure, and hypertension. She also had several episodes of GI bleeding in the past and hence she was maintained on a lower international normalized ratio (INR) goal of 1.3–1.8. Past surgical history included insertion of LVAD, hemiarthroplasty of R hip. Pertinent medications included furosemide, potassium chloride, albuterol-ipratropium inhaler, carvedilol, warfarin, omeprazole, fluticasone-salmeterol, trazodone, aspirin 81 mg, and sildenafil. Physical examination revealed a cachectic female who was 155 cm in height and weighed only 42.3 kg. Her Glasgow Coma Scale (GCS) was 14 and was confused at times. Her vital signs on admission were as follows: heart rate of 83 beats/minute, respiratory rate of 18–20 times/minute, blood pressure of 102/69 mm Hg, and O_2 saturation of 93% on room air. Her neurologic examination was otherwise intact. The neurosurgery service was consulted and recommended surgical resection of the temporal brain lesion. The perioperative planning was multidisciplinary involving neurosurgery, cardiothoracic surgery, cardiology, and the anesthesiology. Her LVAD was interrogated and settings were set at a speed of 8200 rpm, pump power of 4.7, and pulse index of 6.7. She was started on dexamethasone. Her aspirin and coumadin were withheld. On the day of the surgery, her lab values were hemoglobin of 8.8 g/dL, platelet count of 9.7×10^9/L which came up to $134,000 \times 10^9$/L after transfusion of 2 units of platelets, INR 1.6, PTT 27, and PT 19.4. She was also given 2 fresh frozen plasma (FFP) to further decrease the INR intraoperatively. The patient was transported to the operating room by the anesthesiology team and a dedicated VAD nurse.

Intraoperative monitoring included an electrocardiogram, pulse oximetry (SpO_2), invasive arterial pressure, and central venous pressure. Transesophageal echocardiography (TEE) was readily available. Her radial artery was cannulated prior to induction. The anesthesia was induced with 100 mcg of fentanyl, 40 mg of lidocaine, and 100 mg of propofol which was titrated slowly, followed by 50 mg of rocuronium to facilitate intubation with a size 7.0 endotracheal tube. The anesthesia was maintained with 0.8–1 MAC of sevoflurane in 50% FiO_2 and 0.08–0.1 mcg/kg/min of remifentanil. Right internal jugular central line was placed after the induction.

In order to reduce the ICP, she was gradually placed in the reverse Trendelenburg position which she tolerated well. Furosemide 10 mg was administered and she was hyperventilated to maintain $PaCO_2$ in low 30 s as confirmed by the blood gas analysis. Her mean arterial pressure (MAP) was maintained between 80 and 90 mm Hg most of the intraoperative period with only few occasional boluses of phenylephrine. She received 500 mL of crystalloids and 2 packs of FFP. She made 1700 mL of urine. Total duration of anesthesia was about 3 hours. At the end of the case, the patient's neuromuscular blockade was reversed with intravenous neostigmine (2 mg) and glycopyrrolate (0.4 mg) and was extubated deep with the return of spontaneous respiratory activity in order to avoid any coughing and sympathetic stimulation associated with the extubation. She was transported to cardiac intensive care unit in stable condition. She was slightly drowsy but was responding to commands and had a slight left sided weakness. Her GCS was 14. Her postoperative computed tomogram (CT) demonstrated small new intraparenchymal hemorrhages at the resection site. Her neurological exam, however, remained stable and she was kept under close observation with frequent neurological checks. Her repeat CT head was improving. Hence, she was started on heparin drip about 36 hours after the surgery.

The patient tolerated the procedure very well and was discharged from the hospital on postoperative day 10 in stable condition.

3. Discussion

This is the first case report describing successful resection of a brain tumor in an LVAD patient.

The most common neurosurgical procedure performed in LVAD patients is emergency evacuation of the intracranial hemorrhage and the outcome is usually poor. It is estimated that ICH occurs in 2.5% to 10% of patients on VAD therapy [13, 14]. Specific anesthetic considerations secondary to patient's cardiac and neurological status will be discussed in the next section.

4. Preoperative Management

In patients scheduled for elective surgery, thorough preoperative evaluation and optimization should be done which should address any coexisting end organ dysfunction, medications, anticoagulation status, and right ventricular dysfunction. Ideally, these patients should undergo their noncardiac surgery at centers where they received their LVAD under the supervision of the entire LVAD team (cardiac surgeon, LVAD nurses, and perfusionists, among other medical professionals) [7, 8]. The majority of these patients will be on chronic anticoagulants to minimize the risk of thrombosis. In the past, higher levels of anticoagulation were used with a target INR of 2 to 3 along with antiplatelet medications [7]. The Heart Mate II LVAD is associated with an extremely low thromboembolic risk, thereby requiring less stringent anticoagulation [6, 15, 16]. In addition to this, some patients will have acquired Von Willebrand disease secondary to the LVAD placement increasing their risk for bleeding [17]. If the surgery is elective, the patient can be bridged from warfarin to intravenous heparin preoperatively. In emergent situations, FFP can be used to reverse the effect of warfarin; however one should not aim for complete reversal of anticoagulation [6, 18]. Previous case studies have confirmed the rarity of LVAD failure despite correction of anticoagulation [6, 9, 14]. In our patient because of the intracranial surgery we were more aggressive in reversing the anticoagulation. Coumadin and aspirin were stopped preoperatively and since the surgery was relatively urgent due to brain edema and herniation, anticoagulation was reversed with FFP to decrease the INR and was also given 2 units of platelets as recommended by the neurosurgery team.

Attention must be given to electrical power needs of the device including battery back-up during transport. The care must be taken while placing the grounding pad of the electrosurgical unit so that the path of the electrical current from the unit does not go through the LVAD [7, 10]. Many of these patients also have automated internal cardioverter-defibrillators, which should be deactivated during the surgery to avoid any interference with the electrocautery unit, and external defibrillator pads should be applied [7, 10, 11]. Strict aseptic technique is required for all invasive procedures and antibiotic prophylaxis must be administered perioperatively [7, 19].

5. Intraoperative Management

5.1. Monitoring [6, 8, 12]. VAD control consoles continuously display the device output (usually an average of every four beats) which includes 4 different parameters which are as follows: pump flow in liters per minute, pump speed in RPMs, power consumption in watts, and pulsatility index (PI). As such, it provides an important parameter for the assessment and optimization of patient's hemodynamics and end organ perfusion. The Heart Mate II displays a flow based upon pump power consumption and pump rotational speed. The LVAD flow can be used as a substitute of cardiac output. However, pump flow values should be used mostly for trending any changes rather than an absolute estimate of cardiac output as there can be 15% to 20% difference between flow estimate on the display and the actual flow. Pump speed should balance adequate emptying of the left ventricle with adequate end-diastolic volume for aortic valve opening. Pump power refers to the power needed to run the motor. Typical power is 6.8 W and it is within a range of up to 25.5 W. Normally, the power will increase with speed or flow. Power that increases without an increase in speed or flow should raise suspicion for thrombus development on the rotor. The PI is a measure of the size of the flow pulse generated by the pump during the cardiac cycle. During clinical use, the PI usually ranges between 3 and 4. The PI depends on the inter-action among left ventricular preload, contractility, and level of assistance from the device. A high PI indicates an increased preload, an increased ventricular contribution, or a low level of device assistance. A low PI indicates a low preload, a low ventricular contribution, a high device assistance, and inflow or outflow obstruction. In patients with first generation or pulsatile LVADs, noninvasive blood pressure measurement and pulse oximetry can be used [8, 11]. However, due to the lack of adequate pulsatile flow, hemodynamic monitoring is significantly more challenging in patients with continuous-flow LVADs. Hence, invasive blood pressure monitoring may be needed [8, 9]; pulse oximeter might not work very well as well, and serial arterial blood gas measurements or cerebral oximetry can be used as alternatives. The pulse rate on the pulse oximeter and intra-arterial blood pressure monitor reflects VAD ejection and may not be the same as the EKG derived heart rate [6, 9, 19]. Intracranial surgery is not usually associated with significant fluid shifts; hence central venous pressure monitoring is not mandatory. However depending on the patient's right ventricular function, either a central venous catheter or a pulmonary artery catheter may be used to monitor preload, RV function and for drug and volume infusion. The central line was placed because the patient had some underlying RV dysfunction and also to administer any needed vasoactive and/or inotropic agents in. TEE is recommended for procedures in which major hemodynamic changes are anticipated. For all the other cases, TEE should be immediately available [6, 10, 19].

5.2. Hemodynamic Goals. Intraoperative hemodynamic goals should include maintaining sufficient preload, avoiding any abrupt changes in the afterload (SVR), and maintaining RV contractility and the rate and rhythm [7]. The two most important factors that can contribute to decreased pump output are hypovolemia and increased afterload which must be avoided. LVADs are "preload dependent" and the cardiac output and stroke volume generated are limited by the volume received from the right heart [6, 9]. Even though normal or slightly increased intravascular volume is preferred [6], caution must be exercised as this can interfere with the goals of intracranial surgery [14]. It is important to judiciously follow the trends in the hemodynamics and the LVAD parameters. If there is any doubt about the patient's fluid status, TEE should be used.

The reduction in the preload can happen intraopera-tively secondary to surgical blood loss, increased venous capacitance due to vasodilation induced by the anesthetic agents, institution of positive-pressure ventilation, changes in positioning especially reversed Trendelenburg, and RV dysfunction. In our case even though it is a routine practice to administer mannitol for this type of surgery to achieve brain relaxation, mannitol was not used in order to avoid fluid overload and excessive diuresis later. Additionally, positive-pressure ventilation can significantly impede venous return and preload. Hence ventilator settings were adjusted to achieve slight hyperventilation without generating unneces-sarily high intrathoracic pressures. Residual RV dysfunction is common in these patients and attention must be directed at obviating the risks of RV overfilling and increasing pul-monary vascular resistance (PVR) (hypoxia, hypercapnea, overdistension of the lungs, acidosis, and light anesthesia) [10]. TEE is helpful in diagnosing RV failure and in directing therapies to decrease PVR and in initiating pharmacological support of RV dysfunction. Continuous-flow LVADs are afterload sensitive and cannot generally compensate for any abrupt increases in SVR and this can result in a diminished forward flow from the LVAD. Therefore, one must achieve an adequate anesthetic depth to avoid any sympathetic stimulation and acute increases in SVR during laryngoscopy, intense surgical stimulation, and during extubation.

Anesthetic goals from the neuroanesthesia perspective involve preserving the brain from the secondary insult by taking measures to decrease ICP, avoiding hypoxemia, hypercapnia, and hypo- and hypertension, and maximize the brain elastance to decrease the effects of retractor pressure and ischemia [14, 20]. Intracerebral perfusion should be opti-mized along with the conservation of cerebral autoregulation and CO_2 responsiveness. Regarding arterial pressure, it is suggested (although without strong evidence) that the MAP be kept between 70 and 80 mm Hg [10]. Maintaining slightly higher MAP is important in patients with raised ICP in order to optimize cerebral perfusion pressure.

5.3. Anesthetic Agents. There is no one anesthetic technique or agent that is superior to the others. Understanding the unique physiology of the devices and the pathophysiology of the underlying heart failure and intracranial process and following the hemodynamic goals that are discussed before are crucial. Anesthetic induction should be done carefully to prevent any abrupt fall in SVR and cardiac depression. It is also important to maintain adequate depth to avoid excessive sympathetic stimulation which can increase SVR and also ICP. Fall in the SVR due to anesthetic agents can contribute to hypotension and judicious vasoconstriction should be used as necessary.

6. Conclusion

Thus even though anesthetizing patients with VADs can be challenging, by meticulous preparation, monitoring, and vigilance, patients with LVAD can safely undergo some of the most complex surgeries.

References

[1] A. S. Go, D. Mozaffarian, V. L. Roger et al., "Heart disease and stroke statistics—2013 update: a report from the American Heart Association," *Circulation*, vol. 127, no. 1, pp. e6–e245, 2013.

[2] E. A. Rose, A. C. Gelijns, A. J. Moskowitz et al., "Long-term use of a left ventricular assist device for end-stage heart failure," *The New England Journal of Medicine*, vol. 345, no. 20, pp. 1435–1443, 2001.

[3] L. W. Miller, F. D. Pagani, S. D. Russell et al., "Use of a continuous-flow device in patients awaiting heart transplantation," *The New England Journal of Medicine*, vol. 357, no. 9, pp. 885–896, 2007.

[4] F. D. Pagani, L. W. Miller, S. D. Russell et al., "Extended mechanical circulatory support with a continuous-flow rotary left ventricular assist device," *Journal of the American College of Cardiology*, vol. 54, no. 4, pp. 312–321, 2009.

[5] M. S. Slaughter, J. G. Rogers, C. A. Milano et al., "Advanced heart failure treated with continuous-flow left ventricular assist device," *The New England Journal of Medicine*, vol. 361, no. 23, pp. 2241–2251, 2009.

[6] M. E. Stone, W. Soong, M. Krol, and D. L. Reich, "The anesthetic considerations in patients with ventricular assist devices presenting for noncardiac surgery: a review of eight cases," *Anesthesia and Analgesia*, vol. 95, no. 1, pp. 42–49, 2002.

[7] K. A. Slininger, A. S. Haddadin, and A. A. Mangi, "Perioperative management of patients with left ventricular assist devices undergoing noncardiac surgery," *Journal of Cardiothoracic and Vascular Anesthesia*, vol. 27, no. 4, pp. 752–759, 2013.

[8] E. A. Hessel II, "Management of patients with implanted ventricular assist devices for noncardiac surgery: a clinical review," *Seminars in Cardiothoracic and Vascular Anesthesia*, vol. 18, no. 1, pp. 57–70, 2014.

[9] A. C. Nicolosi and P. S. Pagel, "Perioperative considerations in the patient with a left ventricular assist device," *Anesthesiology*, vol. 98, no. 2, pp. 565–570, 2003.

[10] I. El-Magharbel, "Ventricular assist devices and anesthesia," *Seminars in Cardiothoracic and Vascular Anesthesia*, vol. 9, no. 3, pp. 241–249, 2005.

[11] H. Riha, I. Netuka, T. Kotulak et al., "Anesthesia management of a patient with a ventricular assist device for noncardiac surgery," *Seminars in Cardiothoracic and Vascular Anesthesia*, vol. 14, no. 1, pp. 29–31, 2010.

[12] D. J. Ficke, J. Lee, M. A. Chaney, H. Bas, M. F. Vidal-Melo, and M. E. Stone, "Case 6—2010 noncardiac surgery in patients with a left ventricular assist device," *Journal of Cardiothoracic and Vascular Anesthesia*, vol. 24, no. 6, pp. 1002–1009, 2010.

[13] T. N. H. Drews, M. Loebe, M. J. Jurmann et al., "Outpatients on mechanical circulatory support," *Annals of Thoracic Surgery*, vol. 75, no. 3, pp. 780–785, 2003.

[14] F. N. F. Factora, S. Bustamante, A. Spiotta, and R. Avitsian, "Intracranial hemorrhage surgery on patients on mechanical circulatory support: a case series," *Journal of Neurosurgical Anesthesiology*, vol. 23, no. 1, pp. 30–34, 2011.

[15] R. John, F. Kamdar, K. Liao et al., "Low thromboembolic risk for patients with the Heartmate II left ventricular assist device," *Journal of Thoracic and Cardiovascular Surgery*, vol. 136, no. 5, pp. 1318–1323, 2008.

[16] A. J. Boyle, S. D. Russell, J. J. Teuteberg et al., "Low thromboembolism and pump thrombosis with the HeartMate II left ventricular assist device: analysis of outpatient anti-coagulation," *The Journal of Heart and Lung Transplantation*, vol. 28, no. 9, pp. 881–887, 2009.

[17] U. Geisen, C. Heilmann, F. Beyersdorf et al., "Non-surgical bleeding in patients with ventricular assist devices could be explained by acquired von Willebrand disease," *European Journal of Cardio-Thoracic Surgery*, vol. 33, no. 4, pp. 679–684, 2008.

[18] C. A. Thunberg, B. D. Gaitan, F. A. Arabia, D. J. Cole, and A. M. Grigore, "Ventricular assist devices today and tomorrow," *Journal of Cardiothoracic and Vascular Anesthesia*, vol. 24, no. 4, pp. 656–680, 2010.

[19] V. K. Topkara, S. Kondareddy, F. Malik et al., "Infectious complications in patients with left ventricular assist device: etiology and outcomes in the continuous-flow era," *Annals of Thoracic Surgery*, vol. 90, no. 4, pp. 1270–1277, 2010.

[20] J. E. Cottrell and W. L. Young, Eds., *Cottrell and Young's Neuroanesthesia*, Mosby Elsevier, 5th edition, 2010.

46

Complex Perioperative Decision-Making: Liver Resection in a Patient with Extensive Superior Vena Cava/Right Atrial Thrombus and Superior Vena Cava Syndrome

Benjamin Kloesel[1,2] and Robert W. Lekowski[2]

[1]Department of Anesthesia, Perioperative and Pain Medicine, Boston Children's Hospital, Boston, MA 02115, USA
[2]Department of Anesthesia, Perioperative and Pain Medicine, Brigham and Women's Hospital, Boston, MA 02115, USA

Correspondence should be addressed to Robert W. Lekowski; rlekowski@partners.org

Academic Editor: Jian-jun Yang

The perioperative management of patients suffering from extensive superior vena cava (SVC) thrombus complicated by SVC syndrome presents unique challenges. The anesthesiologist needs to be prepared for possible thrombus dislodgement resulting in pulmonary embolism and also has to assess the need for fluid resuscitation given the dangers of massive intravenous fluid application via the upper extremities. We present our perioperative approach in management of a patient scheduled for right hepatectomy who was previously diagnosed with extensive SVC and right atrial (RA) thrombus complicated by SVC syndrome.

1. Introduction

Obstruction of the venous inflow tract to the right heart and the presence of an intracardiac thrombus have multiple implications for anesthesiologists that require careful preparation and communication with the involved subspecialties during the perioperative period. Our case presentation will delineate anesthetic considerations, preoperative preparation, and intraoperative management of a patient with central venous catheter- (CVC-) related SVC and RA thrombus complicated by SVC syndrome who presented for resection of multiple liver metastases from a colorectal primary carcinoma.

2. Case Presentation

A 49-year-old female presented to the oncologic surgery service for right hepatectomy and wedge resection of segment 3 of the left lateral liver to remove four right hepatic lobe and one left hepatic lobe colon cancer metastases. Her past medical history was significant for sigmoid adenocarcinoma status after low anterior resection and four cycles of FOLFOX chemotherapy (leucovorin, 5-fluorouracil, and oxaliplatin) administered via a port-a-cath. Her course was complicated

by development of a port-a-cath associated thrombus comprised of two parts spanning a total length of 8 cm, with extension from the left brachiocephalic vein along the SVC into the RA and RA appendage (Figure 1). Secondary to the thrombus, the patient developed two episodes of SVC syndrome with facial and neck swelling as well as shortness of breath. The first episode at time of diagnosis was managed with discontinuation of her oral contraceptive pill and intravenous heparin with transition to subcutaneous enoxaparin (1.5 mg/kg once daily), a low-molecular-weight heparin (LMWH), in the outpatient setting. Initially, the port-a-cath was scheduled to be removed, but given concerns from interventional radiology in regard to reinsertion of a CVC in the presence of an extensive SVC thrombus and decrease of thrombus burden with therapeutic anticoagulation, the port-a-cath was left in place. During the second episode, which occurred about three months after initial SVC thrombus diagnosis, the patient was admitted for evaluation of possible catheter-based extraction therapies. On further review of her imaging studies and consideration of the clot appearance and time from initial discovery, the interventional cardiology service felt that, due to clot chronicity, an extraction therapy would not be feasible. The recommendation was made to

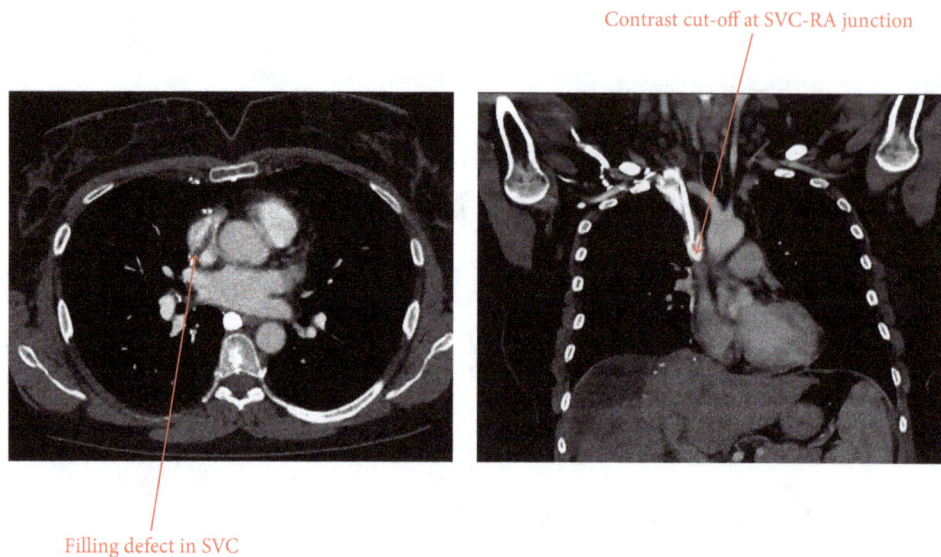

Contrast cut-off at SVC-RA junction

Filling defect in SVC

FIGURE 1: CT angiography of the chest showing a filling defect in the SVC and contrast cut-off at the SVC-RA junction caused by a thrombus.

continue anticoagulation and proceed with surgery after inferior vena cava filter placement. Her surgery was scheduled six months after initial discovery of the port-a-cath associated clot. The patient's anticoagulation management was based on recent guidelines published in 2012 [1]. LMWH was chosen over vitamin K antagonists since clinical trials have shown improved outcomes in patients with solid tumors treated with this regimen [2–4].

A discussion was held with the patient regarding the risks of massive pulmonary embolism and possible therapies. The patient voiced her wish to remain full code and asked for resuscitative efforts to be carried out in the setting of a massive pulmonary embolism. On the day of surgery, a perfusionist and a cardiothoracic surgery team were on stand-by. A perfusion pump was positioned outside of the operating room to allow rapid access to cardiopulmonary bypass capabilities. Arterial access via a 20G catheter was obtained in the right radial artery prior to induction. Anesthesia was induced using a standard induction regimen of midazolam (2 mg) in the preoperative area, followed by fentanyl (100 mcg), propofol (200 mg), and rocuronium (40 mg) via a 20G peripheral intravenous (PIV) catheter in the right upper extremity. No significant lag in medication onset of effect was noted. Bag-mask ventilation was easily achieved. A cuffed 7.0 endotracheal tube was inserted using a MAC 3 blade. Anesthesia was maintained with a volatile agent (sevoflurane) and intermittent fentanyl boluses. After induction, large-bore central venous access was obtained via the right femoral vein under ultrasound guidance to provide means of vasopressor, fluid, and blood product administration. A transesophageal echocardiography (TEE) probe was inserted and images of the right heart thrombus were obtained. The probe was left in place and the thrombus position was periodically checked to confirm the absence of dislodgement. Echocardiography was also used to assess the patient's heart during any signs of hemodynamic alterations. The exam focused on presence of the thrombus, right ventricular systolic function, right

ventricular cavity dilation, presence of new regional wall motion abnormalities, occurrence of new tricuspid insufficiency, and position of the ventricular septum. The surgery was carried out in the reverse Trendelenburg position and the patient's eyes and head were monitored every 20 minutes for evidence of swelling. We aimed at limiting intravenous fluids while maintaining adequate intravascular volume and tissue perfusion. Fluid management was guided by stroke-volume variation obtained from a FloTrac/Vigileo™ monitor (Edwards Lifescience Corp., Irvine, CA). A consistent increase of stroke-volume variation above 12% for five minutes was used as a trigger for a 250 cc albumin 5% bolus. The surgery was uneventful and well tolerated by the patient. Procedure time from patient arrival in the operating room to transfer of the patient who is awake to the postoperative anesthesia care unit was 405 minutes. Estimated blood loss was 400 cc. A total of 750 cc of 5% albumin and 1800 cc of Lactated Ringer's solution were given. Intermittent monitoring of the RA thrombus showed no changes and the patient remained hemodynamically stable. After recovery in the postanesthesia care unit, a 20G PIV catheter was inserted in the lower extremity and both femoral CVCs were removed to reduce the risk of clot formation. The patient's enoxaparin was restarted on postoperative day #6 and she was discharged on postoperative day #7.

3. Discussion

In daily practice, anesthesiologists are not only required to have a good understanding of the patient's comorbidities and the implications of the upcoming surgery; they also need to be able to anticipate possible difficulties and complications. Along this line, the well-prepared clinician has proactively considered management options for the complications and has made sure that the necessary resources are available to respond quickly and appropriately.

Considerations for liver resection surgery include the possible presence of impaired organ function secondary to the malignant process, metastases, and/or chemotherapy. The liver is a highly vascular organ, and its proximity to large vessels carries the risk for significant intraoperative bleeding that necessitates rapid and adequate volume resuscitation. This stands in stark contrast to the initial goal of keeping the patient slightly hypo- to euvolemic in order to avoid increases in central venous pressure which are associated with hepatic congestion and increased blood loss [5, 6].

The presence of an extensive thrombus in the venous system that extended to the RA, leading to previous episodes of SVC syndrome, added another layer of complexity to this case. The incidence of CVC-associated thrombosis in cancer patients varies, depending on the study, between 0–28% for symptomatic and 27–66% for asymptomatic events. Furthermore, 10–15% of those patients develop pulmonary embolism [7]. While the use of upper extremity intravenous access for delivery of drugs and small volumes of fluids was considered possible (in part due to the chronicity of the condition which induced adequate venous collateralization), large volume resuscitation in the setting of massive blood loss could have triggered another episode of superior vena cava syndrome. Sequelae of this might have included significant airway swelling and raised intracranial pressure from venous congestion. Adequate resuscitation via an upper extremity access point might also have proved inadequate. Consequently, we opted for lower extremity access, which, in turn, also had considerable implications: (a) ideally, we would have aimed for multiple large-bore PIV catheters, but the patient's vascular system did not provide adequate targets; (b) the insertion of a CVC in itself increases the risk for clot formation (hence, the decision to remove the catheters as soon as the immediate period with risk for massive blood loss was over).

Another concern in regard to the extensive thrombus was the possibility of dislodgement and propagation to the pulmonary artery. Pulmonary embolism has been described in numerous case reports of RA thrombus [8–10], with most cases arising from hemodialysis catheters. In our case, the patient was evaluated by cardiology, interventional cardiology, and cardiothoracic surgery. While interventional procedures were deemed unlikely to succeed given the clot chronicity, an open thrombectomy was considered to have an unfavorable risk-benefit ratio. The cardiology service considered the time span from detection of the thrombus to the day of surgery to be sufficient to expect clot organization resulting in a low likelihood of embolism. Nevertheless, for the managing anesthesiologist, the question of "what to do in case the patient suffers a massive pulmonary embolism during the case" needed to be addressed.

The presentation of a perioperative pulmonary embolism covers a large spectrum, reaching from no clinical changes in very small emboli to cardiopulmonary arrest with massive embolization. Pathophysiological changes include V/Q mismatch due to an increase in alveolar dead space resulting in right-left shunting, hypoxia, increased right ventricular (RV) afterload, RV ischemia/infarction, and decrease in cardiac output secondary to decreased left ventricular preload and impaired left ventricular filling from displacement of the interventricular septum to the left [11, 12]. A drop in end-tidal CO_2 is related to a decrease in cardiac output. ECG changes can include sinus tachycardia, atrial dysrhythmia, RV strain, right bundle branch block, and SI Q3 T3 pattern (rare) [13]. Transesophageal echocardiography is an excellent tool to diagnose intraoperative pulmonary embolism [14–16]. While direct visualization of thrombus in the pulmonary artery is only sometimes possible (46% of patients in a study by Rosenberger et al. [15]), the echocardiographer can search for evidence of right heart strain such as RV dilation or RV systolic dysfunction [17].

Treatment of pulmonary embolism in the outpatient setting consists of therapeutic anticoagulation with unfractionated or low-molecular-weight heparin followed by transition to warfarin [18]. In the setting of a massive pulmonary embolism leading to hemodynamic instability, thrombolysis with plasminogen-activating fibrinolytic agents [17], catheter-based thrombus reduction via pharmacological and/or mechanical methods [17, 19], or surgical thromboembolectomy [17, 20] can be considered. For sudden cardiovascular collapse, initiation of cardiopulmonary bypass and venoarterial ECMO [21] are considered last resort measures but are limited by their availability and the timeframe to their successful institution.

Thrombus development in the RA has frequently been described in presence of indwelling vascular catheters [10, 22–24] or pacemaker wires [8, 25] and seems to be associated with catheter tip position in the RA as compared to the superior vena cava [26, 27]. A review of six studies by an international working committee identified the following risk factors for CVC-associated thrombosis: CVC tip location above junction between SVC and RA, left-sided CVC insertion, femoral vein access, placement duration of greater than 25 minutes, greater than 1 placement attempt, previous CVC insertion and CVC blockage, and use of triple- (versus double-) lumen CVC and external (versus internal) CVC [7]. Predictors of which atrial thrombi subsequently result in pulmonary embolism are lacking, although there is evidence that this condition is certainly not benign. Kingdon et al. [24] describe a case series composed of 5 patients who developed hemodialysis-catheter associated thrombus. In 3 out of the 5 patients, a pulmonary embolism was documented while another patient suffered a PEA arrest without definitive evidence of pulmonary embolism.

In conclusion, our patient raised multiple considerations for the conduct of safe anesthesia for a liver resection in the setting of SVC syndrome secondary to extensive SVC and RA thrombus. In our report, we delineate our perioperative preparation for possible massive volume loss, vascular access, intraoperative monitoring of thrombus, and an action plan for massive pulmonary embolism.

References

[1] G. H. Guyatt, E. A. Akl, M. Crowther, D. D. Gutterman, and H. J. Schuünemann, "Executive summary: antithrombotic therapy and prevention of thrombosis, 9th ed: American College of Chest Physicians evidence-based clinical practice guidelines," *Chest*, vol. 141, no. 2, supplement, pp. 7S–47S, 2012.

[2] A. Y. Y. Lee, M. N. Levine, R. I. Baker et al., "Low-molecular-weight heparin versus a coumarin for the prevention of recurrent venous thromboembolism in patients with cancer," *The New England Journal of Medicine*, vol. 349, no. 2, pp. 146–153, 2003.

[3] G. Meyer, Z. Marjanovic, J. Valcke et al., "Comparison of low-molecular-weight heparin and warfarin for the secondary prevention of venous thromboembolism in patients with cancer: a randomized controlled study," *Archives of Internal Medicine*, vol. 162, no. 15, pp. 1729–1735, 2002.

[4] R. D. Hull, G. F. Pineo, R. F. Brant et al., "Long-term low-molecular-weight heparin versus usual care in proximal-vein thrombosis patients with cancer," *The American Journal of Medicine*, vol. 119, no. 12, pp. 1062–1072, 2006.

[5] Z. Li, Y.-M. Sun, F.-X. Wu, L.-Q. Yang, Z.-J. Lu, and W.-F. Yu, "Controlled low central venous pressure reduces blood loss and transfusion requirements in hepatectomy," *World Journal of Gastroenterology*, vol. 20, no. 1, pp. 303–309, 2014.

[6] J. T. Huntington, N. A. Royall, and C. R. Schmidt, "Minimizing blood loss during hepatectomy: a literature review," *Journal of Surgical Oncology*, vol. 109, no. 2, pp. 81–88, 2014.

[7] P. Debourdeau, D. Farge, M. Beckers et al., "International clinical practice guidelines for the treatment and prophylaxis of thrombosis associated with central venous catheters in patients with cancer," *Journal of Thrombosis and Haemostasis*, vol. 11, no. 1, pp. 71–80, 2013.

[8] E. L. Kinney, R. P. Allen, W. A. Weidner, W. S. Pierce, D. M. Leaman, and R. F. Zelis, "Recurrent pulmonary emboli secondary to right atrial thrombus around a permanent pacing catheter: a case report and review of the literature," *Pacing and Clinical Electrophysiology*, vol. 2, no. 2, pp. 196–202, 1979.

[9] N. Shammas, R. Padaria, and G. Ahuja, "Ultrasound-assisted lysis using recombinant tissue plasminogen activator and the EKOS EkoSonic endovascular system for treating right atrial thrombus and massive pulmonary embolism: a case study," *Phlebology*, vol. 30, no. 10, pp. 739–743, 2015.

[10] K. E. A. Burns and A. McLaren, "Catheter-related right atrial thrombus and pulmonary embolism: a case report and systematic review of the literature," *Canadian Respiratory Journal*, vol. 16, no. 5, pp. 163–165, 2009.

[11] M. C. Desciak and D. E. Martin, "Perioperative pulmonary embolism: diagnosis and anesthetic management," *Journal of Clinical Anesthesia*, vol. 23, no. 2, pp. 153–165, 2011.

[12] N. Moorjani and S. Price, "Massive pulmonary embolism," *Cardiology Clinics*, vol. 31, no. 4, pp. 503–518, 2013.

[13] K. Somasundaram and J. Ball, "Medical emergencies: pulmonary embolism and acute severe asthma," *Anaesthesia*, vol. 68, supplement 1, pp. 102–116, 2013.

[14] S. K. Shillcutt, T. R. Brakke, C. R. Montzingo, and A. Agrawal, "Intraoperative diagnosis of acute pulmonary embolus by transesophageal echocardiogram," *Journal of Cardiothoracic and Vascular Anesthesia*, vol. 25, no. 3, p. 603, 2011.

[15] P. Rosenberger, S. K. Shernan, S. C. Body, and H. K. Eltzschig, "Utility of intraoperative transesophageal echocardiography for diagnosis of pulmonary embolism," *Anesthesia and Analgesia*, vol. 99, no. 1, pp. 12–16, 2004.

[16] P. Rosenberger, S. K. Shernan, T. Weissmüller et al., "Role of intraoperative transesophageal echocardiography for diagnosing and managing pulmonary embolism in the perioperative period," *Anesthesia and Analgesia*, vol. 100, no. 1, pp. 292–293, 2005.

[17] M. R. Jaff, M. S. McMurtry, S. L. Archer et al., "Management of massive and submassive pulmonary embolism, iliofemoral deep vein thrombosis, and chronic thromboembolic pulmonary hypertension: a scientific statement from the American Heart Association," *Circulation*, vol. 123, no. 16, pp. 1788–1830, 2011.

[18] S. Z. Goldhaber and H. Bounameaux, "Pulmonary embolism and deep vein thrombosis," *The Lancet*, vol. 379, no. 9828, pp. 1835–1846, 2012.

[19] T. M. Todoran and P. Sobieszczyk, "Catheter-based therapies for massive pulmonary embolism," *Progress in Cardiovascular Diseases*, vol. 52, no. 5, pp. 429–437, 2010.

[20] L. Aklog, C. S. Williams, J. G. Byrne, and S. Z. Goldhaber, "Acute pulmonary embolectomy: a contemporary approach," *Circulation*, vol. 105, no. 12, pp. 1416–1419, 2002.

[21] G. Pavlovic, C. Banfi, D. Tassaux et al., "Peri-operative massive pulmonary embolism management: is veno-arterial ECMO a therapeutic option?" *Acta Anaesthesiologica Scandinavica*, vol. 58, no. 10, pp. 1280–1286, 2014.

[22] W. K. Oh, B. H. Lee, and N. K. Sweitzer, "Nonmalignant diagnoses in patients. Case 3. Right atrial thrombus associated with a central venous catheter in a patient with metastatic adrenocortical carcinoma," *Journal of Clinical Oncology*, vol. 18, no. 13, pp. 2638–2639, 2000.

[23] N. Hussain, P. E. Shattuck, M. H. Senussi et al., "Large right atrial thrombus associated with central venous catheter requiring open heart surgery," *Case Reports in Medicine*, vol. 2012, Article ID 501303, 4 pages, 2012.

[24] E. J. Kingdon, S. G. Holt, J. Davar et al., "Atrial thrombus and central venous dialysis catheters," *American Journal of Kidney Diseases*, vol. 38, no. 3, pp. 631–639, 2001.

[25] D. B. Coleman, D. M. DeBarr, D. L. Morales, and H. M. Spotnitz, "Pacemaker lead thrombosis treated with atrial thrombectomy and biventricular pacemaker and defibrillator insertion," *Annals of Thoracic Surgery*, vol. 78, no. 5, pp. e83–e84, 2004.

[26] S. Fuchs, A. Pollak, and D. Gilon, "Central venous catheter mechanical irritation of the right atrial free wall: a cause for thrombus formation," *Cardiology*, vol. 91, no. 3, pp. 169–172, 1999.

[27] D. Gilon, D. Schechter, A. J. J. T. Rein et al., "Right atrial thrombi are related to indwelling central venous catheter position: insights into time course and possible mechanism of formation," *American Heart Journal*, vol. 135, no. 3, pp. 457–462, 1998.

47

Erector Spinae Plane Block for Different Laparoscopic Abdominal Surgeries

Serkan Tulgar ⓘ,[1] Onur Selvi,[1] and Mahmut Sertan Kapakli[2]

[1]Department of Anesthesiology and Reanimation, Maltepe University Faculty of Medicine, Istanbul, Turkey
[2]Department of General Surgery, Maltepe University Faculty of Medicine, Istanbul, Turkey

Correspondence should be addressed to Serkan Tulgar; serkantulgar.md@gmail.com

Academic Editor: Alparslan Apan

The ultrasound guided erector spinae plane (ESP) block is a recent block described for various surgeries for postoperative analgesia. ESP block has effect on both visceral and somatic pain; therefore, its use in laparoscopic cholecystectomy and other abdominal surgeries can be advantageous. We describe successful ESP block application in three different cases for postoperative pain. Two patient were operated on using endoscopic retrograde cholangiopancreatography and laparoscopic cholecystectomy and one patient was operated on using laparoscopic cholecystectomy together with the inguinal hernia operation.

1. Introduction

Ultrasound guided erector spinae (ESP) block is a regional anesthesia technique, recently described by Forero et al. [1] for use in thoracic neuropathic pain. ESP block is reported to lead to analgesic effect on somatic and visceral pain by effecting the ventral rami and rami communicantes that include sympathetic nerve fibers, as LA spreads through the paravertebral space [1, 2]. When performed bilaterally it has been reported to be as effective as thoracic epidural analgesia [2].

ESP block leads to effective postoperative analgesia when performed at T 4-5 level for breast and thoracic surgery, and T 7 level for abdominal surgeries [2–4]. The number of surgeries involving multiple procedures pand/or incisions is increasing [5], with such surgeries requiring complex analgesia protocols for pain management.

As LA widely spreads cranially and caudally when ESP is performed, we hypothesized that ESP can effectively be used as an analgesic method for abdominal surgeries especially those involving more than one procedure and/or incision in a single session. The effectiveness of ESP block as an analgesic method in laparoscopic cholecystectomy (LC), endoscopic retrograde cholangiopancreatography (ERCP), and laparoscopic inguinal hernia repair has not been reported previously.

Herein we report three patients undergoing multiple abdominal procedures in a single surgical session in which ESP was successfully performed for postoperative analgesia.

2. Case Reports

Written informed consent was obtained from patients for this report. Ethics board approval for case reports was not required by our institute.

2.1. Patient 1. A 48-year-old female patient (weight: 66 kg, height: 166 cm) with multiple millimetric gallstones was due to undergo intraoperative ERCP followed by LC. She had a history of caesarean section and appendectomy and had elevated transaminases plus hyperbilirubinemia. She was accepted as being American Anesthesiology Association (ASA) Class 1. ESP block was planned as part of her multimodal analgesia protocol.

After premedication (midazolam 1 mg), anesthesia induction was performed using lidocaine 1 mg/kg, fentanyl 100 mcg, propofol 3 mg/kg, and rocuronium bromide 0.6 mg/kg. Following intubation, anesthesia was maintained with 0.6 MAC sevoflurane in air-oxygen mixture and remifentanil infusion of 0.08–0.1 μg/kg/min. After hemodynamic stability, the patient was placed in the prone position. Bilateral ESP block was performed. After completing ERCP, the patient was positioned supine and LC was performed. Total surgical time was 74 minutes and time under anesthesia was 93 minutes. Perioperative intravenous paracetamol (1 gr) and tenoxicam (20 mg) were given.

She was transferred to the postoperative recovery room after extubation. The patients numeric rating scale (NRS) was 1/10 at rest and when coughing. After follow-up of 1 hour the patient was transferred to the general ward. Postoperative analgesia was ordered as 1 gr intravenous paracetamol every 8 hours. Rescue analgesia was planned as being intramuscular diclofenac sodium 75 mg. The patient's NRS was <3/10 during the first 16 hours of follow-up. Planned analgesia was not applied during this time. At 17th hour, NRS scores were 5/10 when coughing and 4/10 at rest. Rescue analgesia was performed. The patient was externalised home at the 24th hour with prescription pain medication.

2.2. Patient 2. A 54-year-old male patient with multiple millimetric gallstones was due to undergo intraoperative ERCP followed by LC. The patient had a history of smoking 35 pack/years, weighed 84 kg, and was 176 cm tall and ASA class 2. The patient underwent endoscopic sphincterotomy. If ERCP failed, it would go through open surgery. After a successful ERCP, the process was continued with LC. He had high liver function tests, hyperbilirubinemia, and jaundice. Anesthesia, analgesia, and surgical plans were the same as Patient 1. Surgical time and anesthesia time were 92 and 108 minutes, respectively.

In the recovery room, the patients NRS on coughing and at rest was 1/10. Patients NRS was <3/10 during first 12 hours of follow-up. No analgesic medication was applied during this time. On 13th hour, NRS was found to be 5/10 on coughing and 3/10 at rest. Rescue analgesic was performed. The patient was externalised home at the 24th hour with prescription pain medication.

2.3. Patient 3. A 52-year-old male patient was due to undergo LC and right laparoscopic inguinal hernia repair (Transabdominal preperitoneal repair technique). The patient had a history of smoking 30 pack/years and had hypertension. He weighed 96 kg and was 169 cm tall. Anesthesia, perioperative and postoperative analgesia, and ESP block were the same as Patient 1. LC followed by laparoscopic inguinal hernia repair was performed in the supine position. Due to two surgical procedures and the length of surgical time (152 minute), ESP block was added to the multimodal analgesia. The patient was placed in the lateral position and ESP was performed. Total time under anesthesia was 163 minutes. The patients received perioperative 1 gr paracetamol, 20 mg tenoxicam, and 100 mg tramadol intravenously.

The patient's NRS in the recovery room was 5/10 at rest and when coughing. Intravenous fentanyl 25 mg was given. At 20th minute, NRS was found to have decreased to 1/10. He was transferred to the general ward after 1 hour. No additional analgesic was required for the first 15 hours (NRS < 3/10). At 16th hour NRS was found to be 5/10 when coughing

and 4/10 at rest. Rescue analgesic was given. Follow-up was discontinued after 24 hours.

No nausea or vomiting was observed in all patients.

2.4. Performing the ESP Blocks. Local anesthetics mixtures used in ESP blocks were prepared as 20 ml including ten ml bupivacaine 0.5%, five ml lidocaine 2%, and five ml serum physiologic.

Patient 1-2. After anesthesia induction, the patient was placed in prone position for ERCP. Under aseptic conditions, a high frequency linear transducer was placed on the spinous process at T8 level on the parasagittal plane and then slid 2.5–3 cm laterally to visualise the transverse process and erector spinae muscle. Using the in plane technique, the needle was advanced between the transverse process and erector spinae muscle. The correct location was confirmed using 1 ml of LA to view hydrodissection. 19 ml of LA was injected between the muscle and transverse process. The same procedure was performed bilaterally.

Patient 3. The same procedure was performed in the lateral position. The transverse process and erector spinae muscle were more visible on the upper side of the patient.

3. Discussion

ESP was first described having been used for the successful treatment of thoracic neuropathic pain [1]. Later studies demonstrated that ESP was an effective analgesic method in bariatric surgery, pneumothorax surgery, and major abdominal surgery when performed from the thoracic vertebral levels [2–4, 6]. The LA administered during ESP block spreads in the paravertebral space, leading the effective analgesia for somatic and visceral pain [2]. When performed bilaterally ESP block has similar effect as epidural analgesia [2–4].

A cadaver model demonstrated that when 20 ml of fluid was performed at T7 transverse process, the fluid spreads to the level of the C 7-T 2 vertebra levels cranially and L2-3 vertebra levels caudally [7]. ESP block can be performed at T4-5 level for breast and thoracic surgeries and T7-8 levels for abdominal surgeries [3, 7].

Herein we report three cases in which ESP block was successfully performed in patients undergoing various laparoscopic abdominal surgical procedures. Patient 1 and 2 underwent intraoperative ERCP followed by LC. Pain following ERCP is mainly due to visceral pain caused by intestinal distension. Sometimes it can be a painless condition that does not require analgesia, and some surgeons do not even take analgesic order after this procedure. However, there may be differences in pain sensitivity between patients. On the other hand, pain after LC has two causes. The first is visceral pain due to the trauma of gallbladder resection, and the second is parietal pain caused by the skin incision. Other effective analgesic methods have been described for use after LC. Oblique subcostal transversus abdominis plane (OSTAP) block is one of these methods [8, 9]. However, we chose ESP block due to its effect on visceral nerve fibers. We demonstrated that ESP block leads to effective analgesia for both ERCP and LC pain. Frequently oral and intravenous nonsteroidal analgesic drugs (NSAID) are used for LC and are often combined with opioids. Although ESP seems to be a complex regional anesthesia technique for LC and other interventions in combination with LC, regional analgesia techniques can be seen as a technique that can be used to reduce/remove the need for opioid. ESP could been used particularly in patients with comorbidities and/or opioid use, where early mobilization is required. In low pain tolerance patients we could use ESP as a part of multimodal analgesia.

In patient 3, LC and laparoscopic inguinal hernia repair were performed. Preperitoneal CO_2 insufflation is also performed for laparoscopic inguinal hernia repair, in contrast to LC. Considering the insufflation time and that laparoscopic surgery was performed for both an upper and lower abdominal pathology, complementary methods to be added to intravenous postoperative analgesia were limited for this patient. TAP block is an option in laparoscopic inguinal hernia repair [10]. We chose to perform ESP block in our patient undergoing both LC and laparoscopic inguinal hernia repair as it has an effect on somatic fibers carrying pain from the surgical field, and visceral fibers carrying pain caused by widespread peritoneal irritation. Bilateral ESP block was observed to be an effective analgesia method.

The combination of paracetamol, NSAID, and opioid in the form of multimodal regimes may be used in the management of postoperative analgesia for both LC and laparoscopic inguinal hernias. However, it should be considered that different regional anesthesia techniques are used for both surgeries and that multislice analgesia plans that are supposed to be supported by regional anesthesia can use only ESP block and provide effective analgesia instead of using more than one regional anesthesia technique. However a heterogeneous case report series is not really a proper exploration of this subgroup, and this is our limitation.

To our knowledge, ESP block has not been reported previously for LC, ERCP, or laparoscopic inguinal hernia repair. ESP block is effective, easy to perform, and can be performed in a short time. Therefore, we believe that bilateral ESP block may have comparable or improved analgesic effect in upper and lower abdominal surgical procedures when compared to other suitable plane blocks. However, further comparative controlled studies are required.

In conclusion, this case series has demonstrated that ESP block can be successfully used in lower and upper abdominal surgical procedures, especially if these procedures are performed in the same session. However, in homogeneous groups, prospective, randomised studies are needed in different surgical procedures to determine the indications, effective practice points, and segments of the ESP block.

Authors' Contributions

Serkan Tulgar performed the block, set forth the hypothesis, wrote the manuscript, and researched the literature. Onur Selvi helped in searching the literature and reviewing the case reports. Mahmut Sertan Kapakli helped in the revision of discussion.

References

[1] M. Forero, S. D. Adhikary, H. Lopez, C. Tsui, and K. J. Chin, "The erector spinae plane block a novel analgesic technique in thoracic neuropathic pain," *Regional Anesthesia and Pain Medicine*, vol. 41, no. 5, pp. 621–627, 2016.

[2] K. J. Chin, L. Malhas, and A. Perlas, "The erector spinae plane block provides visceral abdominal analgesia in bariatric surgery a report of 3 cases," *Regional Anesthesia and Pain Medicine*, vol. 42, no. 3, pp. 372–376, 2017.

[3] D. Bonvicini, L. Tagliapietra, A. Giacomazzi, and E. Pizzirani, "Bilateral ultrasound-guided erector spinae plane blocks in breast cancer and reconstruction surgery," *Journal of Clinical Anesthesia*, vol. 44, pp. 3-4, 2018.

[4] C. E. Restrepo-Garces, K. J. Chin, P. Suarez, and A. Diaz, "Bilateral Continuous Erector Spinae Plane Block Contributes to Effective Postoperative Analgesia After Major Open Abdominal Surgery," *A & A Case Reports*, vol. 9, no. 11, pp. 319–321, 2017.

[5] M. Jones, M. Johnson, E. Samourjian, K. Slauch, and N. Ozobia, "ERCP and laparoscopic cholecystectomy in a combined (one-step) procedure: A random comparison to the standard (two-step) procedure," *Surgical Endoscopy*, vol. 27, no. 6, pp. 1907–1912, 2013.

[6] H. Ueshima and H. Otake, "Erector spinae plane block provides effective pain management during pneumothorax surgery," *Journal of Clinical Anesthesia*, vol. 40, p. 74, 2017.

[7] K. J. Chin, S. Adhikary, N. Sarwani, and M. Forero, "The analgesic efficacy of pre-operative bilateral erector spinae plane (ESP) blocks in patients having ventral hernia repair," *Anaesthesia*, vol. 72, no. 4, pp. 452–460, 2017.

[8] S. Ozmen, "Analgesia and respiratory function after laparoscopic cholecystectomy in patients receiving ultrasound-guided bilateral oblique subcostal transversus abdominis plane block: A randomized double-blind study," *Medical Science Monitor*, vol. 21, pp. 1304–1312, 2015.

[9] H.-J. Shin, A.-Y. Oh, J.-S. Baik, J.-H. Kim, S.-H. Han, and J.-W. Hwang, "Ultrasound-guided oblique subcostal transversus abdominis plane block for analgesia after laparoscopic cholecystectomy: A randomized, controlled, observer-blinded study," *Minerva Anesthesiologica*, vol. 80, no. 2, pp. 185–193, 2014.

[10] S. Arora, A. Chhabra, R. Subramaniam, M. K. Arora, M. C. Misra, and V. K. Bansal, "Transversus abdominis plane block for laparoscopic inguinal hernia repair: A randomized trial," *Journal of Clinical Anesthesia*, vol. 33, pp. 357–364, 2016.

48

Surdity in the OR: An Unusual Case of Brainstem Anesthesia

Howard D. Palte, Don P. Hoa, and Aldo Pavon Canseco

Department of Anesthesiology, Miller School of Medicine, University of Miami, Miami, FL, USA

Correspondence should be addressed to Howard D. Palte; hpalte@med.miami.edu

Academic Editor: Renato Santiago Gomez

Brainstem anesthesia is a potentially life-threatening complication of regional ophthalmic anesthesia. This case report chronicles an unusual presentation of brainstem anesthesia following an eye block. The unique features of this case were the presenting symptoms of deafness and slurred speech in the absence of loss of consciousness, respiratory depression, or contralateral ophthalmoplegia. This report underscores two key points: first, the importance of ongoing patient monitoring after performance of an eye block; second, the exigency of supportive therapy in suspected cases of brainstem anesthesia.

1. Introduction

Brainstem anesthesia is a potentially life-threatening complication of regional ophthalmic anesthesia. The classic presentation is one of altered states of consciousness in association with permutations of impaired respiratory drive, hemodynamic instability, and contralateral ophthalmoplegia. In general, symptoms manifest only 5 to 20 minutes after completion of the block. We present an atypical case of brainstem anesthesia presenting with hemodynamic volatility, deafness, and slurred speech. In addition, this case was unusual because consciousness was preserved and respiratory effort was not impaired.

2. Case Report

A 42-year-old male sustained a prior penetrating injury to his left eye and now presented for a corneal amniotic membrane graft. He had a background history of hypertension and diabetes mellitus. Current medications included metoprolol, lisinopril, and metformin. Fasting blood sugar on admission was 223 mg%. The patient was transported to the holding area on a chair-bed and standard ASA monitors, peripheral IV, and nasal oxygen cannula were placed. Vital signs included BP 122/83 mmHg, pulse 90/min, and S_pO_2 99%. Following sedation with midazolam (2 mg) and fentanyl (100 mcg), a left-sided inferotemporal transconjunctival eye block was performed using a 27 G 31 mm needle, maintaining the eye in neutral gaze. Nine mL of a local anesthetic (LA) mixture containing lidocaine 2%, ropivacaine 1%, and Hylenex® 7.5 IU/mL was administered. The performance of the block was uneventful. Ten minutes later the patient developed paroxysmal tachycardia (140/min) and acute, severe hypertension (240/140 mmHg) that was immediately treated with intravenous nicardipine (200 mcg) and labetalol (10 mg). At this point, the patient was somewhat somnolent but responded appropriately to verbal command. However, he displayed signs of mild left-sided facial weakness. Within five minutes of treatment, the blood pressure and heart rate returned to baseline levels. The peripheral oxygen saturation (S_pO_2) was always ≥98%. His condition was assessed as stable and he was transferred to the OR.

In the OR monitors were reapplied and the patient was asked to shift towards the head of the bed. He was now unresponsive to verbal command but opened his eyes on manual stimulation and indicated that he was unable to hear. His vital signs remained stable with no evidence of respiratory embarrassment or decline in S_pO_2. In addition to deafness, a repeat neurological examination revealed left-sided facial weakness, slurred speech, and an inability to protrude the tongue. Although the contralateral pupil was dilated, the light reflex and extraocular muscle function remained intact. The blood glucose was reassessed at 271 mg%.

At this stage, the differential diagnosis included brainstem anesthesia and cerebrovascular accident secondary to hypertensive crisis. The planned surgery was aborted and the patient was transferred to a tertiary center for an urgent CT scan to exclude stroke. This was performed within the recommended time constraint for stroke victims and revealed no intracranial pathology. Within three hours there was full return of neurologic integrity, including hearing. A full disclosure of the events was made to the patient. He was discharged home later the same day.

3. Discussion

Brainstem anesthesia is a rare, potentially life-threatening complication of regional ophthalmic anesthesia. The true incidence varies according to the source quoted. However, its prevalence may be on the decline because traditional retrobulbar anesthesia has now been largely superseded by less invasive peribulbar techniques. For example, Riad and Akbar reported only one episode in a case series of over 33000 eye blocks (0.002%) [1], whereas Kumar and Dowd pegged the incidence at 0.03% [2]. However, they opined that the incidence could be as high as 0.8% when retrobulbar blocks are performed with long needles. Lee et al. evaluated the American Society of Anesthesiology (ASA) closed claims database for complications associated with eye blocks from 1980 through 2000 [3]. They found only one claim with cardiorespiratory arrest attributable to eye block although there were another seven instances where cardiac or respiratory arrest followed an eye block. However, the concurrent use of sedation confounded the etiology.

In North America the majority of adult ophthalmic surgical interventions are conducted under topical or regional anesthesia, mostly needle-based techniques. Conversely, in the United Kingdom and Europe, sub-Tenon's block is favored due to the contention that it eliminates risk of needle misadventure. However, no regional technique is entirely safe and major complications have been reported with all techniques [4–7].

Brainstem anesthesia develops secondary to injection of LA within the dural sheath that surrounds the intraorbital segment of the optic nerve. Local anesthetic is subsequently transported towards the optic chiasm and brainstem. Traditionally, the presenting signs include a combination of altered mentation (agitation, confusion, and unresponsiveness), apnea, cardiovascular collapse (hypotension, bradycardia, or asystole), and shivering in association with ophthalmoplegia and amaurosis in the contralateral eye. Convulsions may occur secondary to hypoxia. Typically, symptoms begin 5–10 minutes after the block but presentation may be delayed up to 20 minutes. In general, most cases have favorable outcomes with no long-term sequelae provided that assisted-ventilation and indicated inotropic support are administered.

There is ample evidence that LA injected within the optic nerve dural cuff reaches the brainstem. In 1969, Reed et al. performed orbitography on a patient with an intraorbital tumor and demonstrated injected radiopaque dye within the intracranial subdural space [8]. Wang et al. injected cadaver optic sheaths with methylene blue and traced progression of the dye as far as the middle cranial fossa [9]. In a cadaver model, Drysdale placed a needle within the optic sheath and

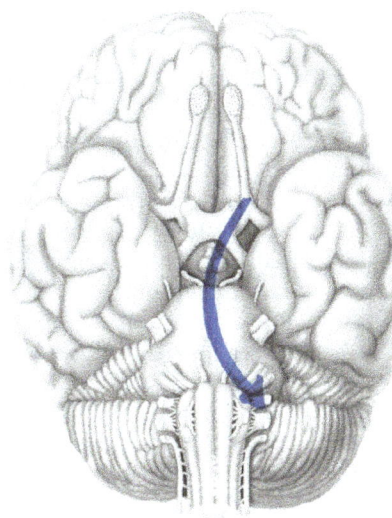

FIGURE 1: Diagrammatic representation of local anesthetic spread along brainstem from CN II to CN VIII.

injected 3 mL radiopaque dye [10]. He demonstrated that contrast material tracked proximally along the nerve to the optic chiasm, ultimately reaching the pons and midbrain. Finally, Kobet retrieved high levels of lidocaine and bupivacaine in the CSF of a case of brainstem anesthesia following retrobulbar block [11].

The clinical course of this case was atypical. The common features of loss of consciousness, respiratory depression, hypotension and contralateral ophthalmoplegia, and amaurosis were absent. Instead, the dominant signs were transient malignant hypertension, hearing loss, and slurred speech. Moreover, pupillary dilation was the only sign in the contralateral eye. We hypothesize that the initial insult was needle penetration of the lateral segment of the dural sheath. Thereafter, local anesthetic tracked in a subdural plane over the lateral optic chiasm and hypothalamus producing a block in parasympathetic efferent activity and overexpression of symapthetic activity and manifesting as hypertensive crisis. We postulate that LA remained confined within this compartment of the optic nerve because there was neither ophthalmoplegia nor amaurosis in the contralateral eye. Ultimately, LA blocked cranial nerves VIII and XII producing deafness and slurred speech (Figure 1). Furthermore, this case is peculiar because brainstem anesthesia followed use of a 31 mm needle. Katsev et al. measured orbital depth in a series of skulls and recommended that 31 mm needles afford greater protection against optic sheath penetration than commonly used 38 mm needle [12].

The peribulbar block deposits LA outside the extraocular muscle cone away from the globe and vital structures. Since successful anesthesia depends on passive diffusion of local anesthetic into the retrobulbar compartment, the technique requires administration of a greater LA volume than for the traditional retrobulbar block. One disadvantage of this technique is that the ultimate needle-tip position in relation to the muscle cone is unconfirmed, raising the specter of intraconal injection. In this case, we contemplate that posttraumatic scar tissue within the orbital cavity produced an aberration of the muscle cone with lateral displacement of the optic nerve.

This case underscores several important take-home points. First, brainstem anesthesia remains a real hazard of regional ophthalmic blockade and may present with atypical features. Second, the latent period between block and symptomatology is variable and influenced by many factors including orbital anatomy, volume of local anesthetic, rate of spread, and constitution of the LA. Also, a prior history of eye trauma or repeat surgeries raises the specter of possible intraorbital scarring and anatomic aberration. Third, the differential diagnosis should include other acute neurologic or cardiovascular insults that produce similar symptomatology, especially cerebrovascular accident. Fourth, beneficial outcomes with no long-term sequelae are expected when assisted-ventilation and inotropic support are instituted in a timely manner. Finally, the temporal relationship between performance of an eye block and onset of neurological, cardiovascular, or respiratory symptomatology should raise suspicion of brainstem anesthesia.

Competing Interests

The authors declare that there is no conflict of interests regarding the publication of this paper.

References

[1] W. Riad and F. Akbar, "Ophthalmic regional blockade complication rate: a single center audit of 33,363 ophthalmic operations," *Journal of Clinical Anesthesia*, vol. 24, no. 3, pp. 193–195, 2012.

[2] C. M. Kumar and T. C. Dowd, "Complications of ophthalmic regional blocks: their treatment and prevention," *Ophthalmologica*, vol. 220, no. 2, pp. 73–82, 2006.

[3] L. A. Lee, K. L. Posner, F. W. Cheney, R. A. Caplan, and K. B. Domino, "Complications associated with eye blocks and peripheral nerve blocks: an American Society of Anesthesiologists closed claims analysis," *Regional Anesthesia and Pain Medicine*, vol. 33, no. 5, pp. 416–422, 2008.

[4] K. R. Edge and J. M. V. Nicoll, "Retrobulbar hemorrhage after 12,500 retrobulbar blocks," *Anesthesia and Analgesia*, vol. 76, no. 5, pp. 1019–1022, 1993.

[5] I. Rahman and S. Ataullah, "Retrobulbar hemorrhage after sub-Tenon's anesthesia," *Journal of Cataract and Refractive Surgery*, vol. 30, no. 12, pp. 2636–2637, 2004.

[6] A. C. Wadood, B. Dhillon, and J. Singh, "Inadvertent ocular perforation and intravitreal injection of an anesthetic agent during retrobulbar injection," *Journal of Cataract and Refractive Surgery*, vol. 28, no. 3, pp. 562–565, 2002.

[7] P. D. Jaycock, C. M. Mather, J. D. Ferris, and J. N. P. Kirkpatrick, "Rectus muscle trauma complicating sub-Tenon's local anaesthesia," *Eye*, vol. 15, no. 5, pp. 583–586, 2001.

[8] J. W. Reed, A. S. Macmillan, and G. W. Lazenby, "Transient neurologic complication of positive contrast orbitography," *Archives of Ophthalmology*, vol. 81, no. 4, pp. 508–511, 1969.

[9] B. C. Wang, B. Bogart, D. E. Hillman, and H. Turndorf, "Subarachnoid injection—a potential complication of retrobulbar block," *Anesthesiology*, vol. 71, no. 6, pp. 845–847, 1989.

[10] D. B. Drysdale, "Experimental subdural retrobulbar injection of anesthetic," *Annals of Ophthalmology*, vol. 16, no. 8, pp. 716–718, 1984.

[11] K. A. Kobet, "Cerebral spinal fluid recovery of lidocaine and bupivacaine following respiratory arrest subsequent to retrobulbar block," *Ophthalmic Surgery*, vol. 18, no. 1, pp. 11–13, 1987.

[12] D. A. Katsev, R. C. Drews, and B. T. Rose, "An anatomic study of retrobulbar needle path length," *Ophthalmology*, vol. 96, no. 8, pp. 1221–1224, 1989.

49

From Bad to Worse: Paraganglioma Diagnosis during Induction of Labor for Coexisting Preeclampsia

Sasima Dusitkasem, Blair H. Herndon, Dalton Paluzzi, Joseph Kuhn, Robert H. Small, and John C. Coffman

Department of Anesthesiology, The Ohio State University Wexner Medical Center, Columbus, OH, USA

Correspondence should be addressed to Sasima Dusitkasem; sasima1308@gmail.com

Academic Editor: Alparslan Apan

Pheochromocytomas and extra-adrenal paragangliomas are catecholamine-secreting tumors that rarely occur in pregnancy. The diagnosis of these tumors in pregnancy can be challenging given that many of the signs and symptoms are commonly attributed to preeclampsia or other more common diagnoses. Early diagnosis and appropriate management are essential in optimizing maternal and fetal outcomes. We report a rare case of a catecholamine-secreting tumor in which diagnosis occurring at the time labor was being induced for concomitant preeclampsia with severe features. Her initial presentation in hypertensive crisis with other symptoms led to diagnostic workup for secondary causes of hypertension and led to eventual diagnosis of paraganglioma. Obtaining this diagnosis prior to delivery was essential, as this led to prompt multidisciplinary care, changed the course of her clinical management, and ultimately enabled good maternal and fetal outcomes. This case highlights the importance of maintaining a high index of suspicion for secondary causes of hypertension and in obstetric patients and providing timely multidisciplinary care.

1. Introduction

Pheochromocytomas and extra-adrenal paragangliomas (PGLs) are catecholamine-secreting tumors that arise from neural-crest derived chromaffin cells [1]. These rare tumors are estimated to occur in 0.1–0.2% of hypertensive adults [2, 3] and 0.002% of pregnant women [4, 5]. Extra-adrenal PGLs have been estimated to account for 19% of chromaffin cell tumors occurring in pregnancy, with pheochromocytomas accounting for the majority of tumors [6]. The classical presentation is associated with episodic catecholamine secretion by the tumor, resulting in paroxysmal hypertension, headaches, sweating, and palpitations [7, 8]. The diagnosis of catecholamine-secreting tumors in pregnancy is challenging given that many of these signs and symptoms are commonly attributed to preeclampsia or other diagnoses that occur more commonly in pregnancy [7–9]. However, it is important to maintain a high level of suspicion for pheochromocytoma or PGL in cases of severe hypertension refractory to conventional antihypertensive treatment, as early diagnosis and appropriate treatment can improve maternal and fetal outcomes [6].

We report an undiagnosed paraganglioma (PGL) in a pregnant woman at 33 weeks of gestation who presented with hypertensive crisis. This complex case presented a unique diagnostic challenge given that the patient had coexisting preeclampsia, though timely diagnosis changed the course of her clinical management and ultimately enabled positive maternal and fetal outcomes.

2. Case Presentation

A 33-year-old G6P3 woman (weight 83.9 kg; height 1.6 m; body mass index 32.8 kg/m^2) presented to our unit at 32 5/7 weeks of gestation with severe headache, palpitations, anxiety, abdominal pain, and hypertensive crisis (blood pressure (BP) 200–230/100–130 mmHg). Her past medical history was significant for viral myocarditis with subsequent cardiomyopathy three years previously. At that time, her left ventricular ejection fraction (LVEF) was <20%, and she

TABLE 1: The results of free plasma and 24-hour urinary and metanephrines and normetanephrines.

	Reference values	Values at 33-week gestation	Values 1 month after tumor excision
Urinary normetanephrines (mcg/24 hrs)	111–419	**11617**	
Urinary metanephrine (mcg/24 hrs)	30–180 (normotensive) <400 (hypertensive)	291	
Total urinary metanephrines (mcg/24 hrs)	149–535 (normotensive) <1300 (hypertensive)	**11908**	
Plasma normetanephrines (pg/mL)	<148	**2920**	110
Plasma metanephrines (pg/mL)	<57	**<25**	41

required extracorporeal membrane oxygenation (ECMO). She was decannulated after normalization of her ejection fraction (LVEF 73%). After decannulation, she developed hypertension and ultimately required initiation of four antihypertensive medications prior to hospital discharge. With hypertension at this level of severity in a 30-year-old woman, a workup for secondary causes of hypertension should have been initiated.

She did not follow up with scheduled outpatient appointments and was lost to follow-up until the current pregnancy. Unfortunately, a more detailed workup for etiologies of her severe hypertension was not completed during the patient's first and only prenatal visit at 14 weeks of gestation. She was no longer taking any antihypertensives prior to this visit, and labetalol 100 mg twice daily was initiated as blood pressure was noted to be 158/72 mmHg. She did not endorse symptoms of headache, palpitations, temperature intolerance, or recent weight changes at that time. She did not attend her other obstetric appointments and was noncompliant with her labetalol.

Upon hospital presentation, she was diagnosed with chronic hypertension with superimposed preeclampsia based on a 24-hour urine protein of 388 mg. Intravenous hydralazine 10 mg and labetalol 20 mg were given for initial control of her BP. She was admitted to the antepartum unit and maintained on oral labetalol 200 mg twice daily for BP control and received betamethasone to enhance fetal lung maturation. Her BP control improved, though she continued to experience intermittent headaches. Urinary and serum metanephrines were collected given the severity of hypertension accompanied by headaches and palpitations, though there was only mild suspicion at this point in time. These samples are processed by an external laboratory which, due to transit times, consequentially causes a delay in the availability of results. Seven days after admission for preeclampsia, labor was induced due to worsening hypertension and headache symptoms. Though the secondary workup had been initiated, the working diagnosis was still superimposed preeclampsia with severe features that could no longer be controlled by medications. Given that catecholamine-secreting tumors were less likely among differential diagnoses at that time, no alpha or calcium channel blockade was initiated prior to induction

of labor (IOL). Intravenous magnesium 4 gm was given, followed by IV infusion of magnesium 2 gm/hr. She had an uneventful epidural placement at L3-4 and obtained effective epidural labor analgesia after an initial dose of 0.125% bupivacaine 10 mL and fentanyl 20 mcg. Labor analgesia was then maintained with a continuous epidural infusion of 0.0625% bupivacaine + 2 mcg/mL fentanyl at 12 mL/hr, with patient-controlled epidural analgesia (8 mL bolus, 15-minute lockout). During her induction, her free plasma and 24-hour urinary and metanephrines and normetanephrines resulted and were found to be significantly elevated (see Table 1). Despite cervical dilation to 5 cm and artificial rupture of membranes, her IOL was stopped and a multidisciplinary meeting consisting of obstetricians, anesthesiologists, endocrinologists, and surgical oncologists was promptly convened to develop appropriate treatment plan. After discussion with the various care teams, a cesarean delivery was planned. Cesarean was determined to be the optimal mode of delivery to avoid rises in intraabdominal pressure and catecholamine releases associated with uterine contractions and vaginal delivery. Due to continued hypertensive urgency, cervical dilation, and ruptured membranes, delivery proceeded in an expedited fashion once patient has been dosed with phenoxybenzamine 10 mg and volume replete with intravenous fluids. The recommendation from the multidisciplinary meeting was to not remove the mass at time of cesarean delivery, as the patient had not been alpha-blocked for a significant amount of time and manipulation of the mass could cause significant morbidity.

A radial arterial line was placed preoperatively for close monitoring of blood pressure. Appropriate emergency medications were prepared for intraoperative administration, including IV phentolamine and nicardipine. IV magnesium 2 gm/hr was continued intraoperatively for prevention of eclamptic seizures and to help manage intraoperative hypertension due to her catecholamine-secreting tumor. Her labor epidural was effectively dosed for cesarean anesthesia with 0.5% ropivacaine 20 mL, given in 3–5 mL increments over fifteen minutes, and fentanyl 100 mcg. Her vital signs were stable during the initial operative course, but she became acutely hypertensive to >220/110 with external abdominal pressure during delivery. This was effectively managed with IV nicardipine 500 mcg in incremental doses. Nicardipine

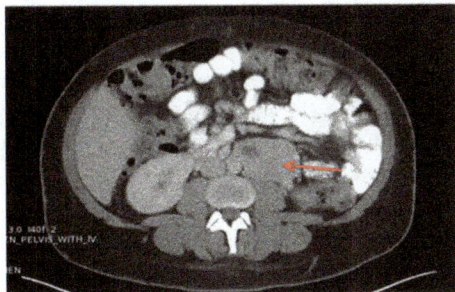

FIGURE 1: CT abdomen/pelvis demonstrating a left para-aortic mass measuring approximately 4.7 × 6.4 cm.

5 mg/hr was initiated toward the end of the procedure and continued for 18 hours. The operation was successful; a 2,570 g female newborn was delivered, with neonatal Apgar scores of 4 at one minute, 3 at five minutes, and 7 at ten minutes. Umbilical arterial pH was 7.28 and umbilical venous pH was 7.36.

The patient was observed in the intensive care unit postoperatively. Her postpartum period was uneventful. CT imaging revealed a left para-aortic mass consistent with PGL (Figure 1). During her ICU stay, oral phenoxybenzamine 10 mg twice daily (BID) and propranolol 10 mg every 8 hours were initiated. Endocrine specialists gradually increased phenoxybenzamine to 60 mg every 8 hours and propranolol to 60 mg every 8 hours, over a two-week period of medical optimization prior to surgical resection of the paraganglioma. An arterial line was placed for careful hemodynamic monitoring. Anesthesia was induced after 4 mg of midazolam with 2% lidocaine 100 mg, propofol 200 mg, fentanyl 200 mcg, and 50 mg rocuronium. Smooth tracheal intubation followed, during which blood pressures peaked at 210/130. This required treatment with 600 mcg of nicardipine given in divided doses. As the surgeons dissected to the tumor, phenylephrine was needed to maintain blood pressure. Pressures reached a nadir of 90/40. Upon manipulation and dissection of the mass, hemodynamics became extremely labile despite the 2-week adrenergic receptor blockade. Intraoperative hemodynamic stability was achieved by careful fluid management, administration of incremental boluses of nicardipine, and esmolol, as well as nitroprusside and remifentanil infusions. Upon removal of the tumor, hemodynamics stabilized and the patient was able to be weaned off the infusions. She required some minimal blood pressure support with phenylephrine during closure. The tumor specimen pathology examination revealed features consistent with the diagnosis of extra-adrenal paraganglioma. She was discharged along with a healthy neonate seven days later without complication. Labs one month after resection showed normalization of her plasma normetanephrine and metanephrine levels (see Table 1). The patient has not been compliant with scheduled follow-up appointments with endocrine, genetics, obstetrics, or surgical oncology specialists.

3. Discussion

Maternal and fetal outcomes in patients with catecholamine-secreting tumors are greatly improved by early antenatal diagnosis and proper management with alpha-adrenergic blockade and sometimes antenatal surgical resection of the tumor [5, 6]. Biggar and Lennard reported that early antenatal recognition of pheochromocytoma/PGL resulted in decreased maternal mortality from 29% to 0% and fetal mortality from 29% to 12% compared with diagnoses made during labor or postpartum [6]. Higher incidence of maternal and fetal mortality has been observed with pheochromocytoma (9.8% and 16%, resp.) compared to extra-adrenal PGL (3.6 and 12%, resp.) in obstetric patients [4], though the tumor location in our case was not determined until after delivery. Regardless of the chromaffin cell tumor location, high maternal, and fetal morbidity and mortality rates underscore the importance of establishing a diagnosis as early as possible. While poor medical compliance of our patient prior to and during pregnancy limited the opportunity of antenatal tumor diagnosis, it is true that hypertension this severe in a young person should have been worked up previously. The lack of workup for 4-drug resistant hypertension after our patient's ECMO decannulation, or during her single prenatal visit, significantly increased mortality risks. She was diagnosed with chronic hypertension with superimposed preeclampsia due to the presence of proteinuria, which is not commonly associated with pheochromocytoma or PGL [5, 6]. Importantly, the physicians involved in her hospital care also searched for secondary causes of hypertension based on modest clinical suspicion given her initial presentation of hypertensive urgency accompanied by headache, sweating, palpitations, and other symptoms. Diagnostic workup revealed the eventual diagnosis of a catecholamine-secreting tumor, which led to prompt multidisciplinary care, altered the course of her clinical management, and ultimately enabled good maternal and fetal outcomes. This case highlights the importance of maintaining a high index of suspicion for secondary causes of hypertension in obstetric patients.

It was essential to have timely involvement and good communication among the obstetricians, anesthesiologists, endocrinologists, and surgical oncologists involved in her care. Based on multidisciplinary discussions, it was decided that cesarean delivery would be the optimal course of action. Obstetric patients with pheochromocytoma or PGL have had successful vaginal deliveries, though cesarean deliveries are more commonly performed [4, 6]. Higher fetal mortality rates have been observed with vaginal delivery compared to cesarean delivery in this setting [10]. The fetus is not directly exposed to the high catecholamine levels due to enzymatic metabolism within the placenta [11], though uncontrolled hypertension can lead to uteroplacental insufficiency, placental abruption, and fetal demise. Hypertension due to catecholamine release may be precipitated by increases in intra-abdominal pressure during uterine contractions, vigorous fetal movements, or second stage pushing with vaginal delivery [12–15]. In addition to potential mechanical disturbance of the tumor, the stresses of labor pain can induce sympathetic stimulation and catecholamine release [6]. Further, this patient was diagnosed during the course of labor and had not been medically optimized on adrenoceptor blockade, which is important prior to both tumor resection and any other procedure that may be associated with catecholamine release from the tumor [16, 17]. Based on these reasons, the multidisciplinary team of physicians caring for this patient agreed that cesarean delivery with delayed surgical resection was the most appropriate course of action. The optimal time for surgical tumor removal is controversial and depends in part upon the gestational age at the time of diagnosis. Tumors can be removed either before 24 weeks of gestation, simultaneously with cesarean delivery, or separately after delivery [18]. In our patient, surgical excision was performed 2 weeks postpartum after inpatient medical stabilization, as there was concern regarding patient compliance as an outpatient.

Undiagnosed chromaffin cell tumors can present with life-threatening complications for both the mother and fetus. Patients presenting with hypertensive crisis, as our patient did, have been reported to have maternal mortality rates of 54.5% [6]. This finding highlights the importance of early diagnosis and also maintaining control of hypertension with adrenoceptor blockade. Preoperative BP control is essential to avoid hypertensive crisis during cesarean delivery or surgical resection of the tumor. Phenoxybenzamine is an irreversible adrenergic antagonist and has been suggested as the preferred treatment of choice in patients with pheochromocytoma or PGL [19]. Our patient was started on phenoxybenzamine for alpha blockade and labetalol was discontinued. Although labetalol has both alpha and beta blocking properties, the ratio of alpha : beta antagonism is approximately 1 : 7 and could lead to unopposed alpha-adrenergic receptor stimulation [20]. Beta-blockade with propranolol was initiated more than 24 hours after treatment with phenoxybenzamine in order to minimize a paradoxical hypertensive response.

The primary goal of her intraoperative anesthetic management for cesarean delivery was to prevent and effectively manage abrupt changes in her hemodynamic measurements. Neuraxial anesthesia was desirable in this patient with PGL given the potential advantage of avoiding hypertension and tachycardia due to sympathetic stimulation and catecholamine secretion associated with laryngoscopy, intubation, and surgical stress [21, 22]. Epidural blockade was gradually induced as IV crystalloid was administered and arterial line BP carefully monitored in order to avoid hypotension and maintain appropriate placental blood flow. Nicardipine was used effectively for treatment of severe hypertension at the time of delivery [23, 24] and was also effectively utilized in the early postdelivery period. Magnesium sulfate was also useful in her hemodynamic management, where the patient was getting this for concomitant preeclampsia. Magnesium sulfate inhibits catecholamine release from the catecholamine-secreting tumor and blocks peripheral catecholamine receptors [9].

After tumor resection, it is important to check plasma or urinary metanephrine levels 2–6 weeks to assess for completeness of resection [25]. It is also important to continue regular surveillance with endocrine specialists, given that tumor persistence or new tumors can occur. For example, 18% of patients with thoraco-abdomen-pelvic PGLs have been reported to have a new tumor event within the first five years after initial surgical resection [25]. Referral for genetic testing is also essential given that a germline mutation in susceptibility genes is identified in approximately 40% of pheochromocytomas or paragangliomas cases [26], which can increase risk of tumor recurrence and also have implications for family members [25]. Unfortunately, the patient described in this case has not arrived for scheduled appointments with endocrine or genetics specialists up to this point.

In conclusion, this case presented a unique diagnostic challenge given that the patient had coexisting preeclampsia, which can share many of the same signs and symptoms as catecholamine-secreting tumors. Diagnosis prior to the patient's IOL would have been ideal, as the patient could have been optimized with alpha adrenergic blockade prior to delivery. Fortunately, multidisciplinary collaboration and planning allowed for a mode of delivery and ultimate tumor resection that enabled good maternal and fetal outcomes.

Competing Interests

The authors confirm that there is no conflict of interests in regard to the publication of this case report.

References

[1] A. S. Tischler, "Pheochromocytoma and extra-adrenal paraganglioma: updates," *Archives of Pathology & Laboratory Medicine*, vol. 132, no. 8, pp. 1272–1284, 2008.

[2] H. Chen, R. S. Sippel, M. S. O'Dorisio, A. I. Vinik, R. V. Lloyd, and K. Pacak, "The north american neuroendocrine tumor society consensus guideline for the diagnosis and management of neuroendocrine tumors: pheochromocytoma, paraganglioma, and medullary thyroid cancer," *Pancreas*, vol. 39, no. 6, pp. 775–783, 2010.

[3] C. M. Kiernan and C. C. Solórzano, "Pheochromocytoma and paraganglioma: diagnosis, genetics, and treatment," *Surgical Oncology Clinics of North America*, vol. 25, no. 1, pp. 119–138, 2016.

[4] L. A. Wing, J. V. Conaglen, G. Y. Meyer-Rochow, and M. S. Elston, "Paraganglioma in pregnancy: a case series and review of the literature," *The Journal of Clinical Endocrinology and Metabolism*, vol. 100, no. 8, pp. 3202–3209, 2015.

[5] J. L. Harrington, D. R. Farley, J. A. Van Heerden, and K. D. Ramin, "Adrenal tumors and pregnancy," *World Journal of Surgery*, vol. 23, no. 2, pp. 182–186, 1999.

[6] M. A. Biggar and T. W. J. Lennard, "Systematic review of phaeochromocytoma in pregnancy," *British Journal of Surgery*, vol. 100, no. 2, pp. 182–190, 2013.

[7] R. Oliva, P. Angelos, E. Kaplan, and G. Bakris, "Pheochromocytoma in pregnancy: a case series and review," *Hypertension*, vol. 55, no. 3, pp. 600–606, 2010.

[8] S. Grodski, C. Jung, P. Kertes, M. Davies, and S. Banting, "Phaeochromocytoma in pregnancy," *Internal Medicine Journal*, vol. 36, no. 9, pp. 604–606, 2006.

[9] K. R. L. Huddle and A. Nagar, "Phaeochromocytoma in pregnancy," *Australian and New Zealand Journal of Obstetrics and Gynaecology*, vol. 39, no. 2, pp. 203–206, 1999.

[10] S. K. Ahlawat, S. Jain, S. Kumari, S. Varma, and B. K. Sharma, "Pheochromocytoma associated with pregnancy: case report and review of the literature," *Obstetrical & Gynecological Survey*, vol. 54, no. 11, pp. 728–737, 1999.

[11] P. L. M. Dahia, C. Y. Hayashida, C. Strunz, N. Abelin, and S. P. A. Toledo, "Low cord blood levels of catecholamine from a newborn of a pheochromocytoma patient," *European Journal of Endocrinology*, vol. 130, no. 3, pp. 217–219, 1994.

[12] L. M. Brunt, "Phaeochromocytoma in pregnancy," *British Journal of Surgery*, vol. 88, no. 4, pp. 481–483, 2001.

[13] P. Lau, M. Permezel, P. Dawson, S. Chester, N. Collier, and I. Forbes, "Phaeochromocytoma in pregnancy," *Australian and New Zealand Journal of Obstetrics and Gynaecology*, vol. 36, no. 4, pp. 472–476, 1996.

[14] M. A. Harper, G. A. Murnaghan, L. Kennedy, D. R. Hadden, and A. B. Atkinson, "Phaeochromocytoma in pregnancy. Five cases and a review of the literature," *British Journal of Obstetrics & Gynaecology*, vol. 96, no. 5, pp. 594–606, 1989.

[15] J. K. Kalra, V. Jain, R. Bagga et al., "Pheochromocytoma associated with pregnancy," *Journal of Obstetrics and Gynaecology Research*, vol. 29, no. 5, pp. 305–308, 2003.

[16] I. Lata and S. Sahu, "Management of paroxysmal hypertension due to incidental pheochromocytoma in pregnancy," *Journal of Emergencies, Trauma and Shock*, vol. 4, no. 3, pp. 415–417, 2011.

[17] K. Pacak, "Approach to the patient: preoperative management of the pheochromocytoma patient," *The Journal of Clinical Endocrinology & Metabolism*, vol. 92, no. 11, pp. 4069–4079, 2007.

[18] J. W. M. Lenders, "ENDOCRINE DISORDERS IN PREGNANCY: pheochromocytoma and pregnancy: a deceptive connection," *European Journal of Endocrinology*, vol. 166, no. 2, pp. 143–150, 2012.

[19] W. M. Manger, "The vagaries of pheochromocytomas," *American Journal of Hypertension*, vol. 18, no. 10, pp. 1266–1270, 2005.

[20] D. A. Richards, B. N. C. Prichard, A. J. Boakes, J. Tuckman, and E. J. Knight, "Pharmacological basis for antihypertensive effects of intravenous labetalol," *British Heart Journal*, vol. 39, no. 1, pp. 99–106, 1977.

[21] S. M. Nimmo, "Benefit and outcome after epidural analgesia," *Continuing Education in Anaesthesia, Critical Care & Pain*, vol. 4, no. 2, pp. 44–47, 2004.

[22] A. Nizamoglu, Z. Salihoglu, and M. Bolayrl, "Effects of epidural-and-general anesthesia combined versus general anesthesia during laparoscopic adrenalectomy," *Surgical Laparoscopy, Endoscopy & Percutaneous Techniques*, vol. 21, no. 5, pp. 372–379, 2011.

[23] E. L. Bravo, "Pheochromocytoma," *Current Therapy in Endocrinology and Metabolism*, vol. 6, pp. 195–197, 1997.

[24] C. Proye, D. Thevenin, P. Cecat et al., "Exclusive use of calcium channel blockers in preoperative and intraoperative control of pheochromocytomas: hemodynamics and free catecholamine assays in ten consecutive patients," *Surgery*, vol. 106, no. 6, pp. 1149–1154, 1989.

[25] P. F. Plouin, L. Amar, O. M. Dekkers et al., "European Society of Endocrinology Clinical Practice Guideline for long-term follow-up of patients operated on for a phaeochromocytoma or a paraganglioma," *European Journal of Endocrinology*, vol. 174, no. 5, pp. G1–G10, 2016.

[26] J. Favier, L. Amar, and A.-P. Gimenez-Roqueplo, "Paraganglioma and phaeochromocytoma: from genetics to personalized medicine," *Nature Reviews Endocrinology*, vol. 11, no. 2, pp. 101–111, 2015.

50

Coccydynia Treated with Dorsal Root Ganglion Stimulation

Nicholas L. Giordano,[1] **Noud van Helmond** [ID],[1] **and Kenneth B. Chapman** [ID][1,2,3]

[1]*Spine & Pain Institute of New York, New York City, NY, USA*
[2]*Department of Anesthesiology, New York University Langone Medical Center, New York City, NY, USA*
[3]*Northwell Health, New York City, NY, USA*

Correspondence should be addressed to Kenneth B. Chapman; chapmanken@spinepainny.com

Academic Editor: Anjan Trikha

Coccydynia can be difficult to resolve with conventional treatment options. Dorsal root ganglion (DRG) stimulation has recently emerged as a treatment for chronic pain, but its application has not been described in the context of coccydynia. We used DRG stimulation treatment in a patient suffering from intractable coccyx pain. At long-term follow-up, the patient experienced a decrease in pain intensity and improvement in function, without any complications. DRG stimulation may be a treatment modality for coccydynia refractory to other approaches.

1. Introduction

Coccydynia, or coccygodynia, is pain in the region of the coccyx. The term was first coined in 1859 by Simpson [1], who also introduced the use of chloroform in anesthesia. Despite the identification of coccygeal pain almost ~150 years ago, its treatment can be difficult in a select patient population in whom the pain becomes chronic and debilitating. Treatment options range from lifestyle modification and cushions, to injections, to treatments as radical as resection of the coccyx [2]. Recent reports have described the use of neuromodulation techniques to treat chronic coccydynia [3]. The aim of this report is to describe the use of dorsal root ganglion (DRG) stimulation to treat chronic coccydynia.

Written informed consent was obtained from the patient for publication of this case report.

2. Case Description

A 37-year-old female from Spain presented to our center in August of 2017 with complaints of chronic intractable pain in the coccyx. The patient suffered from this pain since 2009 when she sustained a coccyx fracture in a work-related slip and fall injury while working as an airline stewardess in Europe. At the time of presentation, the patient endorsed 10/10 coccyx pain on visual analog scale. She described the pain as sharp, stinging, shooting, and radiating throughout her bilateral lower extremities. Due to the injury, she was forced to quit when her pain prevented her from performing her duties. At the time of presentation, she could not sit or walk for more than 10 minutes consecutively and required special cushioning to be brought with her at all times.

Prior to presenting to our center, she had been evaluated and treated by pain management physicians, orthopedic surgeons, and multiple urgent care clinicians in both Spain and the UK. Her past treatments in Europe included multiple coccygeal blocks, trigger point injections, epidural steroid injections, and a conventional spinal cord stimulator in 2011. The spinal cord stimulation therapy consisted of an ANS Genesis (company acquired in 2005 by St. Jude Medical, which was subsequently purchased by Abbot) spinal cord stimulator with one octode lead placed through the sacrococcygeal hiatus. This stimulator was placed in Spain in 2011 and the patient continued to use the stimulator at presentation. Stimulator treatment was previously complicated by an infection, which was treated with IV antibiotics and surgical debridement. The patient reported pain relief from the stimulator, but she was experiencing diminished relief from the stimulator over the last several years and also had inadequate coverage in her most painful region, which was the coccyx itself. She continued to have the stimulator turned on as it provided some relief, but she was still incapacitated from the pain. She was maintained on a pain medication regiment consisting of oxycodone 10 mg PO BID, dexketoprofen 25 mg PO QID, duloxetine 60 mg PO QD, trazodone 100 mg PO QD, and pregabalin 75 mg PO BID. Despite this intensive medical treatment, the patient experienced poor symptom control in addition to side effects from these medications, including constipation and drowsiness.

The patient presented to us seeking other potential options for pain relief, in particular a conventional radiofrequency ablation of the nerves innervating the coccyx or an endoscopic radiofrequency ablation of those nerves. Considering the patient's persistent severe coccydynia and failure of extensive conservative and interventional treatments and the chronicity of her pain, we proposed a DRG stimulator trial in September of 2017. The use of DRG stimulation for coccydynia is an off-label use; the reason we considered DRG stimulation was secondary to our highly successful experiences with DRG stimulation for both complex pelvic and rectal pain, as well as low back and SI joint pain. Our rationale for proceeding with the trial was the potential for better regional coverage versus conventional sacral nerve stimulation, similar to our experience in those cases.

Our proposed approach was a bilateral L1 and S2 DRG stimulator trial. The patient decided to proceed with the DRG stimulator trial and underwent psychological clearance prior to the procedure. During the 7-day trial, the patient rated her pain less than 1/10 on visual analog score, improved sleep hygiene, functioned better in general, and was actually able to ambulate for approximately four miles without limitations. Prior to the trial she could not walk more than a city block without severe pain. She was able to function better in almost all her daily activities and she was able to position herself with minimal limitations and without the aid of her cushion, which she previously carried with her at all times, and claimed to have close to 100% coverage of her pain. After the trial, the patient decided to proceed with permanent lead implantation. She understood she had the option to have the procedure performed in Europe or to have it performed at our institute. After consideration, she decided to proceed with the implantation at our center. We then decided to leave her current spinal cord stimulator system in place rather than to explant the system.

2.1. *Surgical Procedure.* A board-certified anesthesiologist monitored the patient throughout the implant procedure. Thirty minutes prior to the procedure the patient received 2 grams of cefazolin. The patient was placed in the prone position with bolsters under the lumbar/lower thoracic region. After positioning was deemed adequate, the patient received propofol sedation. The lumbar spine and buttocks were prepped and draped in normal sterile fashion with betadine followed by DuraPrep. The L1 vertebral body was then aligned on fluoroscopy and 1.0% lidocaine mixed with 0.5% bupivacaine was used for local anesthesia. A Tuohy needle was inserted at the right side one level below the left L1 target foramen at the level of the pedicle and was then guided toward the midline at the interspace of the target level.

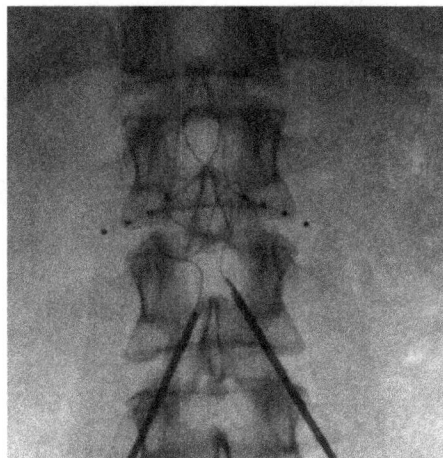

FIGURE 1: Anterior posterior fluoroscopic image of bilateral dorsal root ganglion stimulation leads on the L1 level.

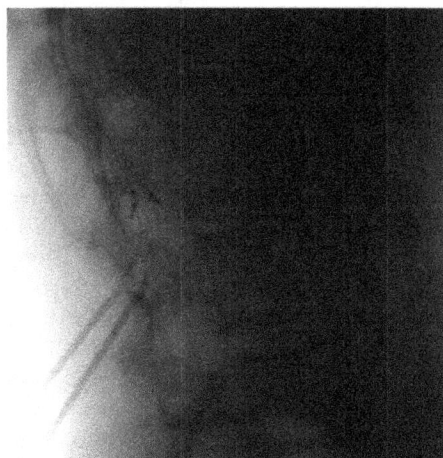

FIGURE 2: Lateral fluoroscopic image of bilateral dorsal root ganglion stimulation leads on the L1 level.

Loss of resistance to air was achieved close to the midline. At this point, the 4-contact DRG lead (Axium™, St. Jude/Abbot, Lake Bluff, IL) was loaded into the introducer catheter with the lead tip approximately 2-3 mm outside of the introducer. The loaded introducer was then passed into the Tuohy needle. The introducer then accessed the epidural space and was directed toward the foramen. The introducer was passed through the target foramen until the middle two contacts were under the level of the pedicle. The introducer was then withdrawn to approximately 5 mm after the proximal contact while applying counterforce on the lead. A strain relief loop was created in the usual fashion [4]. Subsequently, the introducer was removed from the Tuohy needle and the lead was left in place. Fluoroscopy was performed to confirm no displacement of the lead had occurred. The same procedure was performed to place a lead on the right L1 DRG. Figures 1 and 2 depict the position of bilateral leads on the L1 level.

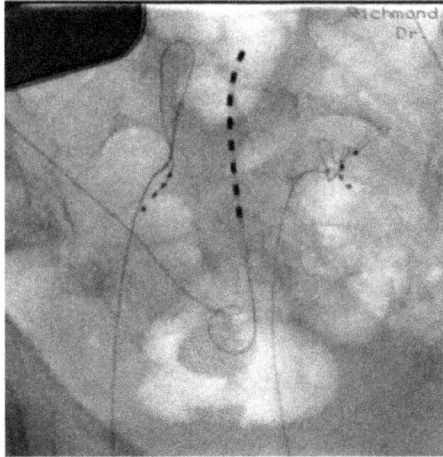

FIGURE 3: Anterior posterior fluoroscopic image of bilateral dorsal root ganglion stimulation leads on the S2 level. The trans-sacral-hiatus octode lead and battery for her previous conventional sacral neuromodulation therapy can be appreciated as well.

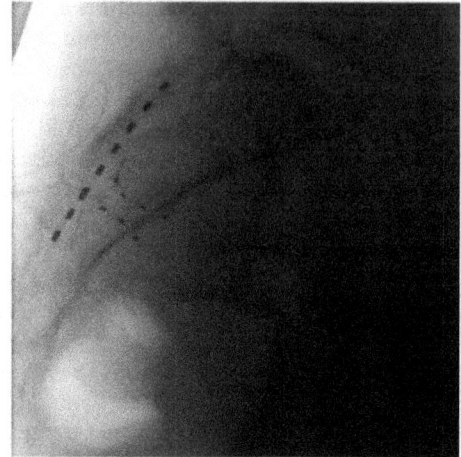

FIGURE 4: Lateral fluoroscopic image of bilateral dorsal root ganglion stimulation leads on the S2 level. The trans-sacral-hiatus octode lead for her previous conventional sacral neuromodulation therapy can be appreciated as well.

At this point the right S2 foramen was aligned under fluoroscopy. A Tuohy needle was directed into the posterior S2 foramen and its position was confirmed on fluoroscopy. The lead loaded introducer was then passed through the anterior foramen and the electrodes were maneuvered such that the final position was with 1 contact anterior to the anterior wall of the sacral vertebral body (extraforaminal), 2 contacts intrasacral, and 1 contact in the sacral epidural space. A strain relief loop was created as previously described [4]. The introducer was then withdrawn into the Tuohy needle with the lead left in place. In withdrawing the Tuohy needle another small loop was placed subcutaneously for additional tensile strength. The lead position was checked again in the AP and lateral position. The same procedure was performed to place a lead on the left S2 DRG. Figures 3 and 4 depict the position of bilateral leads on the S2 level.

All 4 lead positions were then checked again and found to be in good position as well as their tension loops. The leads were then secured with Tegaderm. A marking was placed on the right buttock that was 4 cm transverse in the upper outer quadrant, since the patient's ANS Genesis stimulator was implanted on the left side. 10 cc of 1.0% lidocaine mixed with 0.5% bupivacaine was used to anesthetize the incision site. An incision was made and a pocket was created. The leads were tunneled to the pocket as previously described [5]. The leads were connected to the pulse generator and impedances were confirmed. The incisions were irrigated with Bacitracin solution and the generator was anchored with 2.0 Ethibond. The right buttock wound was closed in layers by using 2.0 Vicryl and the skin was closed with staples. All 4 lead puncture sites were small and the leads were not visualized with manipulation of the puncture site. The lead placement puncture sites and the buttock incision were covered with Steristrips followed by gauze and Tegaderm.

On four-month follow-up, the patient still reports >90% pain relief from the stimulator therapy with concomitant improvements in daily functioning. The improvement in pain

control allowed her to discontinue her oxycodone, which was causing her to suffer from side effects before.

3. Discussion

The aim of this report was to describe the successful application of DRG stimulation for chronic coccydynia. Coccydynia is prevalent and can be difficult to treat in chronic cases. Factors associated with increased risk of developing coccydynia include obesity and female gender [6]; women are 5 times more likely to develop coccydynia than men. The most common etiology of coccydynia is trauma, consistent with the presented case. External trauma usually occurs due to a backwards fall, leading to a bruised, dislocated, or broken coccyx [7]. Patients typically present complaining of "tailbone pain." The pain will usually be worse with prolonged sitting, leaning back while seated, prolonged standing, and rising from a seated position. X-ray and magnetic resonance imaging can be used to evaluate for the presence of fractures, degenerative changes, or masses. Most cases of coccydynia resolve within weeks to months with or without conservative treatment [8]. Conservative treatment consists of cushions, the application of heat and cold, nonsteroidal anti-inflammatory drugs, and transcutaneous electrical nerve stimulation.

For the few cases that do not respond to these conservative treatments, more aggressive treatments may be indicated. Injections around the coccyx, usually at the sacrococcygeal junction or around the sacrococcygeal ligaments, of local anesthetic with steroid can be both diagnostic and therapeutic [9]. Another approach is to target the ganglion impar, also known as the ganglion of Walther [10]. The ganglion impar is the pelvic portion of the sympathetic trunk located in the midline anterior to the sacrococcygeal junction. This block can be useful in refractory cases and cases associated with pelvic pain, as well as for pain associated with malignant neoplasms. Surgical procedures for the treatment of coccydynia have been reported consisting of surgical amputation of the coccyx just proximal to the sacrococcygeal junction [11]. However, this procedure may be associated with a high complication rate and failure to relieve the pain. Consequently, based on current available information, this procedure generally is not recommended [2].

Recent case reports support the use of different neuromodulation techniques to treat refractory coccydynia. In 2008 Haider [12] reported on the use of conventional spinal cord stimulation to successfully treat a patient with chronic coccydynia. Another report by Vajramani et al. [13] described the successful use of high frequency 10 kHz spinal cord stimulation to the conus/cauda region in two patients with chronic coccydynia. Our report adds to this by describing the successful application of DRG stimulation for coccydynia. The DRG has been of interest to pain physicians for years since scientific evidence on spinal structures suggests that the DRG is an integral part of both nociceptive and neuropathic pain states [14]. The suggested mechanism of electrical stimulation of the DRG is a reduction of action potential conduction at the bifurcation (T-junction) of sensory neurons within the DRG, resulting in the reduction of perceived pain [15]. Most studies to date have focused on DRG stimulation for neuropathic pain states [14]. Both neuropathic and nociceptive components are believed to contribute to chronic coccydynia [3], and the instrumental role of the DRG in both pain states may explain the positive results achieved in the present case.

3.1. Conclusion. We successfully used DRG stimulation to treat chronic coccydynia. Future studies need to corroborate the effectiveness of DRG stimulation for this indication.

References

[1] J. Simpson, "Clinical lectures on the diseases of women. Lecture XVII: coccydynia and diseases and deformities of the coccyx," *The Medical Times and Gazette*, vol. 40, pp. 1–7, 1859.

[2] L. S. Lirette, G. Chaiban, R. Tolba, and H. Eissa, "Coccydynia: an overview of the anatomy, etiology, and treatment of coccyx pain," *The Ochsner Journal*, vol. 14, no. 1, pp. 84–87, 2014.

[3] S. Kothari, "Neuromodulatory approaches to chronic pelvic pain and coccygodynia," *Acta Neurochirurgica, Supplementum*, no. 97, pp. 365–371, 2007.

[4] V. van Velsen, N. van Helmond, and K. B. Chapman, "Creating a strain relief loop during S1 transforaminal lead placement for dorsal root ganglion stimulation for foot pain: a technical note," *Pain Practice*, 2017.

[5] V. van Velsen, N. van Helmond, M. E. Levine, and K. B. Chapman, "Single-incision approach to implantation of the pulse generator and leads for dorsal root ganglion stimulation," *A & A Case Reports*, vol. 10, no. 1, pp. 23–27, 2018.

[6] J.-Y. Maigne, L. Doursounian, and G. Chatellier, "Causes and mechanisms of common coccydynia: role of body mass index and coccygeal trauma," *The Spine Journal*, vol. 25, no. 23, pp. 3072–3079, 2000.

[7] S. Schapiro, "Low back and rectal pain from an orthopedic and proctologic viewpoint with a review of 180 cases," *The American Journal of Surgery*, vol. 79, no. 1, pp. 117–128, 1950.

[8] G. H. Thiele, "Coccygodynia: cause and treatment," *Diseases of the Colon & Rectum*, vol. 6, no. 6, pp. 422–436, 1963.

[9] R. Mitra, L. Cheung, and P. Perry, "Efficacy of fluoroscopically guided steroid injections in the management of coccydynia," *Pain Physician*, vol. 10, no. 6, pp. 775–778, 2007.

[10] C. Adas, U. Ozdemir, H. Toman, N. Luleci, E. Luleci, and H. Adas, "Transsacrococcygeal approach to ganglion impar: radiofrequency application for the treatment of chronic intractable coccydynia," *Journal of Pain Research*, vol. 9, pp. 1173–1177, 2016.

[11] R. Perkins, J. Schofferman, and J. Reynolds, "Coccygectomy for severe refractory sacrococcygeal joint pain," *Journal of Spinal Disorders & Techniques*, vol. 16, no. 1, pp. 100–103, 2003.

[12] N. Haider, "Coccydynia treated with spinal cord stimulation: a case report," in *Proceedings of the American Academy of Pain Medicine 24th Annual Meeting*, 2008.

[13] G. Vajramani, J. Hazelgrove, M. Cumming, and N. Berry, "High frequency 10 kHz spinal cord stimulation (HF10 SCS) for coccydynia: report of two cases," in *Proceedings of the 20th Annual Meeting of the North American Neuromodulation Society*, Las Vegas, NV, USA, 2017.

[14] T. R. Deer, E. Krames, N. Mekhail et al., "The appropriate use of neurostimulation: new and evolving neurostimulation therapies and applicable treatment for chronic pain and selected disease states," *Neuromodulation: Technology at the Neural Interface*, vol. 17, no. 6, pp. 599–615, 2014.

[15] L. Liem, E. Van Dongen, F. J. Huygen, P. Staats, and J. Kramer, "The dorsal root ganglion as a therapeutic target for chronic pain," *Regional Anesthesia and Pain Medicine*, vol. 41, no. 4, pp. 511–519, 2016.

51

Thoracic Paravertebral Block, Multimodal Analgesia, and Monitored Anesthesia Care for Breast Cancer Surgery in Primary Lateral Sclerosis

Anis Dizdarevic and Anthony Fernandes

Anesthesiology and Pain Management, Columbia University Medical Center, 622 West 168th Street, PH 5, New York, NY 10032, USA

Correspondence should be addressed to Anis Dizdarevic; ad2689@cumc.columbia.edu

Academic Editor: Renato Santiago Gomez

Objective. Primary lateral sclerosis (PLS) is a rare idiopathic neurodegenerative disorder affecting upper motor neurons and characterized by spasticity, muscle weakness, and bulbar involvement. It can sometimes mimic early stage of more common and fatal amyotrophic lateral sclerosis (ALS). Surgical patients with a history of neurodegenerative disorders, including PLS, may be at increased risk for general anesthesia related ventilatory depression and postoperative respiratory complications, abnormal response to muscle relaxants, and sensitivity to opioids, sedatives, and local anesthetics. We present a case of a patient with PLS and recent diagnosis of breast cancer who underwent a simple mastectomy surgery uneventfully under an ultrasound guided thoracic paravertebral block, multimodal analgesia, and monitored anesthesia care. Patient reported minimal to no pain or discomfort in the postoperative period and received no opioids for pain management before being discharged home. In patients with PLS, thoracic paravertebral block and multimodal analgesia can provide reliable anesthesia and effective analgesia for breast surgery with avoidance of potential risks associated with general anesthesia, muscle paralysis, and opioid use.

1. Introduction

Primary lateral sclerosis (PLS) is a rare degenerative disorder of upper motor neuron function, characterized by progressive spasticity and weakness and affecting the legs, trunk, arms, and bulbar muscles [1]. One of the major clinical challenges in PLS diagnosis is distinguishing it from the more common and fatal ALS, hereditary spastic paraparesis, and other neurodegenerative conditions that may present in similar way early in their course [2]. Progression of neuromuscular degeneration may lead to muscle weakness, atrophy, bulbar dysfunction, muscle denervation, and respiratory compromise (as seen more commonly in ALS), resulting ultimately in aspiration risk, respiratory failure, and death [3]. Patients with neuromuscular disorders presenting for surgery pose an increased risk for surgery and anesthesia related complications and should be very carefully assessed perioperatively [4]. Impairment of respiration, muscle weakness, altered response to muscle relaxants, and aspiration risk may affect safe anesthetic management and postoperative care.

This is the first reported case in English literature of a patient with PLS who underwent a successful mastectomy surgery for breast cancer under an ultrasound guided thoracic paravertebral block, multimodal analgesia, and monitored anesthesia care.

Patient reviewed the case report and gave written permission for the authors to publish the report.

2. Case Report

A 64-year-old woman with a history of PLS was scheduled for a left breast simple mastectomy with axillary level I lymph node dissection for recently diagnosed ductal carcinoma in situ. The patient's PLS symptoms included significant deconditioning and generalized muscle weakness requiring wheelchair use, generalized muscle spasms, and dysarthria. At the time of surgery, the patient had no home oxygen requirement. Her documented peak cough flow rate (measure of respiratory muscle weakness) was 70 liters per minute (indicating ineffective cough). Her comorbidities included an increased body mass index (29.9) and hypertension. Preoperatively, the patient's heart rate was 106 beats per minute, blood pressure 143/73, respiratory rate 20 breaths per minute, and oxygen saturation 95% on room air. EKG and chest XR were within normal limits. No pulmonary function tests were available prior to surgery. The patient's pulmonologist and primary medical doctor strongly recommended avoidance of general anesthesia for the surgery due to concerns about increased risks of prolonged mechanical ventilation and postoperative respiratory complications related to her condition. During the preoperative visit, the patient refused general anesthesia and requested a minimally invasive approach. After discussing with the patient and surgery team all the risks and potential complications associated with general anesthesia, including respiratory depression, postoperative mechanical ventilation, and pulmonary complications, the patient's medical condition, anesthetic requirements for the procedure and alternatives, plan was made to proceed with a peripheral nerve block and multimodal monitored anesthesia care. Discussion was also held regarding general anesthesia not being used as a backup plan and aborting the procedure in case of inadequate anesthesia or patient discomfort.

For the thoracic paravertebral block placement, the patient was positioned sitting upright with the arms resting on a Mayo table for support. Standard American Society of Anesthesiologists monitors and supplemental oxygen via nasal cannula were placed. Intravenous midazolam, 1 mg, and fentanyl, 25 mcg, were administered, prior to starting the procedure. A SonoSite M-Turbo high frequency linear transducer (6–15 MHz) probe was placed transverse to the thoracic vertebral column, parallel to the ribs. Under direct ultrasound guidance, a 21-gauge 100 mm Pajunk Sono TAP needle was inserted parallel to the rib, in a lateral to medial direction, in the plane of the ultrasound beam, and directed toward the paravertebral space between the internal intercostal membrane and pleura (Figure 1). Three single shot left-sided paravertebral blocks were performed at the levels T3, T4, and T5 using a total of 35 mL of 0.5% preservative-free ropivacaine with 6 mg of dexamethasone, to extend the duration of the block. A dexmedetomidine infusion (0.4 mcg/kg/hr) was started, along with additional midazolam, 0.5 mg, fentanyl 25 mcg, and ketamine 10 mg for monitored anesthesia care sedation. Prior to the surgical start, cold temperature sensation was assessed by alcohol swab, demonstrating T3 to T5 dermatome coverage. The patient reported mild discomfort with the surgical incision and received additional 10 mL of 1% lidocaine and 0.25% bupivacaine local anesthetic infiltration into the incision area to reinforce the block. A large elliptical incision was made, and the dissection was performed superiorly to 2 cm below the clavicle, medially to the lateral border of the sternum, inferiorly to the level of the inframammary crease, and laterally to the latissimus muscle. The breast tissue was removed off the pectoralis major and serratus anterior muscles. The patient tolerated the entire surgery reporting no discomfort or pain and remained hemodynamically stable, with no significant change in respiratory rate or oxygen saturation. The pain score on PACU arrival was 0/10 on a numeric rating scale. Vital signs were as follows: heart rate 104, blood

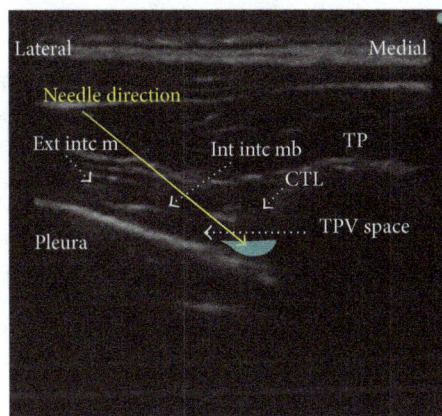

FIGURE 1: Thoracic paravertebral block, transverse in line technique. Needle trajectory: lateral to medial. TP = transverse process. TPV = thoracic paravertebral. Int into mb = internal intercostal membrane. Ext into m = external intercostal muscle. CTL = costotransverse ligament.

pressure 110/78, respiratory rate 19, and oxygen saturation of 98% on 3l nasal cannula. Postoperatively the patient received acetaminophen for pain control with a maximal pain score reported as 2/10 and was discharged home on postoperative day 2. The patient did not require any postoperative opioids.

3. Discussion

PLS is a rare, idiopathic, slowly progressive, nonfamilial, neurodegenerative disorder of the upper motor neuron affecting corticospinal and corticobulbar tracts in the arms, legs, and face. The most common clinical presentation of PLS includes spasticity, hyperreflexia, and mild muscle weakness. Bulbar symptoms can include dysarthria, dysphagia, and emotional lability. The pathophysiologic basis remains unknown, and there is currently no definitive diagnosis or disease marker. Imaging and laboratory testing are used to rule out other diagnoses including metabolic, physiologic, and anatomic confounding processes [5]. PLS classically is described as a pure upper motor neuron neurodegenerative disorder. Newer electrophysiological data may suggest that some patients with PLS may also have concurrent lower motor neuron involvement, similar to amyotrophic lateral sclerosis, ALS, more common and fatal condition [6]. Marked weakness can be absent but patients can progress to debilitating spasticity and have respiratory compromise. It is argued that PLS may be a slowly progressive form of ALS, with subsequent lower motor neuron involvement. A small number of ALS patients initially present with pure upper motor neuron findings but most develop lower motor neuron signs and EMG findings within 4 years [7]. The progression may even occur over several decades. Currently, there is very sparse literature pertaining to the anesthetic management and risks involving patients with PLS. Given some similarities in clinical presentation and pathophysiology between PLS and other neurodegenerative disorders, our discussion of anesthetic management could herein be extrapolated to include those patient populations as well.

The extent of muscle weakness, respiratory dysfunction, and bulbar involvement have been of special importance in patients presenting for surgical procedures. Respiratory complications are a major cause of morbidity and mortality in patients with neurodegenerative conditions. Pure PLS does not involve the same severity and progression of respiratory dysfunction as seen in ALS, but, nevertheless, is of concern [3, 8]. Respiratory failure can result from inability to clear secretions, carbon dioxide retention, and compromised ventilator function. Bulbar muscle dysfunction with tongue fasciculation and pharyngeal muscle weakness may lead to an increased risk of aspiration and related complications [9]. Preoperative pulmonary assessment with pulmonary function tests, if deemed necessary, would be useful in determining a degree of pulmonary dysfunction and potential risk of postoperative respiratory failure. Furthermore, in neurodegenerative conditions, after denervation and prolonged immobilization, upregulation of acetylcholine receptors occurs at the neuromuscular junction and along the skeletal muscle membranes. Administration of depolarizing neuromuscular blockers, such as succinylcholine, can lead to activation of an unpredictably large quantity of receptors resulting in an abnormally high efflux of potassium. Extubation readiness may be difficult to assess as a result of baseline muscle weakness and altered pulmonary function. The intraoperative use of nondepolarizing muscle relaxants should be very carefully weighed against the potential increased likelihood of prolonged weakness and postoperative ventilatory support. Patients with neuromuscular disease, including PLS, may also be sensitive to sedative and analgesic agents, and their judicious use is recommended [10].

Intraoperative recommendations for anesthetic management of patients with PLS and similar neurodegenerative disorders would include the use of rapid reversible short-acting anesthetic and analgesic agents and avoiding (depolarizing) and/or minimizing (nondepolarizing) muscle paralysis. Postoperatively, conservative dosing of opioids and sedatives, enhanced monitoring with continuous pulse oximetry, and use of multimodal analgesia to optimize pain management are recommended.

Regional anesthesia, including local infiltration and peripheral and neuraxial nerve blocks, has been successfully used in patients with neuromuscular disorders to avoid possible respiratory and other complications associated with general anesthesia and opioid use [11, 12]. Agnoletti et al.'s description of a thoracic paravertebral block (TPVB) for breast surgery in a patient with ALS is the only report similar to ours published in the English literature [13]. The authors performed a classic approach to paravertebral blocks at the thoracic T1–T3 levels, using a 3 mL solution of 0.75% ropivacaine at each level.

Paravertebral block can offer specific advantages for patients with neuromuscular disorders, especially when general anesthesia may be unfavorable or relatively contraindicated. By administering local anesthetic near the target somatic nerve roots, unilateral anesthesia and analgesia can be achieved without bilateral sympathectomy and associated side effects. Furthermore, PVB allows for efficient spontaneous breathing and early mobilization, minimizing the risk of postoperative respiratory dysfunction. Schnabel et al. and Tahiri et al., in their meta-analysis, evaluated the efficacy and safety of TPVB in breast surgery and also compared thoracic PVB to general anesthesia [14, 15]. Their results demonstrated that TPVB, combined with sedation, provided effective surgical anesthesia for patients undergoing breast procedures. They also concluded that TPVB alone, or in addition to general anesthesia, provided better postoperative pain control with little adverse effects, when compared to other analgesic options. In addition, when used instead of general anesthesia, TPVB resulted in pain scores that were significantly decreased postoperatively. The potential adverse effects associated with TPVB were Horner's syndrome (most common) and rare cases of accidental intravascular injection of part of the local anesthetic, pneumothorax, epidural spread, hypotension, and intercostal nerve trauma.

In our case, the patient received additional local anesthetic infiltration at the incision site prior to the start of surgery. This was expected for two potential reasons: (1) cutaneous innervation of the anterior chest wall via intercostal nerves may take longer to become anesthetized when using regional technique and (2) the middle supraclavicular nerve, originating from the C3 and C4 cervical nerves, also supplies the skin over the pectoralis major muscle and is not anesthetized with the paravertebral block. We added dexamethasone to the local anesthetic to prolong the analgesic duration of the block [16]. We also added subanesthetic dose of ketamine to our multimodal regimen as it has been reported effective in reducing opioid requirements postoperatively with mild to no adverse effects [17]. Sympathomimetic effects on the cardiovascular system, especially in the presence of dexmedetomidine, would be expected to be minimal, as we observed in our case. Finally, as another part of our multimodal analgesia regimen but also as the main anesthetic in monitored anesthesia care, we chose dexmedetomidine. Dexmedetomidine has been reported to reduce the intra- and postoperative opioid consumption, postoperative pain, and nausea and vomiting, with no effect on the time of recovery [18]. Furthermore, dexmedetomidine, when used for sedation in monitored anesthesia care, has been shown to provide greater hemodynamic stability and less respiratory depression when compared to propofol as well as placebo with rescue midazolam and fentanyl, with the most common side effect of intraoperative bradycardia [19, 20].

4. Conclusion

Patients with primary lateral sclerosis and other similar neurodegenerative disorders presenting for surgery may be at increased risk for surgery and anesthesia related complications and should be carefully assessed perioperatively by all healthcare professionals involved in their care. Special emphasis should be paid to respiratory function, aspiration risk, and muscle dysfunction. Thoracic paravertebral block, along with multimodal analgesia, can provide reliable anesthesia and effective analgesia for breast surgery, with avoidance of potential risks associated with general anesthesia, muscle paralysis, and opioid use.

Competing Interests

The authors declare that they have no competing interests.

Acknowledgments

The authors acknowledge Charles W. Emala, M.D., and Anthony R. Brown, M.D., professors at Department of Anesthesiology and Pain Medicine, Columbia University Medical Center, for their continued guidance, tremendous support, and suggestions for this paper.

References

[1] J. M. Statland, R. J. Barohn, M. M. Dimachkie, M. K. Floeter, and H. Mitsumoto, "Primary lateral sclerosis," *Neurologic Clinics*, vol. 33, no. 4, pp. 749–760, 2015.

[2] M. C. Tartaglia, A. Rowe, K. Findlater, J. B. Orange, G. Grace, and M. J. Strong, "Differentiation between primary lateral sclerosis and amyotrophic lateral sclerosis," *Archives of Neurology*, vol. 64, pp. 232–236, 2007.

[3] R. H. Brown, "Amyotrophic lateral sclerosis and other motor neuron disease," in *Harrison's Principles of Internal Medicine*, D. L. Longo, D. L. Kasper, A. S. Fauci, S. L. Hauser, and J. L. Jameson, Eds., pp. 3345–3351, McGraw-Hill Medical Publishing Division, New York, NY, USA, 18th edition, 2011.

[4] J. A. Giovannitti, *Anesthetic Considerations for Patients with Neurologic Disease. Anesthesia Complications in the Dental Office*, John Wiley & Sons, New York, NY, USA, 1st edition, 2015.

[5] M. A. Singer, J. M. Statland, G. I. Wolfe, and R. J. Barohn, "Primary lateral sclerosis," *Muscle and Nerve*, vol. 35, no. 3, pp. 291–302, 2007.

[6] N. Le Forestier, T. Maisonobe, A. Piquard et al., "Does primary lateral sclerosis exist? A study of 20 patients and a review of the literature," *Brain*, vol. 124, pp. 1989–1999, 2001.

[7] P. H. Gordon, B. Cheng, I. B. Katz et al., "The natural history of primary lateral sclerosis," *Neurology*, vol. 66, no. 5, pp. 647–653, 2006.

[8] L. Lee and R. Kapoor, "Perioperative anesthetic management of a patient with primary lateral sclerosis," *International Journal of Anesthesiology Research*, vol. 3, pp. 76–78, 2015.

[9] A. M. Brambrink and J. R. Kirsch, "Perioperative care of patients with neuromuscular disease and dysfunction," *Anesthesiology Clinics*, vol. 25, no. 3, pp. 483–509, 2007.

[10] A. Romero and G. P. Joshi, "Neuromuscular disease and anesthesia," *Muscle and Nerve*, vol. 48, no. 3, pp. 451–460, 2013.

[11] N. Sertöz and S. Karaman, "Peripheral nerve block in a patient with amyotrophic lateral sclerosis," *Journal of Anesthesia*, vol. 26, no. 2, pp. 314–315, 2012.

[12] K. Hara, S. Sakura, Y. Saito, M. Maeda, and Y. Kosaka, "Epidural anesthesia and pulmonary function in a patient with amyotrophic lateral sclerosis," *Anesthesia and Analgesia*, vol. 83, no. 4, pp. 878–879, 1996.

[13] V. Agnoletti, R. M. Corso, D. Cattano et al., "Thoracic paravertebral block for breast surgery in a patient with amyotrophic lateral sclerosis," *Minerva Anestesiologica*, vol. 79, no. 7, pp. 822–823, 2013.

[14] A. Schnabel, S. U. Reichl, P. Kranke, E. M. Pogatzki-Zahn, and P. K. Zahn, "Efficacy and safety of paravertebral blocks in breast surgery: a meta-analysis of randomized controlled trials," *British Journal of Anaesthesia*, vol. 105, no. 6, pp. 842–852, 2010.

[15] Y. Tahiri, D. Q. H. Tran, J. Bouteaud et al., "General anaesthesia versus thoracic paravertebral block for breast surgery: a meta-analysis," *Journal of Plastic, Reconstructive and Aesthetic Surgery*, vol. 64, no. 10, pp. 1261–1269, 2011.

[16] S. Choi, R. Rodseth, and C. J. L. McCartney, "Effects of dexamethasone as a local anaesthetic adjuvant for brachial plexus block: a systematic review and meta-analysis of randomized trials," *British Journal of Anaesthesia*, vol. 112, no. 3, pp. 427–439, 2014.

[17] R. F. Bell, J. B. Dahl, R. A. Moore, and E. A. Kalso, "Perioperative ketamine for acute postoperative pain. Review," *Cochrane Database of Systematic Reviews*, no. 1, Article ID CD004603, 2006.

[18] A. Le Bot, D. Michelet, J. Hilly et al., "Efficacy of intraoperative dexmedetomidine compared with placebo for surgery in adults: a meta-analysis of published studies," *Minerva Anestesiologica*, vol. 81, no. 10, pp. 1105–1117, 2015.

[19] K. A. Candiotti, S. D. Bergese, P. M. Bokesch, M. A. Feldman, W. Wisemandle, and A. Y. Bekker, "Monitored anesthesia care with dexmedetomidine: a prospective, randomized, double-blind, multicenter trial," *Anesthesia and Analgesia*, vol. 110, no. 1, pp. 47–56, 2010.

[20] B. W. Yon, J. M. Hing, S. L. Hong, S. K. Koo, H. J. Roh, and K. S. Cho, "A comparison of dexmedetomidine versus propofol during drug-induced sleep endoscopy in sleep apnea patients," *The Laryngoscope*, vol. 126, no. 3, pp. 763–767, 2016.

52

Pitfalls in Interventional Pain Medicine: Hyponatremia after DDAVP for a Patient with Von Willebrand Disease Undergoing an Epidural Steroid Injection

Talal W. Khan[1] and Abdulraheem Yacoub[2]

[1]*Department of Anesthesiology and Pain Medicine, University of Kansas Medical Center, Kansas City, KS, USA*
[2]*Division of Medical Oncology, Department of Internal Medicine, University of Kansas Medical Center, Kansas City, KS, USA*

Correspondence should be addressed to Talal W. Khan; tkhan@kumc.edu

Academic Editor: Ilok Lee

Desmopressin (DDAVP), a synthetic analog of vasopressin, has been used in patients with von Willebrand disease (VWD), mild hemophilia A, and platelet dysfunction to reduce the risk of bleeding associated with surgical and interventional procedures. We report the case of a patient with VWD presenting with a bulging disc and radicular pain that underwent transforaminal epidural steroid injections. Her course was complicated with the interval development of headaches and dizziness symptomatic of moderate hyponatremia, likely due to excessive fluid intake. This report highlights a relatively rare side effect of DDAVP when used for prophylaxis in patients with VWD and reinforces the need for vigilance in these patients.

1. Introduction

Von Willebrand disease (VWD) is the most commonly inherited bleeding disorder with a prevalence of at least 0.1% and a global population of approximately 5.8 million affected individuals [1]. The hallmark of this disease includes a qualitative and/or quantitative deficiency in the most active forms of von Willebrand factor (VWF), which results in abnormal platelet adhesion and relative deficiency of factor VIII. Although the majority of cases present with mild disease, the risk of bleeding is proportional to the degree of deficiency of VWF [2]. VWD is classified into three major categories: type 1 (partial quantitative deficiency), type 2 (qualitative deficiency), and type 3 (severe quantitative deficiency). Type 2 is classified further into four variants based upon phenotype [3].

DDAVP, a synthetic analog of L-arginine vasopressin, is the treatment of choice for the perioperative and periprocedural management of VWD, primarily for type 1 patients who respond to the drug and do not have a contraindication for its use. When administered intravenously, this can cause a rapid increase of up to eightfold in circulating levels of factor

VIII and VWF through release of endogenous VWF from endothelial Weibel-Palade bodies [4].

Although neuraxial techniques are commonly avoided in patients with VWD and other bleeding disorders secondary to the risk of hemorrhagic and subsequent neurologic complications, a review by Choi and Brull [5] suggests that even though ideal factor and platelet levels remain undefined for this patient population, the risk of adverse sequelae may be low with appropriate assessment and management of these bleeding diatheses. To our knowledge, only a single abstract reports the management of a lumbar epidural steroid injection in a patient with VWD [6]. The patient reviewed the case report and provided written permission for the authors to publish the report. Both authors participated in the care of the patient described in the case report.

2. Case Presentation

The patient was a 44-year-old woman with a lifetime history of low VWF and clinically significant bleeding manifestations. Her disease manifested with excessive bleeding including menorrhagia and epistaxis. Laboratory evaluation confirmed type 1 VWD with ristocetin cofactor activity of 38%, von Willebrand antigen level of 41%, factor VIII level of 60%, and a normal von Willebrand factor multimer distribution. The patient had type A blood and abnormal Platelet Function Assay (PFA) markedly prolonged clotting times with both collagen/epinephrine and collagen/ADP stimulation. The patient previously underwent a DDAVP challenge test which more than doubled her ristocetin activity after administration of 20 mcg of intravenous DDAVP. This challenge test was not followed by any complications. She presented to the pain clinic with a long-standing history of low back and bilateral lower extremity pain. Over the years, she had tried a variety of medications, multiple episodes of physical therapy, and other conservative care without significant improvement. MRI imaging of the lumbar spine revealed an annular tear and disc bulge at L5-S1. After discussion of risks versus benefits of the procedure and the need for consideration of DDAVP to reduce the risk of bleeding, the patient underwent an infusion of DDAVP 0.3 mcg/kg receiving a total of 22 mcg over a period of 30 minutes immediately before the procedure. The patient was not given any specific instructions for fluid restriction postoperatively. Bilateral L5-S1 transforaminal epidural steroid injections were carried out. Once needle position and good contrast spread along the nerve roots were confirmed, an injection of 1 mL of 0.25% bupivacaine and 40 mg methylprednisolone was carried out on each side. Although the procedure was performed without incident, the patient experienced persistent dizziness and a nonpositional headache early the next day. Thorough investigation, including serial serum and urine electrolyte evaluations, revealed findings consistent with hyponatremia (serum sodium: 125 mmol/L), which was a decrease from baseline serum sodium of 138 mmol/L. Further investigation also revealed excessive water intake of 80 ounces per day that may have contributed to the acute onset of hyponatremia. The electrolyte disorder was gradually corrected over a period of 24 hours through fluid restriction and administration of sodium with complete resolution of symptoms. Serum sodium went from 125 mmol/L to 128 mmol/L at the 6th hour after diagnosis, to 134 mmol/L at the 10th hour, and then to 139 mmol/L at the 18th hour after diagnosis and remained at 136–139 mmol/L for the next several days to weeks on outpatient follow-up.

3. Discussion

Our case demonstrates the potential for serious complications following the administration of DDAVP for mitigation of bleeding risk in a patient with VWD undergoing an interventional spine procedure. DDAVP results in an increase in VWF activity, factor VIII activity, and plasminogen activation in patients with VWD [7]. DDAVP also results in a potent antidiuretic effect through the impairment of free water absorption by the distal tubules, collecting tubules, and collecting ducts by binding to the arginine vasopressin receptor and reducing water permeability [8]. This antidiuretic hormone effect can persist for several hours after DDAVP clearance. During this period of time, the retention of free water and hyponatremia can occur. Williford and Bernstein

TABLE 1: Clinical manifestations of hyponatremia (Na < 135 mmol/L).

Nausea
Vomiting
Headache
Lethargy
Malaise
Muscle cramps
Restlessness
Disorientation/confusion
Depressed reflexes
Seizures
Coma
Respiratory arrest
Brain stem herniation
Irreversible brain damage
Death

TABLE 2: Risk factors for hyponatremia after DDAVP [10].

Stress
Surgery
Administration of anesthesia
Opiates (endogenous release of ADH)
Vomiting (loss of sodium)
Liver disease (impaired metabolism of DDAVP)
Renal tubular acidosis (chronically low sodium)
Multiple doses of DDAVP
Overhydration with hyponatremic fluids

[9] reported the occurrence of severe hyponatremia and seizures in children and adults 1 to 4 days after the administration of DDAVP (Table 1).

Certain physiological changes in the periprocedural phase may potentiate the antidiuretic effect of DDAVP. These include an increase in antidiuretic hormone secretion by the posterior pituitary gland in response to physiological stress, pain, and anxiety related to the primary pain condition, as well as the procedure itself. In addition, this particular patient may have been susceptible to free water overload as the patient was in the habit of drinking over 80 ounces of water per day (Table 2). In addition to excessive water intake that contributed to the symptomatic hyponatremia, the patient also received a dose of DDAVP exceeding 20 mcg. Despite the relatively short half-life of DDAVP of 2 hours, the risk of water intoxication and hyponatremia persisted for several hours after the procedure. This patient also had a history of epilepsy, which was of concern. The patient did not present any epileptic events as a complication but did require hospitalization for observation for 24 hours.

The nature of the disorder of hemostasis, resting factor levels, target factor levels, and the length of time required for maintenance of factor levels for any given procedure dictate the clinical indications for use of DDAVP. When used judiciously, this agent has few troublesome side effects ranging from mild facial flushing to tachycardia and transient headaches. If excessive fluid intake is avoided, signs of more serious hyponatremia and cerebral edema are rare [11]. The authors recommend a thorough discussion of risks versus benefits and alternatives with patients as well as education regarding signs and symptoms that might suggest a more serious problem. Fluids must be restricted to maintenance for 24 hours after any dose of DDAVP. In general, more cautious dosing of DDAVP is recommended. It has been found that sodium nadir occurs within 9–20 hours of DDAVP administration [12]. The healthcare provider, patient, and family should be urged to maintain a high level of vigilance for symptoms suggesting hyponatremia and, if evident, the patient should seek medical treatment promptly to avoid life-threatening complications.

References

[1] F. Rodeghiero, G. Castaman, and E. Dini, "Epidemiological investigations of the prevalence of von Willebrand's disease," *Blood*, vol. 69, no. 2, pp. 454–459, 1987.

[2] G. Castaman, A. B. Federici, F. Rodeghiero, and P. M. Mannucci, "Von Willebrand's disease in the year 2003: towards the complete identification of gene defects for correct diagnosis and treatment," *Haematologica*, vol. 88, no. 1, pp. 94–108, 2003.

[3] K. Hara, N. Kishi, and T. Sata, "Considerations for epidural anesthesia in a patient with type 1 von Willebrand disease," *Journal of Anesthesia*, vol. 23, no. 4, pp. 597–600, 2009.

[4] P. M. Mannucci, M. Aberg, I. M. Nilsson, and B. Robertson, "Mechanism of plasminogen activator and factor VIII increase after vasoactive drugs," *British Journal of Haematology*, vol. 30, no. 1, pp. 81–93, 1975.

[5] S. Choi and R. Brull, "Neuraxial techniques in obstetric and non-obstetric patients with common bleeding diatheses," *Anesthesia and Analgesia*, vol. 109, no. 2, pp. 648–660, 2009.

[6] P. R. Telang and B. M. Vrooman, "Lumbar epidural steroid injection in a patient with Von Willebrand's disease," in *Proceedings of the American Academy of Pain Medicine Annual Meeting*, Palm Springs, Calif, USA, February 2012.

[7] Medical Economics Company, *Physicians' Desk Reference 2002*, Medical Economics Company, Oradell, NJ, USA, 2002.

[8] A. C. Guyton and J. E. Hall, *Textbook of Medical Physiology*, Saunders, Philadelphia, Pa, USA, 10th edition, 2000.

[9] S. L. Williford and S. A. Bernstein, "Intranasal desmopressin-induced hyponatremia," *Pharmacotherapy*, vol. 16, no. 1, pp. 66–74, 1996.

[10] T. J. Smith, J. C. Gill, D. R. Ambruso, and W. E. Hathaway, "Hyponatremia and seizures in young children given DDAVP," *American Journal of Hematology*, vol. 31, no. 3, pp. 199–202, 1989.

[11] P. M. Mannucci, "Desmopressin (DDAVP) for treatment of disorders of hemostasis," *Progress in Hemostasis and Thrombosis*, vol. 8, pp. 19–45, 1986.

[12] H. C. Davidson, A. L. Stapleton, M. L. Casselbrant, and D. J. Kitsko, "Perioperative incidence and management of hyponatremia in vWD patients undergoing adenotonsillectomy," *Laryngoscope*, vol. 121, no. 7, pp. 1399–1403, 2011.

53

Effect of Arm Positioning on Entrapment of Infraclavicular Nerve Block Catheter

Eric Kamenetsky,[1] **Rahul Reddy,**[2] **Mark C. Kendall,**[1] **Antoun Nader,**[1] **and Jessica J. Weeks**[1]

[1]*Department of Anesthesiology, Feinberg School of Medicine, Northwestern University, Chicago, IL, USA*
[2]*Department of Anesthesiology, McGaw Medical Center, Northwestern University, Chicago, IL, USA*

Correspondence should be addressed to Eric Kamenetsky; ekamenet@nm.org

Academic Editor: Alparslan Apan

Continuous brachial plexus nerve block catheters are commonly inserted for postoperative analgesia after upper extremity surgery. Modifications of the insertion technique have been described to improve the safety of placing an infraclavicular brachial plexus catheter. Rarely, these catheters may become damaged or entrapped, complicating their removal. We describe a case of infraclavicular brachial plexus catheter entrapment related to differences in arm positioning during catheter placement and removal. Written authorization to obtain, use, and disclose information and images was obtained from the patient.

1. Introduction

Continuous brachial plexus nerve block catheters are commonly used to prolong postoperative analgesia after painful upper extremity procedures. Removal of these catheters is typically uncomplicated and often can be performed by the patient after hospital discharge. When peripheral nerve block catheters become damaged or entrapped, their removal can be challenging. Most reported cases of catheter entrapment are associated with epidural catheters. In these cases, it is recommended that the spine is flexed and continuous, gentle traction is placed on the catheter [1]. If these recommendations are applied to peripheral nerve block catheters, then, if resistance is met during removal, a patient's extremity should be positioned similar to when the catheter was inserted. We describe a unique case of infraclavicular brachial plexus catheter damage and entrapment related to differences in arm positioning during placement and removal of the catheter.

2. Case Description

A healthy 47-year-old male underwent left wrist radioscapholunate fusion for posttraumatic arthrosis. An infraclavicular brachial plexus nerve block was performed as the primary anesthetic, with an indwelling catheter placed for postoperative analgesia. After sterile preparation and draping of the left upper chest and positioning the left arm in an abducted and externally rotated position, a 2.5 cm linear array ultrasound transducer (13–6 MHz probe, SonoSite, S-Nerve™, Bothell, WA, USA) with sterile covering was used to visualize the infraclavicular brachial plexus. A medial infraclavicular approach was used as described by Bigeleisen and Wilson, with the needle puncture at the apex of the deltopectoral groove [2]. Prior to local anesthetic injection, a distal evoked motor response was obtained with a nerve stimulator, which disappeared at 0.4 mA. After performing a block through the needle with 30 mL 0.5% bupivacaine and 1 : 300,000 epinephrine, the 18 g × 4 cm continuous nerve block needle (Arrow International, Reading, PA, USA) was positioned with the tip between the posterior and medial cords of the brachial plexus. A 20 g × 60 cm continuous nerve block catheter (StimuCath®, Arrow International, Reading, PA, USA) was advanced 5 cm beyond the needle tip without resistance and secured with adhesive bandages with the 9 cm mark at the skin. A test dose of 5 mL 1.5% lidocaine with 1 : 200,000 epinephrine was administered through the catheter and an additional 10 mL of 0.5% bupivacaine was

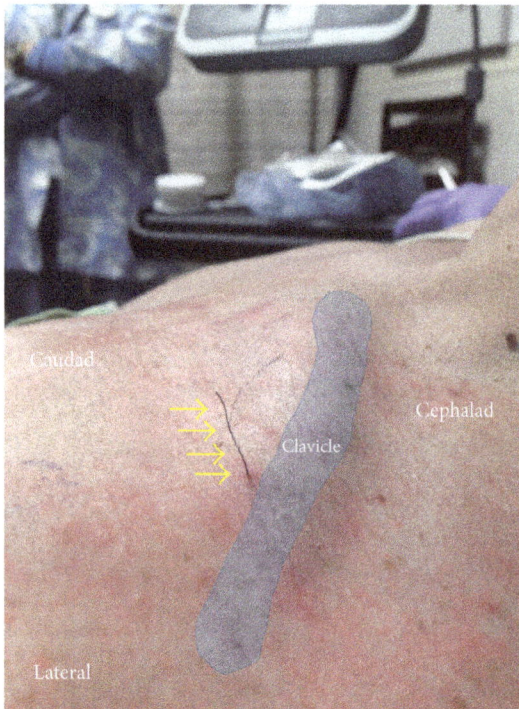

FIGURE 1: Wire fragment extending out of skin. During removal, the central stimulating wire and coil structure were noted to be fractured. Yellow arrows: wire fragment.

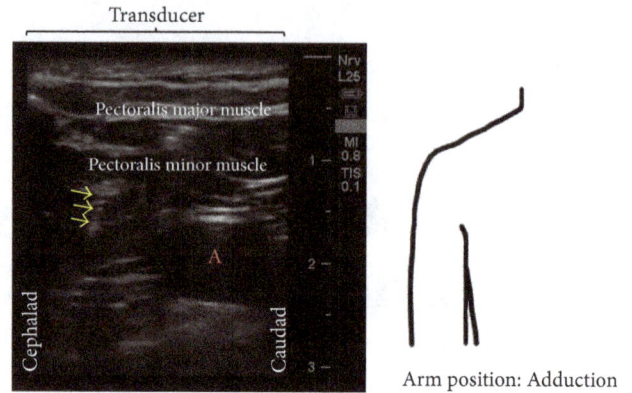

FIGURE 2: Infraclavicular neurovascular sonoanatomy with arm position adducted. The ultrasound image represents a transverse view with the top of the image displaying the ultrasound probe position. Arrows: needle shaft, A = axillary artery.

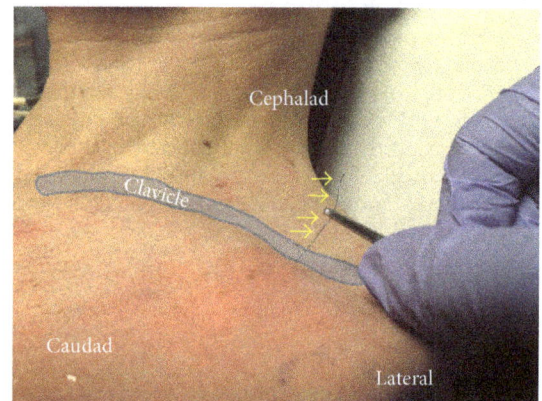

FIGURE 3: Removal of the fractured peripheral nerve catheter fragment. Traction was applied to the fragment while observing real-time removal with ultrasonography. Yellow arrows: wire fragment.

subsequently injected. Perineural spread near the posterior cord was confirmed with ultrasound during injection through the catheter.

The patient successfully underwent the surgical procedure with the peripheral nerve block and intraoperative sedation. He was discharged home with the continuous nerve block catheter infusing 0.2% ropivacaine at 5 mL per hour, plus an additional patient-controlled dose of 2 mL per hour as needed. The patient reported excellent analgesia with 0/10 pain on postoperative days (POD) 1 and 2 and there were no signs of leakage or damage to the catheter. On POD 2, the entire 275 mL 0.2% ropivacaine infusion was completed. On POD 3, the patient went to the surgical office for a scheduled follow-up, at which time the surgeon attempted to remove the catheter with the arm adducted. Prior to removal, the patient reported no residual effects of the nerve block. The surgeon was able to remove the entire polyurethane catheter body without difficulty, but during removal, the central stimulating wire and coil structure were noted to be fractured, with approximately 3 cm remaining above the skin level (Figure 1). The patient reported a transient paresthesia down the left arm at the time of removal.

The patient was referred to the ambulatory surgery center for further evaluation by the anesthesiology team. On physical exam, the patient had normal strength and sensation in the left hand. He did experience sharp, severe, nonradiating pain near the clavicle upon abduction and external rotation of the arm, which resolved with adduction of the arm. Ultrasound evaluation did reveal the wire extending through the pectoralis major and minor muscles and coursing under the clavicle, immediately superficial to the brachial plexus. Since the arm was unable to be abducted, the infraclavicular neurovascular sonoanatomy was more challenging to interpret, as it appeared different than when the catheter was inserted (Figure 2).

A clamp was attached to the wire fragment and gentle traction was applied while observing the wire under real-time ultrasonography (Figure 3). During this process, there was no evidence of tension on the brachial plexus and the patient experienced no paresthesias. There was, however, significant resistance and local discomfort while initially withdrawing the wire. The wire was successfully removed with the tip intact (Figure 4). Of note, the wire fragment was visualized with ultrasound throughout the entire process and no retained fragments were seen after removal. Repeat physical examination showed full left shoulder range of motion without pain or paresthesias. No nerve block related complications were reported at a 2 week follow-up. During this follow-up visit, an ultrasound evaluation (GE Healthcare, Logiq™ P6, 11L probe, Chicago, IL, USA) revealed normal

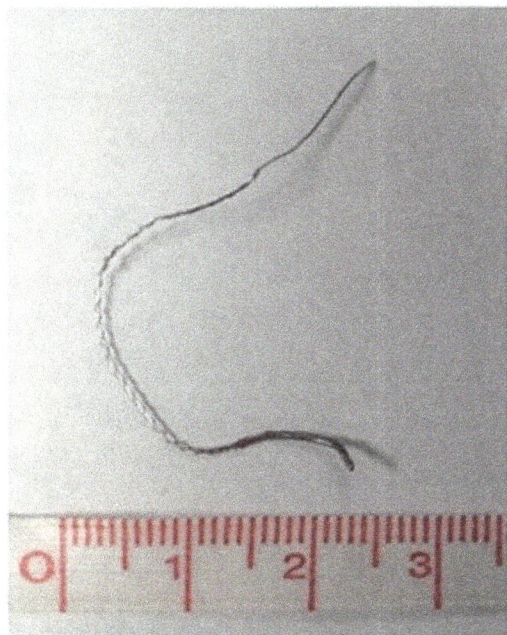

FIGURE 4: The stimulating wire and coil fragment following removal.

infraclavicular brachial plexus anatomy when the patients arm was abducted and externally rotated (Figure 5). No neurological adverse effects or complications were noted.

3. Discussion

Entrapped continuous peripheral nerve block catheters are most often due to a knotted, kinked, or damaged catheter [3–6]. Rarely, a catheter can become sheared, with a fragment remaining inside the patient. When a patient is symptomatic from a retained fragment, surgical exploration and removal may be required, particularly if there is no access to the catheter fragment above the skin level.

We describe a case of a damaged and entrapped infraclavicular nerve block catheter. The entire polyurethane catheter body was removed from the patient, but a fractured part of the stimulating wire and coil structure remained. Ultrasound was used to identify the course of the wire and confirm its position. Although the patient experienced local discomfort while withdrawing the wire fragment, bedside ultrasonography confirmed the fragment was intramuscular and was not causing tension on the brachial plexus or other important structures. The fragment was slowly withdrawn while being visualized in real-time with ultrasonography.

Previous studies described injecting saline through the catheter, to aid in unkinking the catheter or localizing its position in the patient [5]. This was not possible in our case, since the entire catheter body was removed. For the same reason, we were unable to apply electrical stimulation to the catheter to help determine the location of the fragment tip and proximity to the brachial plexus. We were also unable to visually assess the depth, as there were no depth markings. Excessive catheter advancement has been cited as a cause for difficult catheter removal [5]. The catheter in this case was threaded 5 cm beyond the needle tip without resistance and without moving the needle in the process. This was done to avoid leakage and accidental dislodgement of the catheter.

In this patient, the wire may have been entrapped in the costoclavicular space. The infraclavicular catheter was placed with the arm abducted and externally rotated, and the patient was unable to recreate this position due to severe shoulder discomfort. Positioning the arm in abduction and external rotation has been described by both Auyong et al. and Bigeleisen et al. as a means to bring the brachial plexus more superficial, distance the brachial plexus from the pleura, and move the clavicle out of the course of the needle [2, 7, 8]. Recent studies have described the clavicular motion that occurs with the arm abducted, as well as the changes in the costoclavicular space. Ludewig et al. showed that arm abduction to 110° in the coronal plane, similar to the arm position in our case, would result in a 10° increase in clavicular elevation angle, a 14° increase in posterior rotation, and 11° of clavicular retraction compared to a relaxed, neutral position [9]. LaBan et al. used computed tomographic (CT) imaging to evaluate the anatomic changes of the thoracic outlet in patients with clinical evidence of thoracic outlet syndrome. With the arm abducted to 90° and externally rotated, they found an average reduction in the costoclavicular space of 18.2 mm or a 55.6% reduction compared to the neutral position [10].

Several other studies have confirmed that there can be significant changes in clavicular position and space in the thoracic outlet with arm abduction. Although this arm positioning improved our ultrasound view of the brachial plexus during nerve block catheter placement, it may have complicated its removal. The patient was unable to recreate this position after initial catheter removal, due to severe shoulder pain with attempts at arm abduction. We hypothesize that initial catheter removal and subsequent removal of the wire fragment would have been straightforward and uncomplicated with the arm in an abducted position. The remaining fragment was likely entrapped in the costoclavicular space with the arm adducted causing pain with abduction.

Continuous nerve block catheter tip adhesion to the surrounding tissues may be another cause for catheter entrapment. Buckenmaier et al. studied catheter tip adhesion in a rat model using various tip designs provided by Arrow International. The rats randomized to the 19-gauge StimuCath catheter, similar to the catheter used in our case, required a nearly 20-fold greater mean force to remove the catheter tip after one week in a highly inflammatory intraperitoneal environment. In this study, the catheter remained in place for seven days, significantly longer than the three days in our case. Additionally, there was no evidence of adhesion formation on the fragment removed in our patient. A case series from Clendenen et al. described 5 cases of complications related to StimuCath catheter removal in which the polyurethane outer catheter cover became dislodged, while the metal core remained entrapped. In these cases, it is unclear if the catheter was damaged during placement or removal or if the StimuCath catheter tip design increases the propensity for entrapment compared to other catheters.

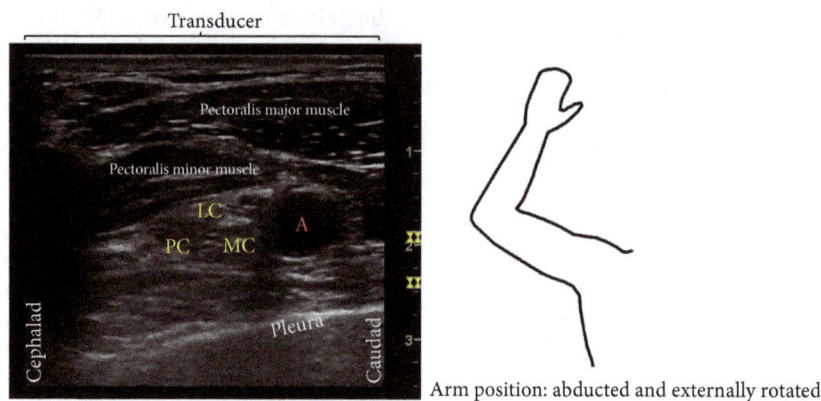

FIGURE 5: Follow-up ultrasound evaluation of the infraclavicular brachial plexus region with arm abducted and externally rotated. The ultrasound image represents a transverse view with the top of the image displaying the ultrasound probe position. A = axillary artery, LC = lateral cord, MC = medial cord, and PC = posterior cord.

Finally, another case reported by Duclas Jr. et al. describes a case of fibrous tissue adhesions complicating infraclavicular stimulating catheter removal. They suggest that a stimulating peripheral nerve catheter should be removed as soon as possible following completion of local anesthetic infusion to avoid the fibrous tissue growth that can occur. Whereas the usual practice at our institution is to instruct patients to remove the catheter at home on the day the local anesthetic is complete, the catheter in this case remained in situ for one additional day, potentially contributing to this complication.

An entrapped infraclavicular brachial plexus nerve block catheter fragment is a rare event and there are limited reports of similar events in the literature. Although previous authors have identified potential causes of nerve block catheter entrapment, our case highlights the importance of arm positioning during brachial plexus catheter removal and the challenges encountered if the arm cannot be repositioned. We also report the utility of ultrasound in this situation, specifically, how it can aid in locating a catheter fragment, confirming its proximity to the brachial plexus and visualizing its complete removal. Since this event, all patients are instructed to elevate their arm above their head prior to removal of the catheter, if their arm was abducted during catheter placement.

Competing Interests

The authors declare that they have no competing interests.

Authors' Contributions

All authors contributed to study design and manuscript preparation. All authors approved the final manuscript and attest to the integrity of the information reported in this manuscript.

References

[1] E. F. Jongleux, R. Miller, and A. Freeman, "An entrapped epidural catheter in a postpartum patient," *Regional Anesthesia and Pain Medicine*, vol. 23, no. 6, pp. 615–617, 1998.

[2] P. Bigeleisen and M. Wilson, "A comparison of two techniques for ultrasound guided infraclavicular block," *British Journal of Anaesthesia*, vol. 96, no. 4, pp. 502–507, 2006.

[3] M. V. Presta, S. W. Byram, C. L. Reis, and M. Sniderman, "Non-invasive removal of an entrapped supraclavicular catheter," *Journal of Clinical Anesthesia*, vol. 24, no. 4, pp. 350–352, 2012.

[4] B. H. S. Lee and C. R. Goucke, "Shearing of a peripheral nerve catheter," *Anesthesia and Analgesia*, vol. 95, no. 3, pp. 760–761, 2002.

[5] M. C. Kendall, A. Nader, R. B. Maniker, and R. J. Mccarthy, "Removal of a knotted stimulating femoral nerve catheter using a saline bolus injection," *Local and Regional Anesthesia*, vol. 3, no. 1, pp. 31–34, 2010.

[6] K. J. Chin and V. Chee, "Perforation of a Pajunk Stimulating Catheter After Traction-Induced Damage," *Regional Anesthesia and Pain Medicine*, vol. 31, no. 4, pp. 389–390, 2006.

[7] D. B. Auyong, J. Gonzales, and J. G. Benonis, "The houdini clavicle: arm abduction and needle insertion site adjustment improves needle visibility for the infraclavicular nerve block," *Regional Anesthesia and Pain Medicine*, vol. 35, no. 4, pp. 403–404, 2010.

[8] A. Ruíz, X. Sala, X. Bargalló, P. Hurtado, M. J. Arguis, and A. Carrera, "The influence of arm abduction on the anatomic relations of infraclavicular brachial plexus: an ultrasound study," *Anesthesia & Analgesia*, vol. 108, no. 1, pp. 364–366, 2009.

[9] P. M. Ludewig, S. A. Behrens, S. M. Meyer, S. M. Spoden, and L. A. Wilson, "Three-dimensional clavicular motion during arm elevation: reliability and descriptive data," *Journal of Orthopaedic and Sports Physical Therapy*, vol. 34, no. 3, pp. 140–149, 2004.

[10] M. M. LaBan, A. T. Zierenberg, S. Yadavalli, and S. Zaidan, "Clavicle-induced narrowing of the thoracic outlet during shoulder abduction as imaged by computed tomographic angiography and enhanced by three-dimensional reformation," *American Journal of Physical Medicine and Rehabilitation*, vol. 90, no. 7, pp. 572–578, 2011.

54

Management of Residual Neuromuscular Blockade Recovery: Age-Old Problem with a New Solution

Michael S. Green, Archana Gundigi Venkatesh, and Ranjani Venkataramani

Department of Anesthesiology and Perioperative Medicine, Drexel University College of Medicine, 245 N. 15th Street, Suite 7502, MS 310, Philadelphia, PA 19102, USA

Correspondence should be addressed to Michael S. Green; michael.green@drexelmed.edu

Academic Editor: Jian-jun Yang

Neostigmine has been traditionally used as the agent of choice to reverse Neuromuscular Blockade (NMB) after muscle paralysis during general anesthesia. However, the use of neostigmine has not been without untoward events. Sugammadex is a novel drug that selectively binds to aminosteroid nondepolarizing muscle relaxants and reverses even a deep level of NMB. Controversy exists regarding the optimal dose of sugammadex that is effective in reversing the NMB after the incomplete reversal with neostigmine and glycopyrrolate. We discuss a case where sugammadex reduced the time of the recovery from NMB in a patient who had incomplete antagonisms following adequate treatment with neostigmine, aiding timely extubation without persistent residual NMB, and hence prevented the requirement of postoperative ventilation and the improvement in patient care. More randomized control studies are needed in order to conclude the appropriate dose of sugammadex in cases of incomplete reversal.

1. Introduction

Neostigmine has been traditionally used as the agent of choice to reverse Neuromuscular Blockade (NMB) after muscle paralysis during general anesthesia. However, the use of neostigmine has not been without untoward events, namely, in the form of postoperative residual paralysis. This residual Neuromuscular Blockade is due to incomplete antagonism of NMB medications. A train of four (TOF) ratios of 0.9 and above is indicative of adequate reversal from NMB. While quantitative assessment of neuromuscular recovery using TOF ratio is considered gold standard [1], most anesthesiologists do not have the ability to perform a quantitative assessment of neuromuscular function [2]. Other factors that influence recovery after NMB, although not exhaustive, are the duration of the paralytic agent, use of single or repeated doses [3], and depth of blockade at the time of administering anticholinesterase [4]. Sugammadex is a novel drug that selectively binds to aminosteroid nondepolarizing muscle relaxants and reverses even a deep level of NMB. There are many studies which proved the effectiveness of sugammadex in reversing the NMB immediately following administration of

NMB. However, there is inadequate evidence of the effectives of sugammadex in cases of incomplete reversal with neostigmine and glycopyrrolate. Furthermore, controversy exists regarding the optimal dose of sugammadex that is effective in reversing the NMB after the incomplete reversal with neostigmine and glycopyrrolate. No standard dosing regimen exists yielding confusion on the management plan of residual curarization. Here, we discuss a case where sugammadex reduced the time of the recovery from NMB in a patient who had incomplete antagonisms following adequate treatment with neostigmine, aiding timely extubation without persistent residual NMB, and hence prevented the requirement of postoperative ventilation and the improvement in patient care. This case highlights sugammadex use in addition to neostigmine as an effective alternative in the management of patients with postoperative residual NMB.

2. Case Report

A 65-year-old female, 5′3″ tall, weighing 52 kilograms with a non-small cell carcinoma of the left upper lobe presented

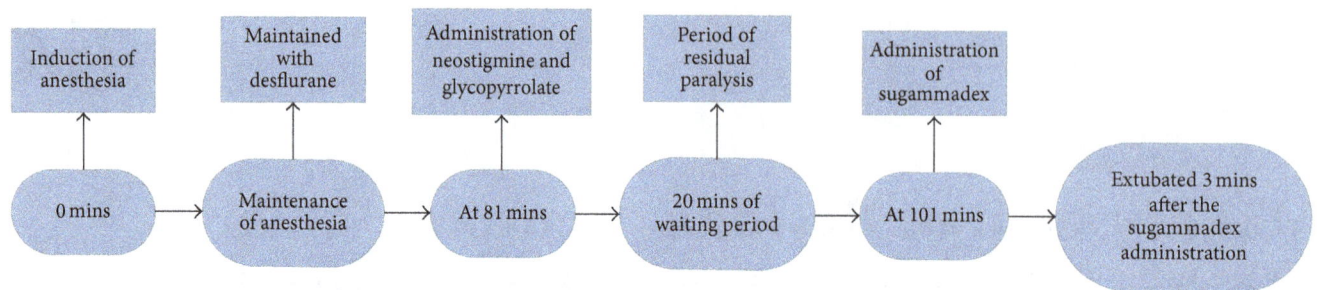

FIGURE 1

for a staging mediastinoscopy and biopsy under general anesthesia. Her medical history was significant for hypertension, COPD, GERD, and hepatitis C. Preoperative laboratory evaluation values were all within normal limits.

Induction of anesthesia was performed with propofol 150 mg, fentanyl 75 mcg, and rocuronium 50 mg. Desflurane provided anesthesia maintenance. The procedure was uneventful with a total time of 81 minutes. Following confirmation of 3 twitches via TOF monitoring the patient received neostigmine 3 mg and glycopyrrolate 0.6 mg intravenously. Persistent fade assessed via visual estimation of the TOF response was still evident even 20 minutes after medication administration. An additional dose of neostigmine 1 mg and glycopyrrolate 0.2 mg was given intravenously. Following a waiting period of 15 minutes the patient still had residual neuromuscular weakness requiring mechanical ventilation support (Figure 1). The decision of mechanical ventilation postoperatively versus a sugammadex trial was considered.

Suspecting residual curarization, sugammadex at 2 mg/kg, total of 100 mg, was given intravenously. A dramatic improvement in clinical response in the form of improved muscle strength, head lift, and tidal volumes were noted. This was coupled with an absence of fade on eliciting a TOF response. Extubation was safely performed within the next 2 minutes and no further recurarization or residual NMB was seen in the PACU.

3. Discussion

Usage of muscle relaxants has brought several advantages in the field of anesthesiology such as optimizing surgical conditions, facilitating tracheal intubation, and improving mechanical ventilation. However, there are several disadvantages of using Neuromuscular Blocking Agents (NMBA) with the most critical one being inadequate recovery of neuromuscular function leading to postoperative pulmonary complications and upper airway muscle weakness. Hence, reversible agents such as acetylcholinesterase inhibitors and sugammadex are used in order to antagonize the effects of nondepolarizing muscle relaxants and to prevent the complications due to residual curarization [5].

Gaszynski et al. conducted a study which included morbidly obese patients undergoing general anesthesia for elective bariatric surgery. A total of 70 patients were allocated randomly into Group SUG where they received sugammadex

for reversal of NMB and Group NEO where they received neostigmine for reversal. They found that mean time to 90% of TOF was 2.7 versus 9.6 minutes ($p < 0.05$) and TOF in the PACU was 109.2% versus 85.5% ($p < 0.05$) in Group SUG and Group NEO, respectively. This study proves that sugammadex is faster in reversing rocuronium-induced Neuromuscular Blockade compared to neostigmine [6].

Jones et al. conducted a study looking at the time taken for the recovery of NMB. This study included 37 patients in each study arm. One group received sugammadex of 4 mg/kg and the other group received neostigmine 70 μg/kg along with glycopyrrolate of 14 μg/kg for reversal of NMB. They found that sugammadex reversed the rocuronium-induced NMB within 2.9 mins as compared to 50.4 mins with neostigmine and glycopyrrolate. The authors concluded that sugammadex is 17-fold faster than the neostigmine and glycopyrrolate [7].

In our case, we used rocuronium of 1.0 mg/kg body weight for NMB at the time of induction. Rocuronium is a steroidal nondepolarizing muscle relaxant with duration of action ranging from 38 to 150 mins [8]. The surgical procedure was over in 81 mins and the patient was reversed with a standard dose of neostigmine and glycopyrrolate. We noticed a residual NMB even after the 20 minutes of neostigmine administration and showed significant fade on TOF stimulation along with inadequate tidal volume, poor respiratory efforts, and incoordination in hand movements. Given the clinical picture, we decided to administer sugammadex 100 mg instead of prolonged ventilation in order to prevent the complications associated with postoperative ventilation. After 2-3 minutes we noticed adequate tidal volume along with good respiratory efforts. There is very little data supporting the use of sugammadex following neostigmine administration. Neostigmine acts as a competitive antagonist at the neuromuscular junction by increasing the level of acetocholine available for binding to nicotinic receptors. Following the binding of the rocuronium by sugammadex there is no longer competition for the receptors thus leaving more available nicotinic and muscuranic receptors free for binding.

Cheong et al. conducted a study to compare the time to recovery of TOF ratio to 90% in four groups, Group S_2 (2 mg/kg of sugammadex), Group S_1 (1 mg/kg of sugammadex), Group SN (1 mg/kg of sugammadex and neostigmine 50 μg/kg and glycopyrrolate 10 μg/kg), and Group N (neostigmine 1 mg/kg + glycopyrrolate 10 μg/kg). Study results showed time for the recovery of TOF to 90% was 182.6 ± 8, 371.1 ± 2, 204.3 ± 103.3, and 953.2 ± 3 seconds, respectively. This shows that 1 mg/kg of sugammadex along with neostigmine 50 μg/kg and glycopyrrolate 10 μg/kg reduced the time to 90% recovery of TOF significantly. Additionally, there was no clinically significant difference between the group which received sugammadex 2 mg/kg and the group which received 1 mg/kg of sugammadex along with neostigmine 50 μg/kg and glycopyrrolate 10 μg/kg. In our case, we used 2 mg/kg of sugammadex, which is a higher dose when compared to effective dose which was proved in this study, that is, 1 mg/kg [9]. However, there is inconclusive evidence supporting one dose versus another with regard to the dosage of combination therapy with sugammadex and neostigmine.

An additional study was conducted in order to see the incidence of residual NMB in patients who are reversed spontaneously, after neostigmine treatment and after sugammadex administration. Interestingly, TOF ratio of <0.9 was present in 4.3% of patients who were treated with sugammadex for reversal as compared to 13% in the spontaneous recovery group and 23.9% in patients who received neostigmine for reversal. This shows that no complete elimination of residual NMB occurs, even after the reversal with sugammadex. Hence, using neuromuscular monitoring plays a key role in diagnosing and treating the residual NMB [10]. Our case is a perfect example showing the importance of utilization of neuromuscular monitoring to diagnose the incomplete reversal from muscle relaxants as well as the need to monitor recovery from residual NMB. Intraoperative use of neuromuscular monitoring allows the anesthesiologist to use adequate muscle relaxants and antagonists during the operation. This is important because 10% of the anesthesiologists in the Europe and 20% of the anesthesiologist in the North America do not use neuromuscular monitoring [8].

In our case, there are many factors responsible for postoperative residual paralysis after rocuronium administration. First, there is an increase in the duration of action of rocuronium with age. A study conducted by Furuya et al. concluded that the duration of time taken for the appearance of posttetanic count (PTC) was twofold longer and variable in older as compared to younger individuals [11]. Secondly, there is a prolongation of rocuronium action in the female gender as compared to males [12]. Thirdly, there is a large variation in the duration of action of rocuronium itself [13]. Fourth, we used desflurane for maintenance of anesthesia which may prolong the action of rocuronium compared to other inhalational agents [14].

There was a similar case reported of a patient who developed postoperative residual NMB after single dose of rocuronium. The patient required ventilation for 125 mins following the end of surgery and was monitored until the complete recovery from NMB [13]. Here, we administered sugammadex 100 mg instead of postoperative ventilation after the diagnosis of incomplete reversal of NMB with neostigmine. The patient developed adequate muscle contraction with good respiratory efforts within 2-3 minutes and we were able to discharge the patient on the same day. This therapy proved to be cost-effective as there is early recovery from the residual NMB which saved the utilization of the anesthesiologists and money spent on ventilator management and prevented the complications of prolonged postoperative ventilation. Hence, this case very well illustrates the role of neuromuscular monitoring and the use of sugammadex in the case of residual paralysis. The best dosing scheme with the use of sugammadex following neostigmine administration still remains to be defined. Our choice of 2 mg/kg proved to be effective in this patient. The aforementioned study showed no difference between sugammadex 2 mg/kg and sugammadex 1 mg/kg along with neostigmine 50 μg/kg and glycopyrrolate 10 μg/kg. Further exploration of the use of sugammadex 2 mg/kg with neostigmine 50 μg/kg for the reversal of neuromuscular blocking medications needs to be completed.

4. Conclusion

Sugammadex for reversing rocuronium-induced NMB has been used extensively in recent years. This novel cyclodextrin is used to reverse rocuronium-induced NMB in doses of up to 16 mg/kg. Recent studies from across the globe have been reporting success in reversing patients with variable depth of NMB by altering the dose of sugammadex.

We used a dose of 2 mg/kg in our patient, who demonstrated fade despite allowing for optimal duration of action of neostigmine. The dramatic recovery in neuromuscular function within 3 minutes of administration suggests that using this drug at lower doses such as 1-2 mg/kg in combination with neostigmine may perhaps prove to be a superior treatment modality. With its elevated price, sugammadex is somewhat cost prohibitive if not used scrupulously. However, if avoidance of postoperative ventilation is possible or postoperative pulmonary complications can be prevented the price of the medication will prove minimal. More studies are needed to pave the way for the administration of lower doses of sugammadex to supplement neostigmine in patients showing lighter levels of NMB or help serve as an alternative in patients showing fade or signs of inadequate NM recovery after reversal.

In our case, we demonstrated the advantages of using sugammadex in the case of residual NMB even after the reversal with neostigmine. In the future, more randomized control studies are need in order to conclude the appropriate dose of sugammadex in cases of incomplete reversal following neostigmine treatment.

References

[1] G. S. Murphy and S. J. Brull, "Residual neuromuscular block: lessons unlearned. Part I: definitions, incidence, and adverse physiologic effects of residual neuromuscular block," *Anesthesia and Analgesia*, vol. 111, no. 1, pp. 120–128, 2010.

[2] L. I. Eriksson, "Evidence-based practice and neuromuscular monitoring: it's time for routine quantitative assessment," *Anesthesiology*, vol. 98, no. 5, pp. 1037–1039, 2003.

[3] G. S. Murphy, J. W. Szokol, M. Franklin, J. H. Marymont, M. J. Avram, and J. S. Vender, "Postanesthesia care unit recovery times and neuromuscular blocking drugs: a prospective study of orthopedic surgical patients randomized to receive pancuronium or rocuronium," *Anesthesia and Analgesia*, vol. 98, no. 1, pp. 193–200, 2004.

[4] G. H. Beemer, A. R. Bjorksten, P. J. Dawson, R. J. Dawson, P. J. Heenan, and B. A. Robertson, "Determinants of the reversal time of competitive neuromuscular block by anticholinesterases," *British Journal of Anaesthesia*, vol. 66, no. 4, pp. 469–475, 1991.

[5] C. Meistelman and F. Donati, "Do we really need sugammadex as an antagonist of muscle relaxants in anesthesia?" *Current Opinion in Anaesthesiology*, vol. 29, no. 4, pp. 462–467, 2016.

[6] T. Gaszynski, T. Szewczyk, and W. Gaszynski, "Randomized comparison of sugammadex and neostigmine for reversal of rocuronium-induced muscle relaxation in morbidly obese undergoing general anaesthesia," *British Journal of Anaesthesia*, vol. 108, no. 2, pp. 236–239, 2012.

[7] R. K. Jones, J. E. Caldwell, S. J. Brull, and R. G. Soto, "Reversal of profound rocuronium-induced blockade with sugammadex: a randomized comparison with neostigmine," *Anesthesiology*, vol. 109, no. 5, pp. 816–824, 2008.

[8] C. C. de Menezes, L. A. M. Peceguini, E. D. Silva, and C. M. Simões, "Use of sugammadex after neostigmine incomplete reversal of rocuronium-induced neuromuscular blockade," *Revista Brasileira de Anestesiologia*, vol. 62, no. 4, pp. 543–547, 2012.

[9] S. H. Cheong, S. Ki, J. Lee et al., "The combination of sugammadex and neostigmine can reduce the dosage of sugammadex during recovery from the moderate neuromuscular blockade," *Korean Journal of Anesthesiology*, vol. 68, no. 6, pp. 547–555, 2015.

[10] Y. Kotake, R. Ochiai, T. Suzuki et al., "Reversal with sugammadex in the absence of monitoring did not preclude residual neuromuscular block," *Anesthesia and Analgesia*, vol. 117, no. 2, pp. 345–351, 2013.

[11] T. Furuya, T. Suzuki, A. Kashiwai et al., "The effects of age on maintenance of intense neuromuscular block with rocuronium,' ' *Acta Anaesthesiologica Scandinavica*, vol. 56, no. 2, pp. 236–239, 2012.

[12] M. Adamus, L. Hrabalek, T. Wanek, T. Gabrhelik, and J. Zapletalova, "Influence of age and gender on the pharmacodynamic parameters of rocuronium during total intravenous anesthesia," *Biomedical Papers of the Medical Faculty of the University Palacký, Olomouc, Czechoslovakia*, vol. 155, no. 4, pp. 347–353, 2011.

[13] C. Claudius, H. Karacan, and J. Viby-Mogensen, "Prolonged residual paralysis after a single intubating dose of rocuronium," *British Journal of Anaesthesia*, vol. 99, no. 4, pp. 514–517, 2007.

[14] N. Kumar, R. K. Mirakhur, M. J. J. Symington, and G. J. Mccarthy, "Potency and time course of action of rocuronium during desflurane and isoflurane anaesthesia," *British Journal of Anaesthesia*, vol. 77, no. 4, pp. 488–491, 1996.

55

Diagnosis and Thrombolytic Management of Massive Intraoperative Pulmonary Embolism Guided by Point of Care Transthoracic Echocardiography

Roman Dudaryk ⓘD, Julio Benitez Lopez, and Jack Louro ⓘD

Department of Anesthesiology, Perioperative Medicine, and Pain Management, University of Miami Miller School of Medicine, Miami, FL, USA

Correspondence should be addressed to Jack Louro; jlouro1@med.miami.edu

Academic Editor: Ilok Lee

Perioperative pulmonary embolism can go undetected until the sudden onset of cardiopulmonary collapse. Point of care echocardiography in such setting can narrow the differential diagnosis of precipitous instability and facilitate tailored, rather than empiric, therapy in the event of a massive pulmonary embolism. We describe the diagnosis and successful multidisciplinary management of intraoperative massive pulmonary embolism aided by both transthoracic and transesophageal echocardiography. Key aspects regarding the classification and treatment of pulmonary embolism are subsequently reviewed.

1. Introduction

Perioperative pulmonary embolism (PE) presents a diagnostic challenge and confers a high risk of mortality due to limited treatment options. Despite advances in imaging modalities and clinical management, overall mortality remains high at approximately 15% [1–3]. For patients with massive pulmonary embolism and cardiac arrest, mortality exceeds 50% [2, 4]. Patients undergoing surgery often have underlying risk factors for thrombosis and embolism, such as obesity, smoking, malignancy, or traumatic injury. Furthermore, the inflammatory response to surgery leads to a prothrombotic state, which further increases the risk in conjunction with postoperative hospitalization, central venous catheterization, and immobilization. These factors account for the fivefold increased incidence of perioperative PE [5].

PE is frequently first suspected following the development of nonspecific signs, which can include hemodynamic instability, hypoxemia, increased alveolar dead space, and electrocardiogram (ECG) changes. However, intraoperatively these findings can be subtle and masked, and the first sign of PE may be sudden cardiopulmonary collapse. Furthermore, typical diagnostic modalities are intended for the hospital ward or emergency department and are impractical in the intraoperative setting. Transesophageal echocardiography (TEE) has

long been recommended to aid in diagnosis of pathologies responsible for persistent hemodynamic compromise, but recently point of care transthoracic echocardiography (TTE) has emerged as a powerful and noninvasive diagnostic tool in perioperative medicine [6]. Use of TTE is very common in the ICU settings but less so in the operating room, which historically was a domain of TEE. Therefore, the use of TTE which currently has greater availability and is less invasive in the operating room for diagnosis and monitoring of the response to hemodynamic intervention in patients with suspected acute cor pulmonale is underappreciated by anesthesiologists. Patients with significant PE can benefit from surgical or pharmacological thrombolysis, and thus rapid diagnosis and treatment are crucial to improve outcomes [3]. Herein, we describe the utility of structured intraoperative TTE and TEE examinations to aid in the diagnosis and management of massive PE. The patient provided signed and witnessed written consent to publish this deidentified case report.

2. Case Description

A 59-year-old male bicyclist with no past medical history presented to the trauma resuscitation unit at the Ryder Trauma Center in Miami, FL, after being struck by a motor vehicle. He sustained a comminuted left subtrochanteric femur fracture

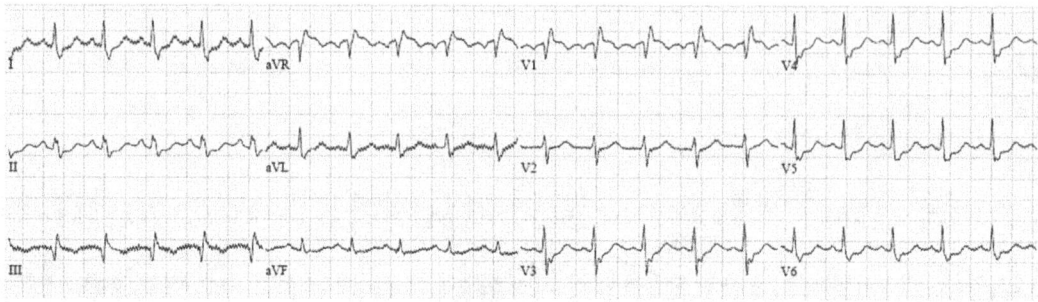

FIGURE 1: Intraoperative 12 lead electrocardiogram demonstrating signs of acute cor pulmonale: S waves in lead 1 and Q waves with the suggestion of T wave inversion in lead 3.

and was taken to the operating room for an open reduction and fixation. Following a rapid sequence induction of general anesthesia with propofol and succinylcholine, the patient was readily intubated via direct laryngoscopy. Approximately 5 minutes after induction, initial skin preparation and positioning were begun by the orthopedic surgery team. Upon initial manipulation of the left lower extremity, the anesthesiologist noticed a precipitous drop in the end-tidal carbon dioxide (EtCO2), heart rate greater than 120 bpm, and systolic blood pressure less than 90 mmHg. The surgical team was informed, and manipulation of the lower extremities was suspended. The patient was immediately treated with phenylephrine and crystalloid fluid boluses. The patient had oxygen desaturation to the low 90s, which responded to an increase in fractional inspired (FiO2), and a transient drop in EtCO2 of greater than 15 mmHg, which were concerning for a sudden increase in dead space ventilation. A 12-lead EKG showed signs of right heart strain, including an S wave in lead 1 and Q waves with T wave inversion in lead 3 (Figure 1). Given this constellation of findings in conjunction with hemodynamic instability, preparations were begun to facilitate a TEE examination. In the interim, a structured TTE examination according to the FATE protocol (Focused Assessed Transthoracic Echocardiography) was immediately performed [7]. The parasternal long axis view was remarkable for massive dilatation and hypokinesia of the right ventricle (RV). In the parasternal short axis, flattening of the intraventricular septum (D-shaped) and paradoxical septal motion were evident. The flattening of interventricular septum at end-systole suggested RV pressure-overload, probably due to distal pulmonary artery obstruction, and enabled us to make differential diagnosis from RV volume overload, as the reason for hemodynamic deterioration. The apical four-chamber view revealed a mobile mass in the right atrium (RA) suspicious for a thrombus (Figure 2, Supplemental Video 1). As this constellation of findings was pathognomonic for massive PE, the surgical procedure was halted.

A TEE was then performed by the anesthesia team, which facilitated more detailed evaluation of the RA. In the midesophageal 4-chamber view, a patent foramen ovale and associated RA thrombus were evident (Figure 3, Supplemental Video 2). Cardiothoracic surgery, interventional radiology, and intensivists from the Trauma Intensive Care Unit (ICU)

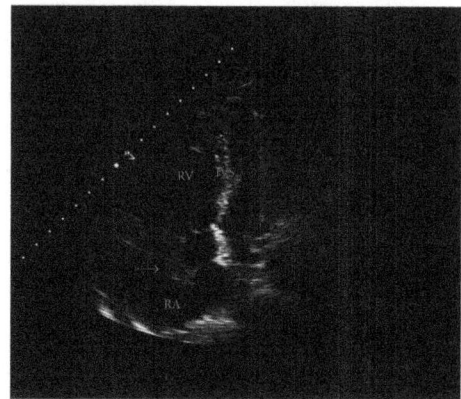

FIGURE 2: Intraoperative transthoracic echocardiography, 4 chamber apical view showing a right atrial thrombus (arrow), right ventricular dilatation, right atrial dilatation, and septal bowing. RV, right ventricle; RA, right atrium; IVS, interventricular septum; LA, left atrium; LV, left ventricle.

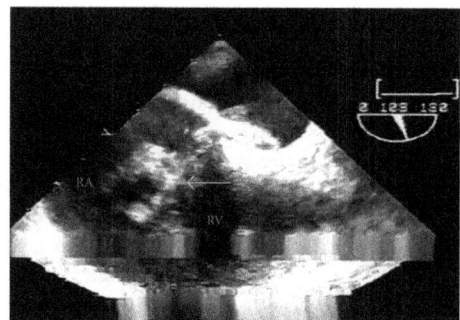

FIGURE 3: Initial intraoperative transesophageal echocardiography; midesophageal 4-chamber view. A large right atrial thrombus was visualized (blue arrow). LA, left atrium; RA, right atrium; RV, right ventricle.

were consulted intraoperatively. A repeat TEE examination after their arrival failed to demonstrate either the previously seen RA clot or any thrombus within the visualized portions of the pulmonary artery (PA). As such, probable migration

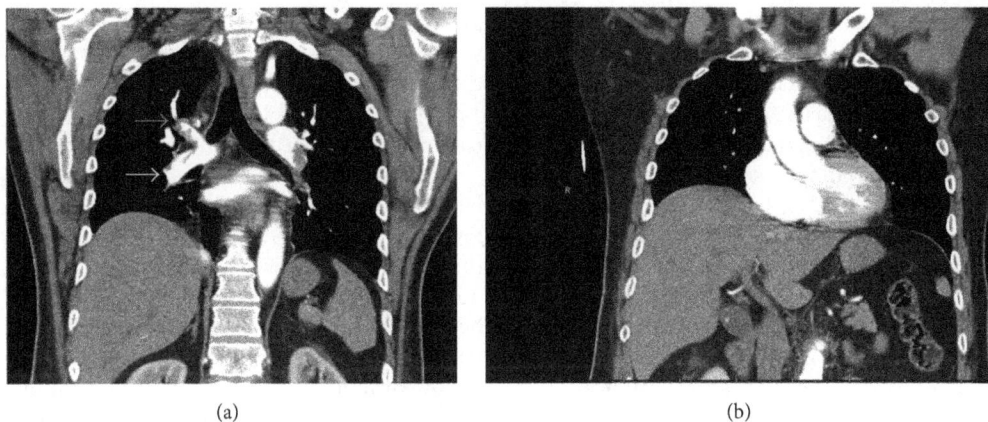

(a)   (b)

FIGURE 4: Perioperative chest computed tomography angiography; coronal reconstructions. (a) Filling defects were noted in right upper (red arrow) and lower lobar (green arrow) pulmonary arteries. (b) Right ventricular dilatation.

was suspected. At this point in time, the contractility of the RV on TEE was noted to be improved with inotropic and vasopressor support despite dilatation and pressure overload. This allowed us to make the decision regarding the transport of the patient to the radiography suite for definitive treatment. No changes in hemodynamics or oxygenation were noted at this time, aside from occasional phenylephrine doses. Following a multidisciplinary discussion, the patient was anticoagulated with a heparin infusion, and a computed tomography (CT) angiogram of the chest was obtained to further evaluate the thrombus and guide the course of treatment. At this juncture, the patient was hemodynamically stable and thus deemed suitable for transport. He was brought intubated and sedated to the radiology department by the anesthesia and surgical team. CT angiography revealed RV dilatation with a large distal right PA thrombus extending into the upper and lower lobar arteries, along with a left upper and lower lobar artery thrombus (Figure 4). Evaluation by cardiothoracic surgery concluded that the thrombi were too distal as they were no longer seen on the repeat TEE exam and only detectable on CT for effective surgical embolectomy. As the patient was still requiring vasopressor and inotropic support with RV dilatation evident on echocardiography, the next step in management required some form of thrombolysis. Interventional radiology deemed him a good candidate for catheter-directed ultrasound accelerated thrombolysis. Ultrasound accelerated thrombolysis catheters measuring 24 and 12 cm were placed into the right and left PA, respectively. The patient was subsequently admitted to the ICU for further monitoring and optimization. Tissue plasminogen activator (tPA) was infused through each catheter at 0.75 mg/hr with a normal saline carrier at 35 ml/hr.

On postoperative day (POD) 2, a formal TTE was performed that demonstrated improved RV function with only slightly increased RV systolic pressures. The patient was extubated on POD 4 and later underwent an uneventful definitive fixation of fractures on hospital day 11. He was bridged to warfarin and discharged to a rehabilitation facility on hospital day 22.

3. Discussion

Rapid and reliable diagnosis of massive PE is critical to identify patients who will benefit from anticoagulation, surgical embolectomy, pharmacological thrombolysis, or catheter directed therapies. As commitment to these treatment options confers a high risk of complications, stratification schemas have been developed to identify patients at a high risk for mortality for whom the benefits of treatment are likely to outweigh the risks. As such, the current classification of PE by the American Heart Association (AHA) as massive, submassive, or low-risk has moved away from the historical model of categorization by degree of clot burden and instead focuses on the presence or absence of symptoms associated with adverse outcomes [8]. The AHA defines massive PE as an acute event coupled with sustained hypotension (systolic blood pressure less than 90 mmHg for more than 15 minutes or requiring inotropic support), pulselessness, or bradycardia in the absence of other causes. Submassive PE, by definition, is not accompanied by sustained hypotension but does involve signs of RV dysfunction or myocardial necrosis as evidenced by certain echocardiographic findings, ECG features, laboratory studies, and clinical scores. These patients are still at a heightened risk for adverse events and require emergent interventions intended to decrease clot burden and improve mortality [8]. Low-risk PE describes patients with the best prognosis, typically those with normal hemodynamics, normal biomarkers, and no signs of RV dysfunction.

Both TEE and TTE have been increasingly utilized to aid in the rapid diagnosis of PE, evaluation of RV strain, and detection of cardiac sequelae. In one case series, the sensitivity of TEE for the detection of massive central PE was found to be about 80% with 100% specificity [9]. However, more distal thromboembolic burden is difficult to visualize via echocardiography, as evidenced by an intraoperative case series wherein PE was directly visualized in only 26% of cases [10]. However, TEE can often reveal extrapulmonary venous or intracardiac emboli, which can easily influence surgical planning [11, 12]. As such, direct visualization of thrombus is specific but not sensitive. Indirect evidence of pulmonary embolism, including RV dysfunction and leftward interatrial septal bowing, has been found in over 96% of patients, and acute tricuspid regurgitation is present in more than 50% of patients undergoing emergent embolectomy [10].

Historically, assessment of RV function by echocardiography is challenging, due its complex geometry, lack of standardized imaging planes, and numerous assumptions required [13, 14]. As such, there is no one single dimension, sign, or parameter that allows for reliable assessment of RV function [14]. Increased evidence of the clinical implications of RV dysfunction and associated outcomes has led to the creation of guidelines and recommendations to standardize RV assessment [13]. In brief, echocardiographic evaluation RV function includes both qualitative assessment and evaluation of quantitative parameters. Patterns describing RV ejection have been shown to be highly specific, including "McConnell's sign" (e.g., RV free wall hypokinesis with preserved contraction of the apex) and the "60-60 sign" (e.g., a tricuspid regurgitation gradient less than 60 mmHg with pulmonary flow acceleration less than 60 milliseconds) [14]. Additional recommended RV evaluation parameters include RV, right atrial, and inferior vena cava dilation, as well as markers of RV systolic function including fractional area change, tricuspid annular plane systolic excursion (TAPSE), RV index of myocardial performance (RIMP), and Doppler estimation of PA pressures [13]. All of these signs and indices must ultimately be combined and interpreted in the context of subjective and clinical assessment.

The treatment of massive PE in the perioperative period typically involves a multidisciplinary discussion to facilitate risk to benefit ratio analysis. Numerous reperfusion therapies are available and include systemic fibrinolysis, catheter directed therapies (fibrinolysis or thrombectomy), and surgical embolectomy. The lack of current consensus, or evidence-driven guidelines in the perioperative period, makes treatment decisions challenging. Systemic anticoagulation and thrombolysis have been used successfully for surgical patients [15–17]. However, pharmacologic treatment may be contraindicated in the setting of recent surgery given a potentially heightened risk of major hemorrhage. Surgical embolectomy is recommended in high-risk PE patients with a contraindication to, or failure of, systemic thrombolysis [14]. Recent evidence suggests low mortality rates in patients undergoing early surgical embolectomy with hemodynamically stable, high-risk PE and echocardiographic signs of RV dysfunction [18, 19]. The signs of right ventricular dysfunction were evident in our patient on TEE. However, the emboli were too distal for effective surgical treatment as they were noted to migrate from the RA on the second echocardiographic evaluation. In the case of this patient, systemic fibrinolysis was deemed to confer a high risk for hemorrhage, but more aggressive thrombolysis was deemed necessary as RV dilatation and dysfunction were clear on TEE. If the patient had normal RV function after supportive therapy and initiation of heparin on echocardiography, management would have involved anticoagulation with heparin in the ICU

as opposed to attempts at thrombolysis. Echocardiography was able to help guide the management approach by revealing the right ventricular dysfunction.

Ultrasound accelerated fibrinolysis catheters are a novel treatment alternative and increasingly available amongst experienced centers. This technology was recently approved by the FDA for the treatment of PE. These catheters deliver low power, high frequency ultrasound waves that hypothetically expose plasminogen receptors sites on the fibrin molecules, which enhances the efficacy of tPA [20]. They have been shown in a small multicenter randomized controlled trial to be more effective than heparin alone in reducing RV strain without an increase in bleeding complications [21].

In the case of this patient, intraoperative TTE and TEE lead to the rapid diagnosis of PE by direct visualization and identification of RV dysfunction, which facilitated immediate multidisciplinary discussion and treatment. Intraoperative diagnosis of the PE led to immediate cessation of manipulation, potentially avoiding further thromboembolic burden from the lower extremity. Due to the changes observed on TEE, systemic anticoagulation was initiated intraoperatively and CT chest angiography was obtained to assess for residual embolism. A multidisciplinary discussion of risks/benefits, PE distribution, and patient condition, along with center-specific resources and experience, facilitated effective treatment. Ultrasound accelerated catheter directed thrombolysis with systemic anticoagulation resulted in normalization of RV function and discharge to rehabilitation without complication.

Disclosure

All authors approved the final manuscript.

References

[1] S. Z. Goldhaber, L. Visani, and M. de Rosa, "Acute pulmonary embolism: clinical outcomes in the International Cooperative Pulmonary Embolism Registry (ICOPER)," *The Lancet*, vol. 353, no. 9162, pp. 1386–1389, 1999.

[2] N. Kucher, E. Rossi, M. De Rosa, and S. Z. Goldhaber, "Massive pulmonary embolism," *Circulation*, vol. 113, no. 4, pp. 577–582, 2006.

[3] K. E. Wood, "Major pulmonary embolism: review of a pathophysiologic approach to the golden hour of hemodynamically significant pulmonary embolism," *CHEST*, vol. 121, no. 3, pp. 877–905, 2002.

[4] I. Kürkciyan, G. Meron, F. Sterz et al., "Pulmonary embolism as a cause of cardiac arrest: presentation and outcome," *Archives of Internal Medicine*, vol. 160, pp. 1529–1535, 2000.

[5] M. C. Desciak and D. E. Martin, "Perioperative pulmonary embolism: diagnosis and anesthetic management," *Journal of Clinical Anesthesia*, vol. 23, pp. 153–165, 2011.

[6] D. M. Thys, R. F. Brooker, M. K. Cahalan et al., "American Society of A, Society of Cardiovascular Anesthesiologists Task Force on Transesophageal E. Practice guidelines for perioperative transesophageal echocardiography. An updated report

by the American Society of Anesthesiologists and the Society of Cardiovascular Anesthesiologists Task Force on Transesophageal Echocardiography," *Anesthesiology*, vol. 112, pp. 1084–1096, 2010.

[7] M. B. Jensen, E. Sloth, K. M. Larsen, and M. B. Schmidt, "Transthoracic echocardiography for cardiopulmonary monitoring in intensive care," *European Journal of Anaesthesiology*, vol. 21, no. 9, pp. 700–707, 2004.

[8] M. R. Jaff, M. S. McMurtry, S. L. Archer et al., "Management of massive and submassive pulmonary embolism, iliofemoral deep vein thrombosis, and chronic thromboembolic pulmonary hypertension: a scientific statement from the american heart association," *Circulation*, vol. 123, no. 16, pp. 1788–1830, 2011.

[9] P. Pruszczyk, A. Torbicki, R. Pacho et al., "Noninvasive diagnosis of suspected severe pulmonary embolism: Transesophageal echocardiography vs spiral CT," *CHEST*, vol. 112, no. 3, pp. 722–728, 1997.

[10] P. Rosenberger, S. K. Shernan, S. C. Body, and H. K. Eltzschig, "Utility of intraoperative transesophageal echocardiography for diagnosis of pulmonary embolism," *Anesthesia and Analgesia*, vol. 99, no. 1, pp. 12–16, 2004.

[11] O. Langeron, J. P. Goarin, J. L. Pansard, B. Riou, and P. Viars, "Massive intraoperative pulmonary embolism: diagnosis with transesophageal two-dimensional echocardiography," *Anesthesia and Analgesia*, vol. 74, no. 1, pp. 148–150, 1992.

[12] P. Rosenberger, S. K. Shernan, T. Weissmüller et al., "Role of intraoperative transesophageal echocardiography for diagnosing and managing pulmonary embolism in the perioperative period," *Anesthesia & Analgesia*, vol. 100, no. 1, pp. 292-293, 2005.

[13] L. G. Rudski, W. W. Lai, J. Afilalo et al., "Guidelines for the echocardiographic assessment of the right heart in adults: a report from the American Society of Echocardiography endorsed by the European Association of Echocardiography, a registered branch of the European Society of Cardiology, and the Canadian Society of Echocardiography," *Journal of the American Society of Echocardiography*, vol. 23, no. 7, pp. 685–713, 2010.

[14] S. V. Konstantinides, A. Torbicki, and G. Agnelli, "2014 ESC Guidelines on the diagnosis and management of acute pulmonary embolism: The Task Force for the Diagnosis and Management of Acute Pulmonary Embolism of the European Society of Cardiology (ESC) Endorsed by the European Respiratory Society (ERS)," *European Heart Journal*, vol. 35, no. 43, pp. 3033–3073, 2014.

[15] M. Wenk, D. M. Pöpping, S. Hillyard, H. Albers, and M. Möllmann, "Intraoperative thrombolysis in a patient with cardiopulmonary arrest undergoing caesarean delivery," *Anaesth Intensive Care*, vol. 39, pp. 671–674, 2011.

[16] K. Zhang, X. Zeng, C. Zhu et al., "Successful thrombolysis in postoperative patients with acute massive pulmonary embolism," *Heart, Lung and Circulation*, vol. 22, no. 2, pp. 100–103, 2013.

[17] R. V. Sondekoppam, M. Kanwar, Y. S. Latha, and B. Mandal, "High dose streptokinase for thrombolysis in the immediate postoperative period: a case report," *Middle East Journal of Anaesthesiology*, vol. 22, pp. 207–211, 2013.

[18] E. M. Carvalho, F. I. B. MacEdo, A. L. Panos, M. Ricci, and T. A. Salerno, "Pulmonary embolectomy: recommendation for early surgical intervention," *Journal of Cardiac Surgery*, vol. 25, no. 3, pp. 261–266, 2010.

[19] M. Leacche, D. Unic, and S. Goldhaber, "Modern surgical treatment of massive pulmonary embolism: results in 47 consecutive patients after rapid diagnosis and aggressive surgical approach," *The Journal of Thoracic and Cardiovascular Surgery*, vol. 129, no. 8, pp. 1018–1023, 2005.

[20] C. W. Francis, A. Blinc, S. Lee, and C. Cox, "Ultrasound accelerates transport of recombinant tissue plasminogen activator into clots," *Ultrasound in Medicine & Biology*, vol. 21, no. 3, pp. 419–424, 1995.

[21] N. Kucher, P. Boekstegers, and O. J. Muller, "Randomized, controlled trial of ultrasound-assisted catheter-directed thrombolysis for acute intermediate-risk pulmonary embolism," *Circulation*, vol. 129, pp. 479–486, 2014.

56

Ultrasound-Guided Interscalene Catheter Complicated by Persistent Phrenic Nerve Palsy

Andrew T. Koogler and **Michael Kushelev**

Department of Anesthesiology, The Ohio State University Wexner Medical Center, 410 W. 10th Ave., Columbus, OH 43210, USA

Correspondence should be addressed to Andrew T. Koogler; andrew.koogler@osumc.edu

Academic Editor: Pavel Michalek

A 76-year-old male presented for reverse total shoulder arthroplasty (TSA) in the beach chair position. A preoperative interscalene nerve catheter was placed under direct ultrasound-guidance utilizing a posterior in-plane approach. On POD 2, the catheter was removed. Three weeks postoperatively, the patient reported worsening dyspnea with a subsequent chest X-ray demonstrating an elevated right hemidiaphragm. Pulmonary function testing revealed worsening deficit from presurgical values consistent with phrenic nerve palsy. The patient decided to continue conservative management and declined further invasive testing or treatment. He was followed for one year postoperatively with moderate improvement of his exertional dyspnea over that period of time. The close proximity of the phrenic nerve to the brachial plexus in combination with its frequent anatomical variation can lead to unintentional mechanical trauma, intraneural injection, or chemical injury during performance of ISB. The only previously identified risk factor for PPNP is cervical degenerative disc disease. Although PPNP has been reported following TSA in the beach chair position without the presence of a nerve block, it is typically presumed as a complication of the interscalene block. Previously published case reports and case series of PPNP complicating ISBs all describe nerve blocks performed with either paresthesia technique or localization with nerve stimulation. We report a case of a patient experiencing PPNP following an ultrasound-guided placement of an interscalene nerve catheter.

1. Introduction

Interscalene blocks (ISB) are frequently used as an adjuvant therapy for shoulder surgery to optimize postoperative pain, decrease the length of hospitalization, and minimize the time in the postanesthesia care unit [1]. Up to 100% of patients receiving an ISB can anticipate transient phrenic nerve palsy with full recovery following nerve block resolution [2].

Prolonged phrenic nerve paresis (PPNP) resulting from interscalene catheters is rare. One previous investigation identified cervical degenerative disc disease as a potential risk factor for developing PPNP following ISB [3]. Otherwise, there have been few other proposed risk factors thought to contribute to the development of PPNP. We present a case of PPNP following placement of an interscalene nerve catheter for a patient undergoing reverse total shoulder arthroplasty (TSA) with previously undiagnosed cervical degenerative disc disease. This case report is to help highlight risk factors for the development of PPNP, as well as the appropriate workup and treatment of PPNP.

2. Case Report

Verbal and written permission was obtained from the patient for the publication of this report. Written permission was obtained for the use of the patient's medical records.

A 76-year-old male of average body habitus with history of hypertension, chronic obstructive pulmonary disease (COPD), coronary artery disease, and myocardial infarction status after three percutaneous coronary interventions presented for reverse TSA in the beach chair position under general anesthesia with an interscalene nerve catheter for postoperative pain management. After obtaining surgical and anesthetic consent, the patient was placed in a semirecumbent position with his head turned slightly toward the nonoperative shoulder with care to avoid neck discomfort. Intravenous midazolam and fentanyl were administered to achieve moderate sedation for the placement of an inter-scalene nerve catheter under direct ultrasound-guidance utilizing a lateral-to-medial in-plane approach as described by Antonakakis et al. [4]. A 17-gauge 5 cm Tuohy needle (Arrow International, Reading, PA, USA) was inserted at the anterior edge of the trapezius muscle and advanced using an in-plane technique, passing through the middle scalene muscle and entering the interscalene groove. An initial bolus of 30 cc of 0.5% ropivacaine was delivered in the interscalene groove on the posterior edge of the C5 and C6 nerve roots, followed by the advancement of a 19-gauge Arrow Stimucath Catheter (Teleflex Medical, Reading, PA, USA) without resistance 3 cm past the needle tip. The Tuohy needle was subsequently removed. A 5 ml test dose of 1.5% lidocaine with 1 : 200,000 epinephrine was administered followed by injection of 10 cc of 0.5% ropivacaine with direct ultrasound visualization of the injectate along the posterior edge of the interscalene groove. The catheter was secured with Der-mabond liquid adhesive (Ethicon, Somerville, NJ, USA) and covered with a Tegaderm dressing (3M Company, St. Paul, MN, USA). The patient was responsive to verbal stimulation and denied paresthesia or shortness of breath immediately after catheter placement. He was then brought to the oper-ating room and connected to standard anesthesia monitors. General anesthesia was induced with fentanyl, propofol, and rocuronium followed by an uneventful placement of a 7.0 endotracheal tube with direct laryngoscopy. Intraoperatively the patient was placed in the beach chair position with his neck in a neutral position with the combination of a head rest and towels below the jaw line after the endotracheal tube was secured. Neutral head positioning was reconfirmed throughout the course of the surgery by the anesthesia provider. Total surgery time was exactly three hours. Patient was extubated and transferred to the recovery room. One hour postoperatively in the postanesthesia recovery unit, the interscalene catheter was attached to an Elastomeric ON-Q pump (I-Flow Corporation, VQ OrthoCare, Irvine, CA, USA) followed by a 2-day infusion of 0.2% ropivacaine at 10 ml/hour. The patient's surgical course was uneventful, and he was seen on postoperative days (POD) 1 and 2 during acute pain rounds. The patient did not endorse any significant changes in his baseline exertional dyspnea, and his pain was well controlled. On POD 2, the catheter was removed, and he was discharged without significant complaints.

Three weeks postoperatively, the patient presented to his PCP with a complaint of worsening dyspnea. He was diag-nosed with bronchitis and prescribed a course of antibiotics and inhalers. After completing his antibiotic regimen, the patient continued to experience dyspnea and was referred to a pulmonologist for consultation. Further investigation revealed that the patient had both orthopnea and worsened dyspnea on exertion. The physical exam revealed decreased breath sounds in the right lower lobe lung field and bilateral upper airway expiratory wheezing. A chest X-ray (CXR) demonstrated an elevated right hemidiaphragm with a small right-sided pleural effusion.

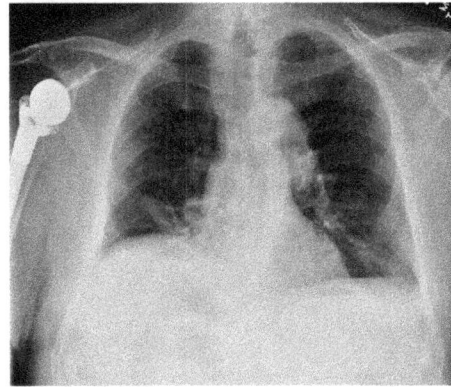

FIGURE 1: Chest X-ray 6 weeks postoperatively.

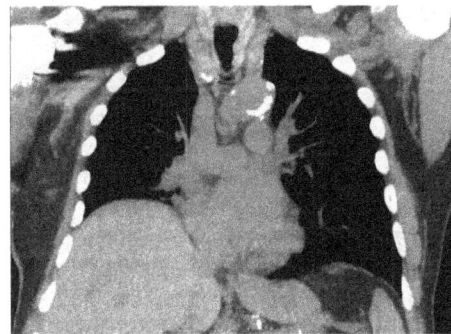

FIGURE 2: Chest CT scan 6 weeks postoperatively.

A repeat CXR six weeks postoperatively continued to demonstrate an elevated right hemidiaphragm and right-sided pleural effusion, unchanged from his previous CXR (Figure 1). A diaphragm fluoroscopy (sniff test) confirmed a paralyzed right hemidiaphragm. Chest (Figure 2) and neck CT scans demonstrated an elevated right hemidiaphragm with overlying right lower lobe atelectasis and degenera-tive changes in his cervical spine (C4–7) consistent with cervical spinal stenosis (Figure 3). The patient had repeat pulmonary function testing, which demonstrated a wors-ening deficit from presurgical values (Table 1). The patient decided to continue conservative management consisting only of close follow-up with his pulmonologist and declined further invasive testing or treatment, such as an EMG or surgical intervention. The patient was followed for one year postoperatively with moderate improvement of his exertional dyspnea. A repeat CXR at 1 year postoperatively no longer demonstrated an elevated right hemidiaphragm, although the patient continued to endorse mildly worsened exertional dyspnea compared to preoperative levels (Figure 4).

3. Discussion

The anatomical proximity of the brachial plexus and phrenic nerve leads to a nearly universal transient blockade of the phrenic nerve with large volume ISB; however, PPNP is a rare complication with a reported incidence to be 1 out of every 2069 single shot ISB or 0.048% [3]. The close proximity

TABLE 1: Pulmonary function tests pre- and postoperatively.

	Preoperative			Postoperative		
	Pred	Actual	% Pred	Pred	Actual	% Pred
Forced vital capacity (FVC; L)	3.86	3.39	88	3.59	2.12	59
Forced expiratory volume 1 (FEV1; L)	2.81	2.18	78	2.56	1.29	50
% FEV1/FVC	73.0%	64.3%		72.0%	61.0%	
Mid-expiratory flow (FEF25–75; L/sec)	2.10	0.99	47	1.71	0.58	32
Peak flow (PF; L/sec)	7.49	6.46	86	6.84	6.01	88

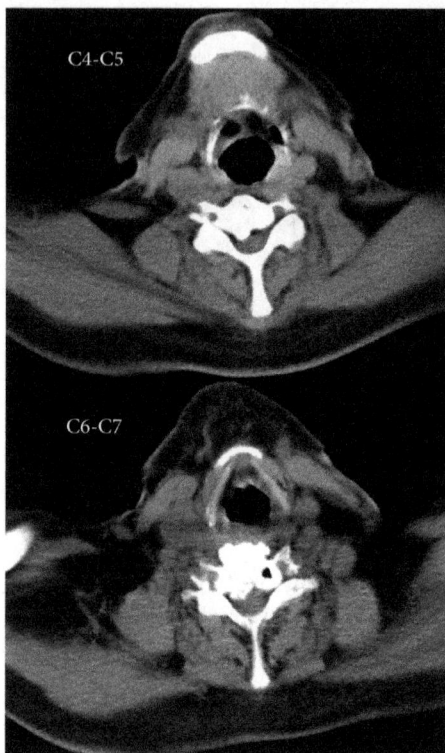

FIGURE 3: Neck CT scan C4-C5, C6-C7.

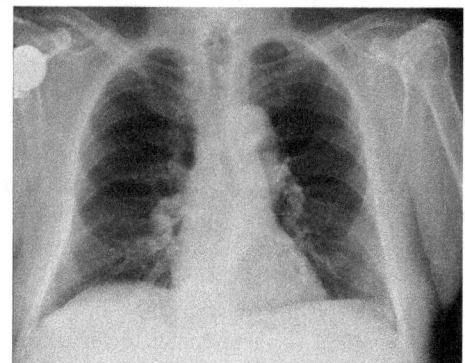

FIGURE 4: Chest X-ray 1 year postoperatively.

of the phrenic nerve to the brachial plexus in combination with its frequent anatomical variation can lead to unintentional mechanical trauma, intraneural injection, or chemical injury during performance of ISB [5]. Our patient's phrenic nerve was not readily identifiable on a brief preprocedure ultrasound (US) examination. Various in-plane and out-of-plane techniques have been described for performance of the continuous interscalene block without any clear consensus as to the technique that is most efficacious [6]. The needle trajectory for the in-plane technique can be either lateral-to-medial or medial-to-lateral. Neither approach eliminates risk of nerve injury as the dorsal scapular nerve (DSN) and the long thoracic nerve (LTN) travel through the middle scalene muscle, while the phrenic nerve may be placed at risk of injury while traversing along the anterior scalene muscle. Out-of-plane approaches place the needle trajectory in closer proximity to the phrenic nerve, potentially increasing the risk of mechanical trauma. US guidance may allow for

visualization of the DSN, LTN, and phrenic nerve, therefore limiting the risk of nerve injury [7].

Although decreasing the volume of local anesthetic utilized for interscalene blockade has been shown to decrease the incidence transient phrenic nerve palsy [8], total dose or volume of local anesthetic has not been identified as a risk factor for developing PPNP [3]. Additionally, relatively large initial block volumes of 40 to 65 mL are routinely used to establish interscalene blockade in the era of US guidance [9]. With the use of relatively large initial volumes, our patient must have certainly experienced phrenic nerve palsy during the course of his interscalene catheter infusion (approximately 50 hours); however, his baseline preoperative dyspnea, relative inactivity as an inpatient, and accessory muscle utilization during his 2-day postoperative hospitalization are thought to have masked a worsening of his exertional dyspnea. Although partially compensated phrenic nerve palsy was to be anticipated, there were no indications to suggest development of PPNP prior to discharge from the hospital.

Proposed mechanisms for PPNP complicating an ISB include compression neuropathy from needle trauma, intraneural injection, chemical toxicity, or neuronal ischemia [10, 11]. Shoulder arthroplasty as well as beach chair positioning, separate from regional anesthesia, has been associated with nerve injury at a rate of 0.6–3.6%, most commonly involving the axillary or musculocutaneous nerves. Mechanism of injury is often related to direct trauma, retraction, hematoma formation, or neck positioning during surgical manipulation [12]. Incidentally, TSA in the beach chair position without a regional nerve block has been reported to result in a PPNP in a case that did not involve a regional anesthetic [13]. Ultimately the definitive cause of PPNP cannot be determined without electromyography or a pathological analysis of the phrenic nerve. One hypothesis describing such an unexpected persistent nerve injury is the "double-crush" phenomenon [14]. Our patient may have suffered a neural insult secondary to the regional anesthetic technique, combined with compression of the phrenic nerve at the root level secondary to surgical positioning, traction, or underlying (at the time unknown) C4–C7 cervical degenerative disease.

Previously published case reports and case series of PPNP complicating ISBs all describe nerve blocks performed with either paresthesia technique or localization with nerve stimulation (NS). Of note, this patient's interscalene catheter was performed with only US guidance and did not rely on NS or paresthesia techniques. Although the use of US guidance for regional anesthesia has not demonstrated a reduction in peripheral nerve injury, routine use of US guidance allows practitioners many practical advantages [15]. A recent review demonstrated a decreased number of needle passes, decreased procedural time, and decreased procedure pain for US guided blocks as compared to NS guided blocks [16]. Furthermore, the ability to observe "real-time" needle advancement suggests the potential for US guidance to decrease nerve injury, including the phrenic nerve, compared to other localization techniques. In support of such a hypothesis, a letter to the editor in response to the case-control series identifying risk factors for PPNP speculated that persistent phrenic nerve dysfunction may disappear as a complication of ISB with the transition to US guided needle localization [17]. Unfortunately, we report that exclusive US guidance for performance of interscalene catheter placement did not eliminate the rare complication of PPNP following ISB. Utilizing NS in addition to US guidance would have potentially elicited a diaphragmatic muscular contraction during catheter placement. However, NS has demonstrated low sensitivity for detecting direct needle-to-nerve contact; therefore, NS may not have made a significant difference in this case in preventing PPNP [18]. In addition, relying partially on NS may lead to a greater number of needle passes making the patient more susceptible to potential phrenic nerve trauma [16].

We attempt to add to the body of literature describing the phenomenon of PPNP following ISB. The only previously identified risk factor for PPNP is cervical degenerative disc disease [3]. Our patient was diagnosed with degenerative disc disease following development of postoperative PPNP. Various diagnostic studies including CXR, diaphragm fluoroscopy, spirometry, nerve conduction testing, and electromyography can be used to diagnose phrenic nerve palsy, as well as assessing respiratory improvement during recovery. The long course of the phrenic nerve and slow rate of nerve regeneration may allow for improvement of PPNP up to 24 months after initial injury [19]. Surgical decompression with or without nerve grafting has shown to improve 69% of PPNP cases that did not improve with conservative treatment [20]. The time course for nerve regeneration coincides with this patient's slow resolution of dyspnea over 12 months and supports the case of phrenic nerve disruption with eventual regeneration. Anesthesiologists should be aware of the risk factors that may place patients at a higher likelihood of developing PPNP. Cautious patient selection and close postoperative monitoring should be considered given the significant consequences patients may face from persistent phrenic nerve palsy.

Disclosure

This case report did not receive any specific grant from funding agencies in the public, commercial, or not-for-profit sectors.

References

[1] N. A. Bryan, J. D. Swenson, P. E. Greis, and R. T. Burks, "Indwelling interscalene catheter use in an outpatient setting for shoulder surgery: Technique, efficacy, and complications," *Journal of Shoulder and Elbow Surgery*, vol. 16, no. 4, pp. 388–395, 2007.

[2] W. F. Urmey, K. H. Talts, and N. E. Sharrock, "One hundred percent incidence of hemidiaphragmatic paresis associated with interscalene brachial plexus anesthesia as diagnosed by ultrasonography," *Anesthesia & Analgesia*, vol. 72, no. 4, pp. 498–503, 1991.

[3] S. R. Pakala, J. D. Beckman, S. Lyman, and V. M. Zayas, "Cervical spine disease is a risk factor for persistent phrenic nerve paresis following interscalene nerve block," *Regional Anesthesia and Pain Medicine*, vol. 38, no. 3, pp. 239–242, 2013.

[4] J. G. Antonakakis, B. D. Sites, and J. Shiffrin, "Ultrasound-guided posterior approach for the placement of a continuous interscalene catheter," *Regional Anesthesia and Pain Medicine*, vol. 34, no. 1, pp. 64–68, 2009.

[5] A. G. Prates Júnior, L. C. Vasques, and L. S. Bordoni, "Anatomical variations of the phrenic nerve: An actualized review," *Journal of Morphological Sciences*, vol. 32, no. 1, pp. 53–56, 2015.

[6] E. S. Schwenk, K. Gandhi, J. L. Baratta et al., "Ultrasound-guided out-of-plane vs. in-plane interscalene catheters: A randomized, prospective study," *Anesthesiology and Pain Medicine*, vol. 5, no. 6, Article ID e31111, 2015.

[7] H. Sehmbi and U. J. Shah, "In-plane interscalene block: A word of caution," *Journal of Anaesthesiology Clinical Pharmacology*, vol. 31, no. 1, pp. 129-130, 2015.

[8] P. Gautier, C. Vandepitte, C. Ramquet, M. Decoopman, D. Xu, and A. Hadzic, "The minimum effective anesthetic volume of 0.75% ropivacaine in ultrasound-guided interscalene brachial plexus block," *Anesthesia & Analgesia*, vol. 113, no. 4, pp. 951–955, 2011.

[9] S. S. Liu, V. M. Zayas, M. A. Gordon et al., "A prospective, randomized, controlled trial comparing ultrasound versus nerve stimulator guidance for interscalene block for ambulatory shoulder surgery for postoperative neurological symptoms," *Anesthesia & Analgesia*, vol. 109, no. 1, pp. 265–271, 2009.

[10] K. R. Ediale, C. R. Myung, and G. G. Neuman, "Prolonged hemidiaphragmatic paralysis following interscalene brachial

plexus block," *Journal of Clinical Anesthesia*, vol. 16, no. 8, pp. 573–575, 2004.

[11] S. Deruddre, D. Vidal, and D. Benhamou, "A case of persistent hemidiaphragmatic paralysis following interscalene brachial plexus block," *Journal of Clinical Anesthesia*, vol. 18, no. 3, pp. 238-239, 2006.

[12] T. Dwyer, P. D. G. Henry, P. Cholvisudhi, V. W. S. Chan, J. S. Theodoropoulos, and R. Brull, "Neurological complications related to elective orthopedic surgery: part 1: common shoulder and elbow procedures," *Regional Anesthesia and Pain Medicine*, vol. 40, no. 5, pp. 431–442, 2015.

[13] N. M. Lynch, R. H. Cofield, P. L. Silbert, and R. C. Hermann, "Neurologic complications after total shoulder arthroplasty," *Journal of Shoulder and Elbow Surgery*, vol. 5, no. 1, pp. 53–61, 1996.

[14] P. M. Kane, A. H. Daniels, and E. Akelman, "Double crush syndrome," *Journal of the American Academy of Orthopaedic-Surgeons*, vol. 23, no. 9, pp. 558–562, 2015.

[15] J. M. Neal, M. J. Barrington, R. Brull et al., "The second ASRA practice advisory on neurologic complications associated with regional anesthesia and pain medicine: executive summary 2015," *Regional Anesthesia and Pain Medicine*, vol. 40, no. 5, pp. 401–430, 2015.

[16] S. Choi and C. J. L. McCartney, "Evidence base for the use of ultrasound for upper extremity blocks: 2014 update," *Regional Anesthesia and Pain Medicine*, vol. 41, no. 2, pp. 242–250, 2016.

[17] A. De and J. E. Hayes, "Persistent phrenic nerve paresis after interscalene block a "triple crush" hypothesis of nerve injury," *Regional Anesthesia and Pain Medicine*, vol. 38, no. 6, article 553, 2013.

[18] A. Perlas, A. Niazi, C. McCartney, V. Chan, D. Xu, and S. Abbas, "The sensitivity of motor response to nerve stimulation and paresthesia for nerve localization as evaluated by ultrasound," *Regional Anesthesia and Pain Medicine*, vol. 31, no. 5, pp. 445–450, 2006.

[19] P. G. Wilcox, P. D. Pare, and R. L. Pardy, "Recovery after unilateral phrenic injury associated with coronary artery revascularization," *CHEST*, vol. 98, no. 3, pp. 661–666, 1990.

[20] M. R. Kaufman, A. I. Elkwood, M. I. Rose et al., "Surgical treatment of permanent diaphragm paralysis after interscalene nerve block for shoulder surgery," *Anesthesiology*, vol. 119, no. 2, pp. 484–487, 2013.

57

Airway Management during Thyroidectomy for a Giant Goitre due to McCune-Albright Syndrome

Hiroyuki Nakao (iD)

Department of Emergency and Critical Care Medicine, Hyogo College of Medicine, Hyōgo Prefecture, Japan

Correspondence should be addressed to Hiroyuki Nakao; nakaonakaokobe@yahoo.co.jp

Academic Editor: Kuang-I Cheng

There have been no case reports to date describing the technical aspects of tracheal intubation in a patient with a goitre associated with McCune-Albright syndrome (MAS), even though goitre is frequently observed in this condition. I describe a case of resection of a giant goitre in a patient with MAS, with difficult airway management. Preoperative investigation showed that the trachea was shifted to the right by the goitre, with the narrowest part of the tracheal lumen 4 mm in diameter. There was dome-shaped protuberance of the posterior pharyngeal wall into the airway. The patient had an S-shaped total spine, a short neck, and a relatively large jaw, which interfered with airway visualisation during intubation. Anaesthesia was induced with light sedation and supplemental oxygen. Endotracheal intubation was successfully performed using a fiberoptic laryngoscope and a flexible, spiral-wound, obtuse-tipped tracheal tube.

1. Introduction

General anaesthesia in high-risk patients with anatomical anomalies of airway needs careful airway management, especially in cases undergoing prolonged neck surgery. I describe anaesthesia in a case of McCune-Albright syndrome (MAS) undergoing thyroidectomy. MAS is thought to be due to a point mutation of the GNAS1 gene on chromosome 20q13.2 and is characterised by polyostotic fibrous dysplasia, autonomous endocrine hyperfunction, and abnormal skin pigmentation (café-au-lait spots) [1, 2]. Patients may demonstrate precocious puberty, pathological fractures, bone malformations, pituitary gigantism, Cushing syndrome, or hypophosphatemia. In some cases, hyperplasia of the thyroid gland may compress the trachea [1–3]. However, there are no previous reports of general anaesthesia management in a MAS patient with a giant goitre.

I report a MAS patient with difficult airway management due to giant goitre, craniofacial deformities, extreme spinal deformities, and tracheal displacement and compression.

2. Case Presentation

A 33-year-old male who was diagnosed with MAS suffered from dyspnoea at bedtime for several months and was diagnosed with giant goitre at another clinic.

Physical examination showed a height of 145 cm and weight of 50 kg. He had skeletal abnormalities including craniofacial deformities, short neck, enlarged and greatly deformed thorax, scoliosis, and kyphosis (Figure 1(a)). He was unable to walk without help and could not be with face-up position for an airway obstruction. Patient's ASA physical status was class 3. His range of cervical spine movement was flexion 4° and extension 84° with measurement in his surface of a body. Palpation revealed a huge thyroid gland, but more specific thyroid examination was not possible due to his enlarged thorax and short neck.

Complete blood count, biochemistry, and arterial blood gas tests were normal. Thyroid hormone levels were mildly elevated (fT4 1.62 (0.7–1.48) ng/dl, fT3 3.50 (1.71–3.71) pg/ml, TSH 4.03 (0.35–494) μg/dl, and T4 12.5 (4.87–11.7) μg/dl). Lateral neck X-ray showed a dome-shaped protuberance of the posterior pharyngeal wall. The oral, pharyngeal, and tracheal axes were measured (Figure 2). Preoperative computed tomography (CT) scan showed that the trachea was shifted to the right and compressed by a giant goitre, with a lumen of 4 mm × 14 mm at its narrowest point in the subglottic region. The narrow portion extended over a length of about 20 mm (4 slices at 5 mm width) (Figure 1(b)). The cross-sectional oval area was $2 \times 7 \times 3.14 = 43.96$ mm^2.

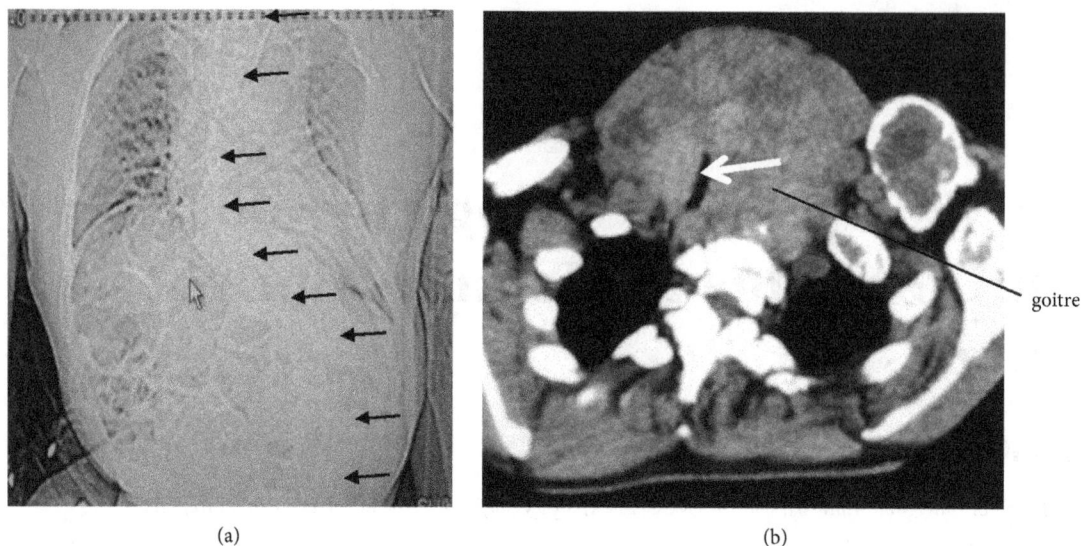

(a)

(b)

FIGURE 1: Preoperative CT scan. (a) Lateral curvature of the spine. (b) Narrowest portion of the trachea was 4 mm in diameter in lying down.

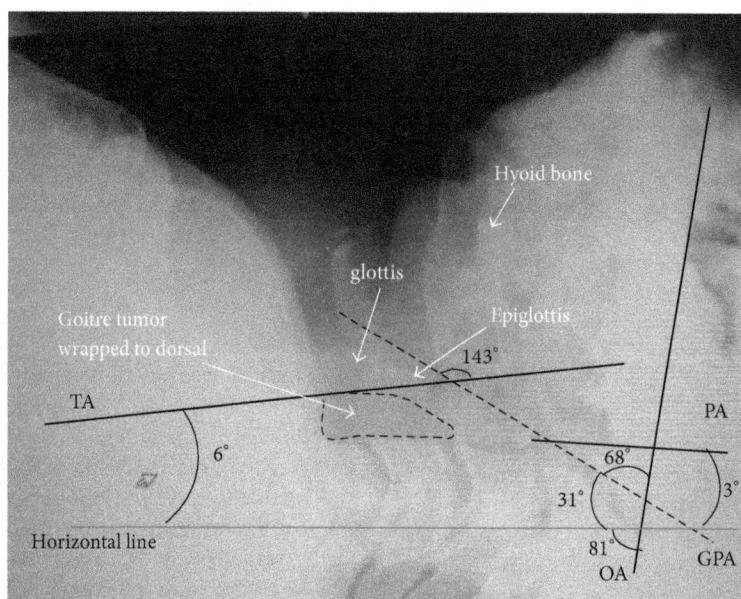

FIGURE 2: Preoperative lateral neck X-ray with the head resting on the bed in a neutral position. X-ray shows short neck with limited extension. The glottis is elevated by the dorsally located goitre. OA: oral axis, PA: pharyngeal axis, TA: tracheal axis, and GPA: glottis- pharyngeal axis.

The cross-sectional orbicular area was $4.35 \times 4.35 \times 3.14 = 59.42\,mm^2$. The goitre had a benign appearance on ultrasonography and I assumed that goiter was softer than malignant tumor. I could anticipate that an endotracheal tube could enlarge a narrow soft tumor. In laryngeal fiberscope of the preoperative examination, I recognized his elevated lesion in the posterior pharyngeal wall and his vocal cord shifted to right side. Total thyroidectomy was scheduled and was expected to take approximately 8 hours.

Intraoperative monitoring included ECG, noninvasive and invasive blood pressure, end-tidal CO_2, bispectral index (BIS), and pulse oximetry. Because this case was predicted to have a difficult intubation, general anaesthesia was cautiously induced with oxygen and fentanyl (0.1 mg of the total dose), and intubation was performed with the patient semiawake. No muscle relaxants were used, and spontaneous ventilation was preserved. The patient was given a sufficient preoperative explanation of semiawake intubation to eliminate anxiety. After the operation, I confirmed that he did not remember the intubation even though the BIS was maintained within the 95–98 range.

Our plans for intubation were (1) attempt intubation with conventional laryngoscopy, (2) attempt intubation with flexible fiberscope laryngoscopy and a variety of endotracheal tubes, and (3) laryngeal mask airway (LMA) for ventilation if the operation was abandoned.

Tracheal Tube: RUSCHELIT

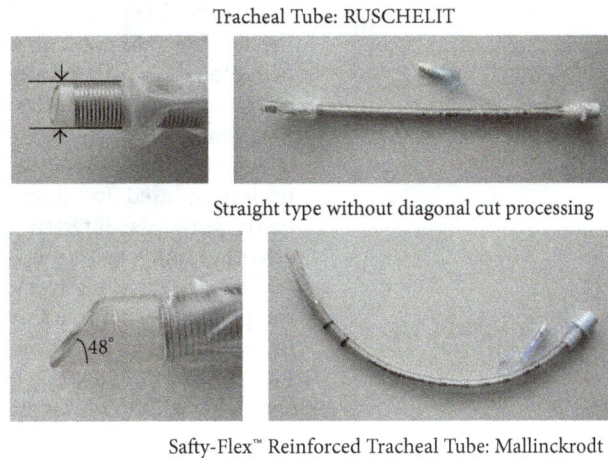

Straight type without diagonal cut processing

Safty-Flex™ Reinforced Tracheal Tube: Mallinckrodt

FIGURE 3: Straight type without diagonal tip. The Rüschelit tube has an obtuse-angled tip; the Safety-Flex Reinforced tube has a slanted tip.

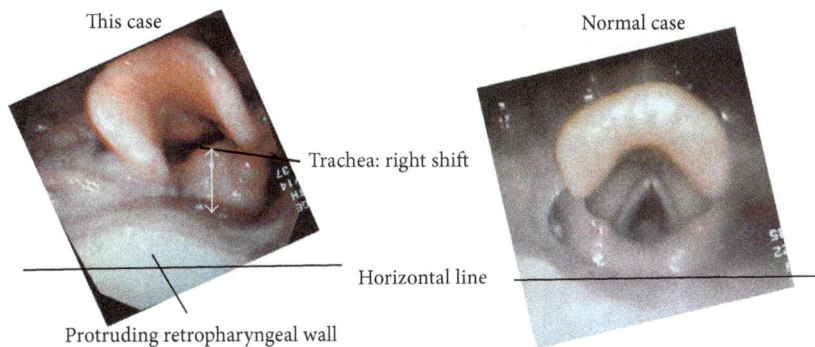

This case

Normal case

Trachea: right shift

Horizontal line

Protruding retropharyngeal wall

FIGURE 4: Preoperative laryngeal fibroscopy showing the trachea shifted to the right, and the posterior pharyngeal wall and glottis were pushed forward.

LMA is not used in thyroidectomy at the thyroid position that the neck is greatly extended increasing the space between the clavicles and the jaws for his giant goiter, or with risk of bilateral recurrent nerve paralysis on operating. The operation cannot be carried out if plans 1 and 2 did not succeed. Plan 3 was prepared for his safety based on ASA difficult ventilation guideline until he wakes up.

Oral intubation could not be accomplished using a conventional laryngoscope (Macintosh curved blade) as it was impossible to elevate the protruded epiglottis (Cormack and Lehane Grade 3). It was very difficult to identify intraoral structures by fiberscope. I chose a fiberscope for high torque capability (Olynpus laryngofiberscope ENF-V2: OD 3.2 mm, Up/Down 130°/130°). I attempted nasotracheal fiberoptic intubation with a standard endotracheal tube (Lo-counter™ Muphy Tracheal Tube Mallinckrodt, 5.5 mm internal diameter (ID)) and a spiral-wound tube (Safety-Flex™ Reinforced Tracheal Tube Mallinckrodt, 5.5 mm ID) (Figure 3). Both tubes have angled tips. Even though I were able to introduce the fiberscope into the trachea, I were unable to perform tracheal intubation as I could not pass the tip of the endotracheal tube beyond the arytenoids (Figure 4).

I proceeded to orotracheal intubation with fiberoptic laryngoscopy and a spiral-wound tube (Rüschelit Tracheal Tube, 5.5 mm ID) with an obtuse-angled tip (Figure 3). This method allowed us to successfully perform intubation without being blocked by the arytenoids. The slight rightwards shifts of the trachea by the goitre did not increase the difficulty of intubation using the fiberoptic laryngoscope. The tumour was soft and permitted easy placement of the tracheal tube. The total anaesthetic time was 8 hours 32 minutes, with 33 minutes' tracheal intubation from induction of anaesthesia and 6-hour 49-minute operation (Figure 5). I did not extubate the patient immediately after the operation because of the risk of postoperative oedema of the glottis and neck. Examination by fibroscopy showed intact recurrent laryngeal nerve function. Extubation the following day was uneventful. The extirpated tumour weighed 515 g and measured 15 cm × 13 cm (Figure 6).

3. Discussion

Mastorakos and colleagues reported that goitre is observed in 71.4% of MAS cases [1]. The combination of goitre and skeletal malformations in MAS requires special attention to securing the airway during general anaesthesia [4, 5]. However, there are no previous reports describing general anaesthesia in an MAS patient undergoing thyroidectomy for

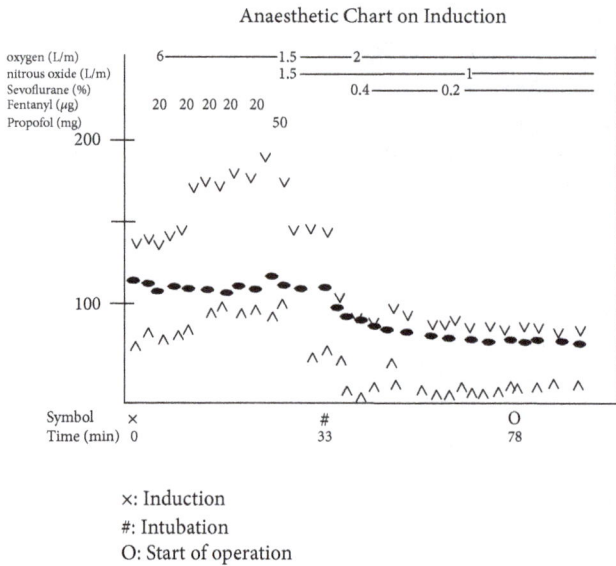

Anaesthetic Chart on Induction

FIGURE 5: Anaesthetic chart of patient undergoing thyroidectomy. ×: induction, #: intubation, and O: start of operation.

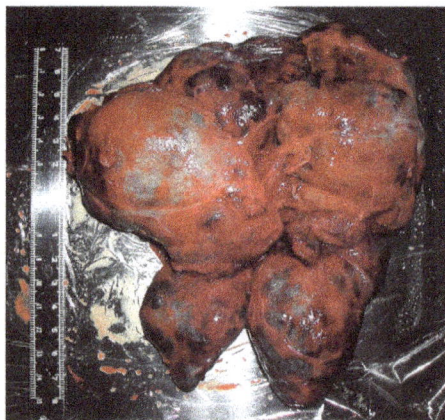

FIGURE 6: The extirpated tumour (515 g, 15 cm × 13 cm).

a giant goitre. Bouaggad and colleagues reported that difficult tracheal intubation was likely in thyroid surgery cases with thyroid cancer, tracheal compression, or dyspnea [6]. This case demonstrates that a goitre which extends dorsally also causes difficult tracheal intubation because of elevation of the glottis. Careful preoperative evaluation by CT scan is therefore important in cases of giant goitre.

Short neck, obesity, round back, limited neck extension, enlarged thorax which encroaches on the face, abnormal facial structure, tracheal deviation, and tracheal compression may all contribute to technical difficulties with intubation in patients with MAS. All of these except for obesity were present in this case. Preoperative assessment included neck CT scan, neck X-rays, and fiberoptic laryngoscopy to check the entire length of the trachea. As a result, it was expected that technical intubation difficulties might be encountered and I undertook preoperative planning to secure the airway [7, 8]. The difficult airway algorithm of the American Society

of Anesthesiologists (ASA) suggests the use of mask anaesthesia, laryngeal mask airway anaesthesia, local anaesthesia, or regional anaesthesia not requiring tracheal intubation in cases with technical intubation difficulties [9]. However, in a patient with a giant goitre, tracheal intubation is essential to secure the airway during a prolonged procedure with the neck retroflexed. In this case, the remarkably large size of the goitre would also interfere with the ability to perform prompt cricothyrotomy or tracheostomy.

When severe malformation of the face is present as in the present case, the use of a muscle relaxant may increase the difficulty of airway management due to relaxation of the muscles in the oral cavity [10, 11]. I also hoped that spontaneous respiration might help to localize the vocal cords due to air currents moving the saliva.

And novel video assisted device can observe the epiglottis and is useful for an expected intubation difficulty [12, 13]. These devices may fast observe his epiglottis in this case too. However, the trachea tube must get over the tumor around his glottides because a tumor piled up the glottides to a ventral from the dorsal. Therefore, as for Reinforce Tracheal Spiral Tube that the tip was cut keenly, the tube cut surface touched the trachea ventral wall, and the tube could no longer advance.

It is important to consider the oral, pharyngeal, and tracheal axes during endotracheal intubation. Bannister and Macbeth reported that alignment of these three axes is important for successful intubation [14]. In this case, the goitre pushed the glottis ventrally, and I had to consider four axes during intubation: the oral axis which was 81° to the horizontal on X-ray at maximum retroflexion, the pharyngeal axis (3°), the tracheal (6°), and the glottic-pharyngeal axis (31°) (Figure 1). The endotracheal tube therefore had to be passed around the protrusion caused by the tumour.

Horton and colleagues reported the "ideal angles" for upper cervical flexion and lower cervical extension as 15° and 35°, respectively, which they determined by reviewing various values from previous research [15]. The upper cervical flexion angle of 4° in this case indicated restricted mouth opening, and the lower cervical extension angle of 84° indicated restricted neck extension.

I attempted to intubate with the patient's head elevated on a pad and his neck extended but was unable to align the axes due to his large jaw, short and inflexible neck, abnormally shaped thorax, and kyphosis. The fiberscope had to follow an S-shaped path with a 68° angle followed by a 143° angle, and the endotracheal tube then followed the path of the fiberscope. Successful intubation was helped by the pliability of the endotracheal tube and the shape of the tip which eventually enabled it to pass through the glottis.

Some researchers have reported on a variety of tracheal tubes with their tips designed especially for fiberoptic intubation of difficult airways [16–19]. Among them, the Rüschelit tracheal tube is flexible enough to follow the path of a laryngeal fiberscope and is able to get past protrusion in the subglottis because of the obtuse-angled tip (Figure 4) [20].

In general, the difficulty of tracheal intubation in cases with thyroid disease is affected by compression of the trachea and the position and hardness of the tumour [21, 22]. In this case, the position of the tumour posterior to the trachea increased the difficulty of intubation. However, the soft texture of the tumour made it easy to pass the tube through the narrowed part of the trachea.

In the present case with MAS complicated by giant goitre and skeletal malformations, successful intubation was achieved with detailed assessment, careful induction, and appropriate selection of endotracheal tube. The most useful tool in achieving this difficult intubation case was the fiberoptic laryngoscope which helped to identify the glottis.

References

[1] G. Mastorakos, N. S. Mitsiades, A. G. Doufas, and D. A. Koutras, "Hyperthyroidism in McCune-Albright syndrome with a review of thyroid abnormalities sixty years after the first report," *Thyroid*, vol. 7, no. 3, pp. 433–439, 1997.

[2] M. T. Collins, N. J. Sarlis, M. J. Merino et al., "Thyroid carcinoma in the McCune-Albright syndrome: Contributory role of activating Gsα mutations," *The Journal of Clinical Endocrinology & Metabolism*, vol. 88, no. 9, pp. 4413–4417, 2003.

[3] R. A. Langer, I. Yook, and L. M. Capan, "Anesthetic considerations in McCune-Albright syndrome: Case report with literature review," *Anesthesia & Analgesia*, vol. 80, no. 6, pp. 1236–1239, 1995.

[4] H. Ayabe, K. Kawahara, Y. Tagawa, and M. Tomita, "Upper airway obstruction from a benign goiter," *Surgery Today*, vol. 22, no. 1, pp. 88–90, 1992.

[5] T. O'Donnell, M. Karetzky, D. K. Brief, J. Nahmias, and R. Jhaveri, "Treatment of upper airway obstruction associated with goiter," *New Jersey Medicine*, vol. 90, pp. 450–456, 1993.

[6] A. Bouaggad, S. E. Nejmi, M. A. Bouderka, and O. Abbassi, "Prediction of difficult tracheal intubation in thyroid surgery," *Anesthesia & Analgesia*, vol. 99, no. 2, pp. 603–606, 2004.

[7] D. K. Rose and M. M. Cohen, "The airway: problems and predictions in 18,500 patients," *Canadian Journal of Anesthesia*, vol. 41, no. 5, pp. 372–383, 1994.

[8] M. F. Rozen, *Anesthetic Implications of Concurrent Diseases*, Curchill Livingstone, New York, NY, USA, 3rd edition, 1990.

[9] J. L. Apfelbaum, C. A. Hagberg, R. A. Caplan et al., "Practice guidelines for management of the difficult airway: an updated report by the American Society of Anesthesiologists Task Force on Management of the Difficult Airway," *Anesthesiology*, vol. 118, no. 2, pp. 251–270, 2013.

[10] D. Sharma, P. K. Bithal, G. P. Rath, and M. P. Pandia, "Effect of orientation of a standard polyvinyl chloride tracheal tube on success rates during awake flexible fibreoptic intubation," *Anaesthesia*, vol. 61, no. 9, pp. 845–848, 2006.

[11] D. M. Johnson, A. M. From, R. B. Smith, R. P. From, and M. A. Maktabi, "Endoscopic study of mechanisms of failure of endotracheal tube advancement into the trachea during awake fiberoptic orotracheal intubation," *Anesthesiology*, vol. 102, no. 5, pp. 910–914, 2005.

[12] P.-Y. Chang, P.-Y. Hu, Y.-C. Lin et al., "Trachway video intubating stylet allows for optimization of electromyographic endotracheal tube placement for monitored thyroidectomy," *Gland Surgery*, vol. 6, no. 5, pp. 464–468, 2017.

[13] K.-Y. Tseng, S.-W. Chau, M.-P. Su, C.-K. Shih, I.-C. Lu, and K.-I. Cheng, "A comparison of Trachway intubating stylet and Airway Scope for tracheal intubation by novice operators: A manikin study," *Kaohsiung Journal of Medical Sciences*, vol. 28, no. 8, pp. 448–451, 2012.

[14] F. Bannister and R. Macbeth, "Direct laryngoscopy and tracheal intubation," *The Lancet*, vol. 244, no. 6325, pp. 651–654, 1944.

[15] W. A. Horton, L. Fahy, and P. Charters, "Defining a standard intubating position using 'angle finder'," *British Journal of Anaesthesia*, vol. 62, no. 1, pp. 6–12, 1989.

[16] J. R. Greer, S. P. Smith, and T. Strang, "A comparison of tracheal tube tip designs on the passage of an endotracheal tube during oral fiberoptic intubation," *Anesthesiology*, vol. 94, no. 5, pp. 729–731, 2001.

[17] M. S. Kristensen, "The Parker Flex-Tip tube versus a standard tube for fiberoptic orotracheal intubation: A randomized double-blind study," *Anesthesiology*, vol. 98, no. 2, pp. 354–358, 2003.

[18] K. F. Barker, P. Bolton, S. Cole, and P. A. Coe, "Ease of laryngeal passage during fibreoptic intubation: A comparison of three endotracheal tubes," *Acta Anaesthesiologica Scandinavica*, vol. 45, no. 5, pp. 624–626, 2001.

[19] H. E. Jones, A. C. Pearce, and P. Moore, "Fibreoptic intubation: Influence of tracheal tube tip design," *Anaesthesia*, vol. 48, no. 8, pp. 672–674, 1993.

[20] P. Hakala, T. Randell, and H. Valli, "Comparison between tracheal tubes for orotracheal fibreoptic intubation," *British Journal of Anaesthesia*, vol. 82, no. 1, pp. 135–136, 1999.

[21] I. K. Kolawole and G. A. Rahman, "Emergency thyroidectomy in a patient with severe upper airway obstruction caused by goiter: Case for regional anesthesia," *Journal of the National Medical Association*, vol. 98, no. 1, pp. 86–89, 2006.

[22] T. Krishan Thusoo, U. Gupta, K. Kochhar, and H. Singh Hira, "Upper airway obstruction in patients with goiter studied by flow volume loops and effect of thyroidectomy," *World Journal of Surgery*, vol. 24, no. 12, pp. 1570–1572, 2000.

58

Unexpected Exacerbation of Tracheal Stenosis in a Patient with Hunter Syndrome Undergoing Cardiac Surgery

Nobue Terabe,[1] **Soichiro Yamashita ⓘ,**[2] **and Makoto Tanaka**[2]

[1]*Department of Anesthesiology, University of Tsukuba Hospital, Tsukuba, Japan*
[2]*Department of Anesthesiology, Faculty of Medicine, University of Tsukuba, Tsukuba, Japan*

Correspondence should be addressed to Soichiro Yamashita; soichi2003@aol.com

Academic Editor: Pavel Michalek

We report unexpected exacerbation of tracheal stenosis during general anesthesia in a 50-year-old patient with Hunter syndrome undergoing cardiac surgery for valvular disease. He had undergone cervical laminoplasty 3 months previously; at that time, his airway had been uneventfully managed. Preoperative flexible fiberoptic laryngoscopy showed a normal upper respiratory tract, but chest computed tomography showed tracheal stenosis that had flattened the lumen. The narrowest part above the tracheal bifurcation was 2 cm long and the anteroposterior diameter was ≤6 mm. Cardiac surgery was uneventfully performed. After weaning from cardiopulmonary bypass, the tidal volume suddenly decreased from 450 to 120 ml at sternal closure. The end-expiratory carbon dioxide pressure increased from 39 to 71 mmHg. Bronchoscopic examination showed that the part of tracheal bifurcation was almost occluded. A tidal volume of 400 ml was obtained after the transesophageal echocardiography probe was removed and the peak inspiratory pressure increased. Although extubation was performed on the second postoperative day, procaterol inhalation and noninvasive positive-pressure ventilation were needed for 3 days because of wheezing and dyspnea. In conclusion, the risk of lower respiratory tract obstruction should be considered during general anesthesia in patients with Hunter syndrome with collapsible tracheal stenosis undergoing cardiac surgery.

1. Introduction

Hunter syndrome is characterized by a deficiency of the iduronate-2-sulfatase required for mucopolysaccharide degradation [1]. Various complications should be considered in patients with Hunter syndrome undergoing surgery because intracellular accumulation of glycosaminoglycans (GAGs) causes progressive damage to various organs and tissues [2, 3]. We herein report unexpected exacerbations of tracheal stenosis during general anesthesia in an adult patient with Hunter syndrome undergoing cardiac surgery and discuss some problems derived from pathological changes in the lower respiratory tract. Written informed consent was obtained from the patient for publication of this case report and accompanying images.

2. Case Presentation

A 50-year-old, 50-kg, 152-cm man with aortic and mitral valvular disease was scheduled for a double valve replacement. He had been diagnosed with Hunter syndrome at the age of 40 years and had received enzyme replacement therapy with idursulfase infusion. He had undergone general anesthesia 3 months previously for cervical laminoplasty at another hospital, and his airway had been managed uneventfully at that time with a reinforced tracheal tube of 7-mm inner diameter (ID). He showed the distinctive features of a short neck, jaw deformation, and macroglossia, and he had slight cervical motor restriction and a Mallampati classification of III. Preoperative flexible fiberoptic laryngoscopy 2 week previously showed that the patency of the upper respiratory tract was kept though oropharyngeal soft tissue thickening was recognized. However, chest computed tomography (CT) 1.5 months previously showed tracheal stenosis that had flattened the lumen (Figure 1). The narrowest part above the tracheal bifurcation was 2 cm long and the anteroposterior diameter was ≤6 mm, but the patency of the upper part of the trachea was adequate for insertion of a tracheal tube of 7-mm ID. Cardiac ultrasound demonstrated severe aortic valve stenosis, moderate aortic valve regurgitation, and mild mitral valve regurgitation. The aortic valve area was 0.53 cm². The

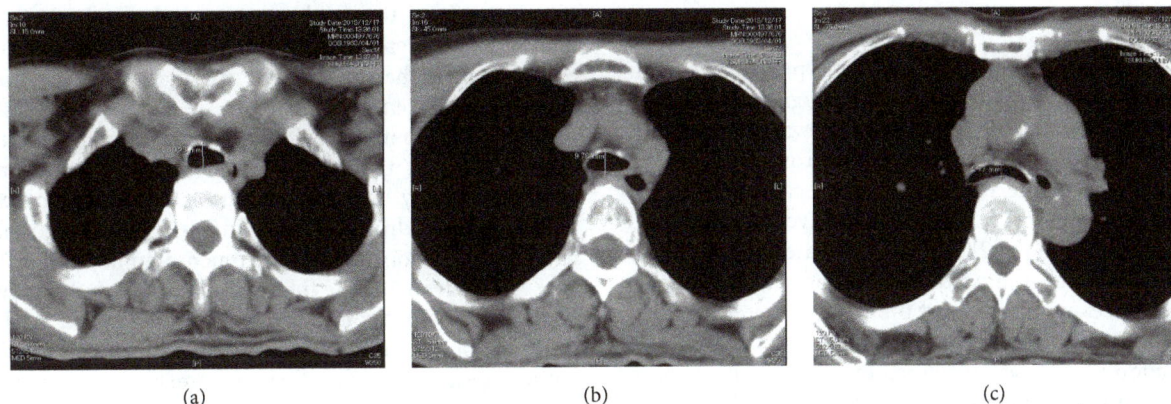

(a)   (b)   (c)

FIGURE 1: Chest computed tomography 1.5 months previously. (a) The anteroposterior diameter of the trachea at 3 cm away from the glottis was 10.3 mm. (b) The anteroposterior diameter of the trachea at 6 cm away from the glottis was 9.8 mm. (c) The anteroposterior diameter of the tracheal bifurcation at 9 cm away from the glottis was 5.8 mm.

maximum and mean aortic valve pressure gradients were 106 and 67 mmHg, respectively. The left ventricle was generally enlarged and the ejection fraction was 71% (Simpson's method). Abdominal CT showed hepatosplenomegaly. All blood parameters were within the normal ranges. During a preoperative conference, we assessed that his airway could be managed in the same way as during the previous anesthetic procedure because the patient had not felt difficulty in breathing.

At the time of admission, his blood pressure was 139/47 mmHg, heart rate was 65 beats/min, and peripheral oxygen saturation was 97%. After cannulation to the left radial artery for continuous monitoring of arterial blood pressure, 3 mg of midazolam and 200 μg of fentanyl were administered for induction of anesthesia. After confirming mask ventilation, 60 mg of rocuronium bromide was provided for neuromuscular blockade. The glottis was easily confirmed using the Airway Scope (Pentax-AWS®; Hoya, Tokyo, Japan), and a tracheal tube of 7-mm ID was inserted into the trachea. However, the tube could not be advanced more than 3 cm from the glottis. The tube was removed. The upper airway was then secured using an i-gel #4 (Nihon Kohden, Tokyo, Japan), and bronchoscopic examination was performed through the breathing channel of the i-gel. Tracheal stenosis that gradually became more severe from under the glottis was revealed (Figure 2). Therefore, a tracheal tube of 6-mm ID was inserted using the Airway Scope. We felt slight resistance during insertion of the tube, but an audible leak around the tube with an inspiratory pressure of 20 cmH$_2$O was heard when the cuff was deflated. The tube was secured at the 22-cm mark at the alveolar ridge. Pressure-controlled ventilation was started with a peak inspiratory pressure of 20 cmH$_2$O and a respiratory rate of 12 breaths/min, and a tidal volume of about 450 ml was obtained. Although a transesophageal echocardiography (TEE) probe was inserted, the tidal volume did not change.

The aortic and mitral valve replacement was uneventfully performed under cardiopulmonary bypass. After aortic declamping, the patient was easily weaned from cardiopulmonary bypass with a 5-μg/kg/min dopamine infusion.

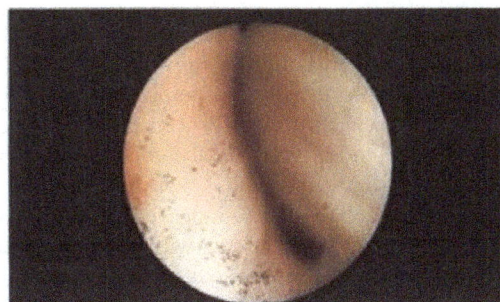

FIGURE 2: Bronchoscopy after induction of anesthesia revealed tracheal stenosis that gradually became more severe from under the glottis.

Cardiac function after weaning was good. However, the tidal volume suddenly decreased from 450 to 120 ml at sternal closure, and the end-expiratory carbon dioxide pressure increased from 39 to 71 mmHg. Bronchoscopic examination showed that the stenosis became more severe than that after induction of anesthesia, and the part of the tracheal bifurcation was almost occluded. The tidal volume was hardly obtained in spite of a peak inspiratory pressure of >30 cmH$_2$O. Therefore, we tried to remove the TEE probe because it might have been exacerbating the tracheal stenosis by pushing the trachea adjacent to the esophagus. As a result, a tidal volume of 400 ml was obtained with a peak inspiratory pressure of 25 cmH$_2$O by improving the severe stenosis of the tracheal bifurcation, and the end-expiratory carbon dioxide pressure decreased to 43 mmHg. In addition, 125 mg of methylprednisolone was administered intravenously to reduce edema in the lower respiratory tract. Extubation was performed on the second postoperative day. After extubation, the patient's oxygenation was good but wheezing and dyspnea were noted. Procaterol inhalation and noninvasive positive-pressure ventilation were administered for 3 days. After his breathing had become stable, the patient was discharged from the hospital on the 25th postoperative day.

3. Discussion

Intracellular accumulation of GAGs causes progressive damage to various organs and tissues. Although the extent of organ damage and disease progression are variable, approximately 75% of patients with Hunter syndrome are severely affected and die in the first or second decade of life. The remaining patients have normal cognitive function and survive into adulthood [2]. Valvular disease is frequent in patients with Hunter syndrome but cardiac surgery remains uncommon because of the short lifespan of severely affected patients [4–6]. However, various complications due to GAGs accumulation should be considered in patients with Hunter syndrome undergoing cardiac surgery [2, 3]. In the present case, we encountered unexpected exacerbation of tracheal stenosis at sternal closure after weaning from cardiopulmonary bypass. This critical episode highlights the risk of lower respiratory tract obstruction during general anesthesia in patients with Hunter syndrome undergoing cardiac surgery.

Accumulation of GAGs in the lower respiratory tract causes softening and weakness of the supporting cartilage, resulting in tracheobronchial stenosis and malacia [7]. In the present case, the trachea had already been affected by malacia because tracheal stenosis that had flattened the lumen was observed on the preoperative CT. In such a condition, the trachea might be collapsed by increased intramediastinal pressure at sternal closure. Patients with Hunter syndrome have several factors which might contribute to the lower respiratory tract obstruction caused by this mechanism. Myocardial edema and increased intraventricular filling pressure due to volume load after cardiopulmonary bypass might increase the intramediastinal pressure because the hypertrophic myocardium had been already occupying the intramediastinal space [8]. Stiffness of the chest wall and reduced thoracic volume due to hepatosplenomegaly might also enhance the intramediastinal pressure [2, 3]. In addition, mucosal edema related to systemic inflammation due to cardiopulmonary bypass might contribute to exacerbation of the tracheal stenosis because of mucosal thickening [2, 9]. Increased sputum production due to reduced mucociliary clearance might increase the airway resistance [10]. Moreover, TEE probe might also contribute to exacerbation of the tracheal stenosis by pushing the collapsible trachea [11]. Therefore, we must consider that patients with Hunter syndrome with collapsible tracheal stenosis have the risk of lower respiratory tract obstruction during cardiac surgery. Checking the change in airway diameter during respiration in dynamic chest CT may be useful to predict the collapsibility of the tracheobronchial wall [10].

On the other hand, a tracheal tube of the same size as that used during general anesthesia only 3 months previously could not be advanced more than 3 cm from the glottis after induction of anesthesia. Although the patency of the upper part of the trachea was still adequate for insertion of a tracheal tube of 7-mm ID based on the preoperative CT performed 1.5 months previously, the tracheal stenosis gradually progressed. Increased intramediastinal pressure by cardiac dilation due to valvular disease might contribute to

exacerbation of the tracheal stenosis because the trachea had already been affected by malacia. Another possible explanation is that mechanical stimulation by the tracheal tube that had been used during the recent general anesthetic procedure 3 months previously might have contributed to exacerbation of the tracheal stenosis. A previous report showed that any instrumentation of the airway in patients with Hunter syndrome might induce increased mucopolysaccharide deposition and that the mucosal injury and ischemia caused by advancing the tube or inflating the cuff might lead to disease progression [12]. However, the speed of disease progression is definitively unknown. In the review article, the authors describe the fact that the interval between multiple planned surgical procedures should be sufficiently short because of the progressive nature of Hunter syndrome [2]. Therefore, the possibility of disease progression in the lower respiratory tract should be considered even if the airway was uneventfully managed during a recent general anesthetic procedure in patients with Hunter syndrome, and a smaller tracheal tube should be selected.

The anesthetic management of patients with tracheal stenosis is one of the most clinical challenges for the anesthesiologist [13, 14]. If patients have critical airway obstruction, maintenance of spontaneous ventilation is theoretically important as conversion to positive-pressure ventilation can lead to an aggravation of the obstruction or complete airway collapse. In those patients, an inhalational anesthetic agent (sevoflurane) which maintains spontaneous ventilation is preferred over intravenous anesthetic agents for induction of anesthesia. Otherwise, an awake intubation under sedation or rapid induction with using an extracorporeal membrane oxygenator can be selected according to the risk of airway collapse [3]. In the present case, a conventional rapid induction was performed because the patient had not felt difficulty in breathing. A muscle relaxant was administrated after checking whether a trachea stenosis was worsened by a cessation of the spontaneous ventilation.

I-gel is designed for airway maintenance during general anesthesia and is also useful as a rescue device in unpredicted difficult airway [15]. The conduit of i-gel facilitates the fiberoptic examination of the vocal cord and trachea while improving oxygenation by intermittent ventilation and reducing our stress associated with difficult airway situations. Because wide bore of the conduit allows passage of a tracheal tube, fiberoptic-guided tracheal intubation is possible if necessary.

Various anesthetic risks other than tracheobronchial stenosis and malacia should also be considered during general anesthesia in patients with Hunter syndrome [2, 3]. GAGs accumulations in the mucosa and soft tissues of the upper respiratory tract cause enlargement of the larynx, tonsils, adenoids, and tongue, leading to a difficult airway or obstruction during general anesthesia [16, 17]. Spinal cord compression may occur due to spinal canal narrowing. A short neck and reduced cervical joint mobility also contribute to a difficult airway. Restrictive pulmonary disease can develop due to thoracic-cage abnormalities or compromised excursion of the diaphragm secondary to an enlarged liver and spleen. Cardiac risks other than valvular disease include diastolic dysfunction from the hypertrophied myocardium, or complete atrioventricular block.

4. Conclusion

Patients with Hunter syndrome with collapsible tracheal stenosis have the risk of lower respiratory tract obstruction during cardiac surgery. Careful airway evaluation and management are required while considering the pathological changes of the lower respiratory tract in patients with Hunter syndrome undergoing cardiac surgery.

Acknowledgments

The authors thank Angela Morben, DVM, ELS, from Edanz Group (https://www.edanzediting.com/ac) for editing a draft of this manuscript.

References

[1] M. Scarpa, "Mucopolysaccharidosis type II," in *GeneReviews*, R. A. Pagon, M. P. Adam, H. H. Ardinger, S. E. Wallace, A. Amemiya, and L. J. H. Bean, Eds., University of Washington, 2007.

[2] J. Muenzer, M. Beck, C. M. Eng et al., "Multidisciplinary management of Hunter syndrome," *Pediatrics*, vol. 124, no. 6, pp. e1228–e1239, 2009.

[3] R. Walker, K. G. Belani, E. A. Braunlin et al., "Anaesthesia and airway management in mucopolysaccharidosis," *Journal of Inherited Metabolic Disease*, vol. 36, no. 2, pp. 211–219, 2013.

[4] E. A. Braunlin, P. R. Harmatz, M. Scarpa et al., "Cardiac disease in patients with mucopolysaccharidosis: presentation, diagnosis and management," *Journal of Inherited Metabolic Disease*, vol. 34, no. 6, pp. 1183–1197, 2011.

[5] K. Bhattacharya, S. C. Gibson, and V. L. Pathi, "Mitral valve replacement for mitral stenosis secondary to Hunter's syndrome," *The Annals of Thoracic Surgery*, vol. 80, no. 5, pp. 1911-1912, 2005.

[6] S. H. Lee, J. Kim, J. H. Choi, K. W. Yun, C. B. Sohn, and D. C. Han, "Severe mitral stenosis to Hunter's syndrome," *Circulation*, vol. 128, pp. 1269-1270, 2013.

[7] J. M. Morehead and D. S. Parsons, "Tracheobronchomalacia in Hunter's syndrome," *International Journal of Pediatric Otorhino-laryngology*, vol. 26, no. 3, pp. 255–261, 1993.

[8] C. A. Mestres, J. L. Pomar, M. Acosta et al., "Delayed sternal closure for life-threatening complications in cardiac operations: An update," *The Annals of Thoracic Surgery*, vol. 51, no. 5, pp. 773–776, 1991.

[9] R. Sánchez-Véliz, M. J. Carmona, D. A. Otsuki et al., "Impact of cardiopulmonary bypass on respiratory mucociliary function in an experimental porcine model," *PLoS ONE*, vol. 10, no. 8, Article ID e0135564, 2015.

[10] M. Rutten, P. Ciet, R. Van Den Biggelaar et al., "Severe tracheal and bronchial collapse in adults with type II mucopolysaccharidosis," *Orphanet Journal of Rare Diseases*, vol. 11, article 50, 2016.

[11] T. B. Gilbert, F. G. Panico, W. A. McGill, G. R. Martin, D. G. Halley, and J. E. Sell, "Bronchial obstruction by transesophageal echocardiography probe in a pediatric cardiac patient," *Anesthesia & Analgesia*, vol. 74, no. 1, pp. 156–158, 1992.

[12] H. Steven Sims and J. J. Kempiners, "Special airway concerns in patients with mucopolysaccharidoses," *Respiratory Medicine*, vol. 101, no. 8, pp. 1779–1782, 2007.

[13] I. A. Hobai, S. V. Chhangani, and P. H. Alfille, "Anesthesia for Tracheal Resection and Reconstruction," *Anesthesiology Clinics*, vol. 30, no. 4, pp. 709–730, 2012.

[14] S. Ahuja, B. Cohen, J. Hinkelbein, P. Diemunsch, and K. Ruetzler, "Practical anesthetic considerations in patients undergoing tracheobronchial surgeries: A clinical review of current literature," *Journal of Thoracic Disease*, vol. 8, no. 11, pp. 3431–3441, 2016.

[15] P. Michalek, P. Hodgkinson, and W. Donaldson, "Fiberoptic intubation through an I-Gel supraglottic airway in two patients with predicted difficult airway and intellectual disability," *Anesthesia & Analgesia*, vol. 106, no. 5, pp. 1501–1504, 2008.

[16] P. Busoni and G. Fognani, "Failure of the laryngeal mask to secure the airway in a patient with Hunter's syndrome (mucopolysaccharidosis type II)," *Pediatric Anesthesia*, vol. 9, no. 2, pp. 153–155, 1999.

[17] R. W. M. Walker, V. Colovic, D. N. Robinson, and O. R. Dearlove, "Postobstructive pulmonary oedema during anaesthesia in children with mucopolysaccharidoses," *Pediatric Anesthesia*, vol. 13, no. 5, pp. 441–447, 2003.

59

Anesthetic Considerations in a Patient with Myotonic Dystrophy for Hip Labral Repair

Ramon Go, David Wang, and Danielle Ludwin

Department of Anesthesiology, New York-Presbyterian, Columbia University Medical Center, New York, NY, USA

Correspondence should be addressed to Ramon Go; rvg002@gmail.com

Academic Editor: Jian-jun Yang

Myotonic Dystrophy (DM) affects multiple organ systems. Disorders such as hyperthyroidism, progressive musculoskeletal weakness, cardiac dysrhythmias, hypoventilation, and cognitive-behavioral disorders may be present in these patients. Thorough preoperative assessment and anesthetic planning are required to minimize the risk of anesthetic complications. Patients with DM can exhibit exquisite sensitivity to sedatives, neuromuscular blocking agents, and volatile anesthetics, resulting in potential postoperative complications. There is limited literature available on successful anesthetic techniques for the DM patient. We present this case report to add to our current fund of knowledge.

1. Introduction

Myotonic muscular dystrophy (dystrophia myotonica) (DM) is a rare musculoskeletal disease with a prevalence of 1 in 8,000 [1]. This genetic disease requires significant considerations for patients in the perioperative period. Here we discuss the case of a patient with DM for labral hip repair and review the literature on the management and anesthetic concerns of DM.

2. Case Report

Our patient is a 58-year-old Caucasian man weighing 92.9 kg, 175 cm tall, with a history of type 1 DM who presented for repair of a hip labral tear. His past medical history was significant for obstructive sleep apnea (OSA), gastroesophageal reflux disease, bicuspid aortic valve, bipolar disorder, obsessive-compulsive disorder, and cataracts. His only prior anesthetic exposure was for cataract surgery and he had no complications. However, the patient's daughter, who also had DM, experienced severe respiratory depression following general anesthesia, requiring intensive care unit (ICU) admission postoperatively. Primary considerations in relation to anesthesia include the disease's association with cardiomyopathy and cardiac conduction abnormalities, sensitivity to respiratory depression and ventilatory weakness,

prolonged gastric emptying, and myoclonus triggered by stimuli such as hypothermia and specific medications.

Following the application of standard ASA monitors, a combined spinal and epidural anesthetic technique was performed successfully. Fifteen mg of isobaric bupivacaine was injected into the subarachnoid space at the L4-L5 interspace and an epidural catheter was inserted immediately. The spinal level was tested and found to be at a T10 dermatomal level. External pacer/defibrillator pads were applied and an arterial line was used for continuous blood pressure monitoring and to facilitate arterial blood gas measurements in the event of pulmonary compromise. A thermometer was placed in the patient's axilla for continuous monitoring. The operating room's ambient temperature was increased, a forced-air warming blanket was applied to the patient, and a fluid warmer was connected to his intravenous line. Intraoperatively, the patient received small (0.5 to 1 mg) boluses of midazolam titrated for a Richmond Agitation-Sedation Scale (RASS) of −3. For the 3 hour and 43 minute procedure, the patient received a total of 10 mg of midazolam and 50 mcg of fentanyl. Forty-five minutes into the surgical procedure the surgeon requested further relaxation of the patient's hip muscles and the epidural catheter was subsequently bolused with 5 mL of 2% lidocaine. Two hours into the procedure, another 5 mL of 2% lidocaine was bolused into the epidural.

No complications were noted in the intraoperative period. The patient was transported to the postanesthesia care unit (PACU) with continuous SpO_2, ECG, and blood pressure monitoring. A written consent was obtained from the patient for this case report.

3. Discussion

Two genes have been identified as playing a role in the development of DM. A CTG expansion in *DMPK* gene results in type 1 (DM1), while an expansion in the ZNF gene results in type 2 (DM2) [1, 2]. Although the functions of these genes are unknown, the CTG expansion of either gene results in faulty communication within the cell. The severity of the disease appears to correlate with the expansion repeats. DM affects multiple organ systems and patients may present with different symptomatology (see Table 1). A thorough assessment of the patient is critical to successful perioperative management (see Table 2). Poor preoperative assessment or undiagnosed DM in a surgical patient can lead to morbidity and mortality in the perioperative period.

4. Central Nervous System and Behavioral

DM is associated with cognitive impairment, anxiety, and bipolar disorder which may limit perioperative cooperation and preparation [1]. Patients commonly demonstrate hypersomnia or excessive daytime somnolence independent of neuromuscular respiratory compromise [3]. Together, these CNS effects increase sensitivity to sedatives, anxiolytics, and analgesics that put the patient at high risk for compromised ventilatory drive and potential for aspiration. Patient's sensitivity to short-acting opioids should be assessed prior to administering long-acting opioids.

5. Pulmonary

Lee and Hughes demonstrated abnormalities in lung function tests in 90% of patients. In severe cases, an obstructive pattern is seen [4]. A diminished response of respiratory muscles to respond to increasing carbon dioxide (CO_2) levels has also been observed, suggesting that the shift in the CO_2 response curve may perhaps not only be due to increased sensitivity to opiates [4]. Radiological evidence of abnormal swallowing has also been observed, likely explaining episodes of aspiration pneumonia [4]. The pulmonary effects of DM can be significant as shown in a clinical study of 219 patients undergoing surgical procedures by Mathieu; 89% of all complications were pulmonary in nature [1, 5]. Furthermore, patients with DM2 who have less pulmonary involvement have been shown to have less perioperative involvement as compared with DM1 [6]. Both DM1 and DM2 are associated with a high prevalence of sleep-disordered breathing. Sleep studies have documented OSA in 69% of DM1 and 43% of DM2 [3]. Careful monitoring in the postoperative period and assessing the patient's ability to protect his/her airway and aggressive pulmonary hygiene are crucial to preventing anesthetic complications in the DM patient.

6. Cardiovascular

The cardiovascular effects of DM have been well established. Dense granules in the mitochondria of cardiac myocytes result in necrosis, fatty infiltration, and fibrosis resulting in hyperexcitability of the cardiac conduction system [7]. Atrioventricular conduction abnormalities in patients with DM have been shown to increase the risk of ventricular arrhythmias. Benhayon et al. found 32% of DM patients with atrial fibrillation [8]. Patients with DM1 are more likely to have conduction disease and have higher all-cause mortality as compared with DM2 [8]. In a 20-year study of 171 patients with DM, sudden death was the most common cause of patient demise at 41.7%, while respiratory complications were associated with 29.2% of deaths [9]. Hypertension, presence of palpitations, right bundle branch blocks, bifascicular blocks, and a "severely abnormal" EKG were identified as risk factors for sudden cardiac death (SCD) in DM patients [9]. In a 2004 study of 382 DM1 patients by Bhakta et al., abnormal electrocardiographic findings correlated structural heart abnormalities such as left ventricular hypertrophy (19.8%), left ventricular dilatation (18.6%), and left ventricular systolic dysfunction (14%) [10].

Anesthetic considerations for the DM patient must involve a thorough assessment of the patient's cardiac status. Patients with cardiac involvement may have an implantable cardioverter defibrillator (ICD) and require interrogation prior to surgery. A defibrillator along with external pads should be available in the perioperative setting.

7. Musculoskeletal

DM can affect multiple muscle groups including cardiac, smooth, and skeletal muscle. In a retrospective analysis of 320 patients with DM, Kirzinger et al. found that 14.6% of the patients who underwent general anesthesia had a worsening of musculoskeletal symptoms. This is in part from the effect of hypothermia on exacerbating the myotonia and the prolonged effect of muscle relaxants. Although a majority of these symptoms were reversible, a small group of 9 patients had irreversible aggravation of their disease [6].

8. Endocrine

There is an increased incidence in insulin resistance and diabetes particularly in DM2 which should be managed perioperatively with blood glucose measurement as usual for diabetics [1].

9. Gastrointestinal

Involvement of the gastrointestinal (GI) system occurs frequently in patients with DM [1, 11]. Dysphagia is prevalent in 25% to 80% of patients with DM. Delayed gastric emptying, choledocholithiasis, irritable bowel syndrome, and elevated gamma glutamyl transferase levels have been associated [11]. The etiology may be from abnormal smooth muscle cells in the alimentary and/or a neurological component. Whether

TABLE 1: Summary of DM effects on organ systems.

Organ system	Effect	
Musculoskeletal	(i) Myopathy, atrophy, myalgias (ii) Myotonia: triggers include stress and cold as well as specific medications	(i) DM1: tends to affect facial muscles e.g. distal muscles (ii) DM2: tends to affect proximal muscles e.g. hip flexors
Nervous System	(i) Cognitive impairment (ii) Mental retardation more common in DM1	(i) Axonal sensorimotor polyneuropathy (ii) Sensorineural hearing loss
Eye	(i) Cataracts (ii) Proptosis	

Cardiac	(i) Arrhythmias
	  (a) AV block, bundle branch block most common
	  (b) Atrial flutter and fibrillation
		(i) Cardiomyopathy: Hypertrophy, dilation, systolic dysfunction

Pulmonary	(i) OSA (ii) Hypersomnia/excessive daytime somnolence (iii) Increased risk of aspiration pneumonia	(i) Respiratory muscle weakness (ii) Increased sensitivity to respiratory depressants
Gastrointestinal	(i) Dysphagia (ii) GERD (iii) IBS-like symptoms	(i) Gallstones
Endocrine	(i) Primary Hypogonadism (ii) Diabetes, Insulin resistance (iii) Hyperthyroidism	(i) Hyperparathyroidism (ii) Hyperhidrosis (iii) Male pattern baldness
Reproductive	(i) Low sperm count secondary to hypogonadism	(i) Higher risk of miscarriage, preterm labor
Cancer	(i) Increased risk for cancers of endometrium, brain, ovary, colon, and skin	

TABLE 2: Summary of DM effects and practice suggestions for perioperative management of patients with DM.

Organ system	Effect	Plan
Central Nervous System	(i) Temperature regulation (ii) Increased risk of corneal abrasions from proptosis	(i) Keep patient warm (ii) Increase temperature in operating room (iii) Careful taping of eyes, ophthalmic ointment

Behavioral issues	(i) Cognitive dysfunction
	(ii) Behavioral issues
	  (a) Anxiety
	  (b) Bipolar disorder
	  (c) Obsessive- compulsive disorder
		(i) Check for mood altering medications
		(ii) Use small 0.5 mg to 1 mg boluses of benzodiazepines to assess patient's sensitivity

Endocrine	(i) Diabetes (ii) Hyperthyroid (iii) Hyperparathyroid	(i) Check AM blood sugar (ii) Preop thyroid function testing (iii) Check calcium level preoperatively

Cardiac	(i) Arrhythmias:
	  (a) Atrial flutter
	  (b) Atrial fibrillation
		(i) Have defibrillator available and pads on patient
		(ii) Interrogate AICD if present

Pulmonary	(i) Impairment of ventilation and sensitivity to respiratory depressants (ii) Ineffective coughing (a) Aspiration pneumonia	(i) Minimize use respiratory depressants (ii) Aggressive postoperative pulmonary hygiene

Musculoskeletal	(i) Involuntary muscle contraction, progressive weakness	(i) Avoid triggering agents:
		  (a) Succinylcholine
		  (b) Neostigmine

Gastrointestinal	(i) Prolonged gastric emptying	(i) Consider rapid sequence induction and intubation

rapid sequence induction and intubation is necessary for all DM patients is unknown.

10. Anesthetic Agents and DM

In 2010, Kirzinger et al. published a retrospective study of 134 patients with DM and side effects of anesthesia. 116 of these patients underwent a total of 342 surgical procedures with regional anesthesia over the course of several years [7]. Only 35 of these procedures were performed under spinal or peripheral nerve block. The rest were performed under local anesthesia. From this study, regional anesthetic techniques appear less likely to result in anesthetic complications in the DM patient [7]. This study however did not risk stratify the patients in terms of disease severity. The Myotonic Dystrophy Foundation has provided formalized suggestions for the anesthetic management of patients with Myotonic Dystrophy (see the following).

Practical Management

Chart Adapted from Myotonic Dystrophy Foundation. Suggestions for Perioperative Management of Patients with DM

(1) Check preoperative blood sugar.

(2) Keep patient warm. Use forced-air warming device and increase ambient temperature in OR.

(3) Have defibrillator available in the operating room and defibrillator pads on patient.

(4) Avoid succinylcholine and neostigmine.

(5) Utilize continuous pulse oximetry and EKG monitoring.

(6) Plan for possible prolonged postoperative stay.

11. Conclusion

DM is a rare genetic disease affecting multiple organs. Here we present a case of a patient with established diagnosis of DM for hip labral arthroscopy. The severity of the patient's disease must be elucidated on preoperative evaluation and is critical for successful anesthetic management. Important considerations and suggestions for management of DM in the preoperative period are presented in this literature review.

Disclosure

This case report was presented at the 41st Annual Regional Anesthesiology and Acute Pain Medicine Meeting.

Competing Interests

The authors declare that they have no competing interests.

References

[1] J. Zhou, "Neuromuscular disorders and malignant," in *Miller's Anesthesia*, R. D. Miller, Ed., pp. 1181–1195, Churchill Livingstone/Elsevier, Philadelphia, Pa, USA, 7th edition, 2010.

[2] C. Toth, C. Dunham, O. Suchowersky, J. Parboosingh, and K. Brownell, "Unusual clinical, laboratory, and muscle histopathological findings in a family with myotonic dystrophy type 2," *Muscle and Nerve*, vol. 35, no. 2, pp. 259–264, 2007.

[3] M. L. A. E. Bianchi, A. Losurdo, C. Di Blasi et al., "Prevalence and clinical correlates of sleep disordered breathing in myotonic dystrophy types 1 and 2," *Sleep & Breathing*, vol. 18, no. 3, pp. 579–589, 2014.

[4] F. I. Lee and D. T. D. Hughes, "Systemic effects in dystrophia myotonica," *Brain*, vol. 87, no. 3, pp. 521–536, 1964.

[5] J. Mathieu, P. Allard, L. Potvin, C. Prévost, and P. Begin, "A 10-year study of mortality in a cohort of patients with myotonic dystrophy," *Neurology*, vol. 52, no. 8, pp. 1658–1662, 1999.

[6] L. Kirzinger, A. Schmidt, C. Kornblum, C. Schneider-Gold, W. Kress, and B. Schoser, "Side effects of anesthesia in DM2 as compared to DM1: a comparative retrospective study," *European Journal of Neurology*, vol. 17, no. 6, pp. 842–845, 2010.

[7] R. M. Ludatscher, H. Kerner, S. Amikam, and B. Gellei, "Myotonia dystrophica with heart involvement: an electron microscopic study of skeletal, cardiac, and smooth muscle," *Journal of Clinical Pathology*, vol. 31, no. 11, pp. 1057–1064, 1978.

[8] D. Benhayon, R. Lugo, R. Patel, L. Carballeira, L. Elman, and J. M. Cooper, "Long-term arrhythmia follow-up of patients with myotonic dystrophy," *Journal of Cardiovascular Electrophysiology*, vol. 26, no. 3, pp. 305–310, 2015.

[9] V. R. Stojanovic, S. Peric, T. Paunic et al., "Cardiologic predictors of sudden death in patients with myotonic dystrophy type 1," *Journal of Clinical Neuroscience*, vol. 20, no. 7, pp. 1002–1006, 2013.

[10] D. Bhakta, M. R. Lowe, and W. J. Groh, "Prevalence of structural cardiac abnormalities in patients with myotonic dystrophy type I," *American Heart Journal*, vol. 147, no. 2, pp. 224–227, 2004.

[11] M. Bellini, S. Biagi, C. Stasi et al., "Gastrointestinal manifestations in myotonic muscular dystrophy," *World Journal of Gastroenterology*, vol. 12, no. 12, pp. 1821–1828, 2006.

60

Anesthetic Considerations for an Adult Patient with Freeman-Sheldon Syndrome Undergoing Open Heart Surgery

S. Viehmeyer,[1] P. Gabriel,[1] K. Bauer,[2] S. Bauer,[2] R. Sodian,[2] and J. N. Hilberath ⓘ [1]

[1]*Department of Anesthesiology and Critical Care Medicine, MediClin Heart Institute Lahr/Baden, Lahr, Germany*
[2]*Department of Cardiac Surgery, MediClin Heart Institute Lahr/Baden, Lahr, Germany*

Correspondence should be addressed to J. N. Hilberath; jan.hilberath@mediclin.de

Academic Editor: Anjan Trikha

Freeman-Sheldon syndrome (FSS) or "whistling face" syndrome is a rare congenital disorder complicated by characteristic facial deformities and muscular contractures. We report on a 64-year-old male patient presenting for surgical replacement of his aortic valve and review the available literature on anesthetic considerations and perioperative management principles. FSS frequently poses a significant challenge to airway management and gaining vascular access. Moreover, these patients are reportedly at risk for developing malignant hyperthermia (MH) or neuroleptic malignant syndrome.

1. Introduction

Freeman-Sheldon syndrome (FSS) was first described in 1938 [1] and is part of a group of pathologies referred to as distal arthrogryposis (DA). FSS has been categorized as a specific subtype of DA type 2A in 2006 [2] and is due to a mutation in embryonic myosin, mostly Myosin Heavy Chain 3 (MYH3) [3]. The defect leads to abnormal contraction and relaxation patterns of myocytes frequently already recognized in utero by decreased or absent fetal movement. This mismatch of muscular tonicity directly affects proper skeletal and overall fetal growth, and the facies and distal extremities appear heavily deformed (Figure 1). Patients typically show a distinct physiognomy, initially also described as craniocarpotarsal dysplasia [1, 4]: contractures of musculature and soft tissues lead to characteristic circumoral fibrosis, microstomia, pursed lips, micrognathia, and a short webbed neck with severely limited range of motion. FSS is therefore also described as whistling face syndrome. The distal extremities show malformations like camptodactyly, ulnar deviation, and clubfoot. Kyphoscoliosis and spina bifida occulta can also occur, while strabism and hearing loss are less frequently encountered. Mental retardation is only rarely associated with FSS.

Written consent was provided for publication and photographs of this case.

2. Case Report

Our patient was referred from another hospital with newly diagnosed critical aortic valve stenosis (aortic valve area (AVA); 0.7 cm^2) in combination with a severely decreased left ventricular function (left ventricular ejection fraction (LVEF); 25%). He had a known long-standing history of coronary artery disease and acute coronary syndromes and had undergone coronary stenting procedures repeatedly in recent years. Twice he suffered ST-segment elevation myocardial infarctions (STEMI). Admission chest X-rays showed cardiac congestion with bilateral pulmonary infiltrates. His blood work showed signs of systemic infection including elevated markers of inflammation and leukocytosis. After initiation of antibiotic and heart failure therapy his symptoms improved and he was scheduled for aortic valve replacement. A calculated EuroSCORE II of 2.08% lead to our center's interdisciplinary heart team decision for surgical aortic valve replacement (SAVR).

His past medical history was otherwise significant for type 2 diabetes, colonic diverticulosis, and COPD. During

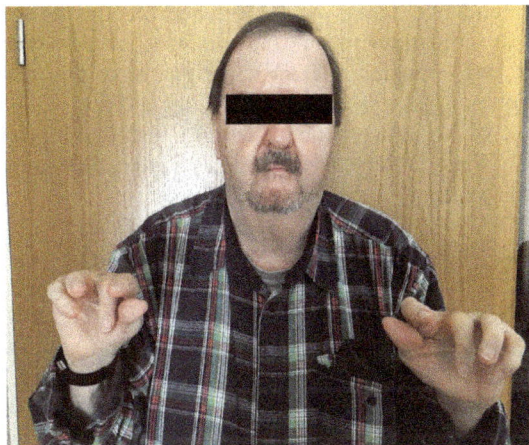

FIGURE 1

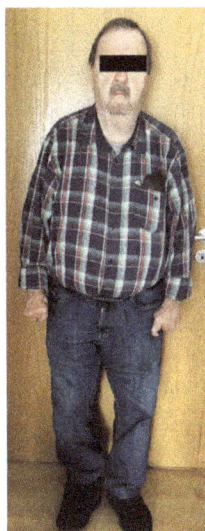

FIGURE 2

childhood and adolescence he had undergone numerous surgical procedures to correct skeletal deformities. Despite significant physical disabilities the patient had remained ambulatory and able to sufficiently perform activities of daily living (ADL) without assistance (Figure 2).

3. Anesthetic Management

The patient did not report problems with previous anesthetics on preoperative evaluation. Written records of previous anesthetics could not be obtained. Given his orofacial anatomy including microstomia, retrognathia, and limited mobility of his neck, his airway was secured via awake nasal fiberoptic intubation (AFOI) (Figure 1). After local anesthesia of his naso- and oropharynx with aerosolized lidocaine (4%) and decongestant treatment of the nasal mucosa (xylometazoline 1%), he received small incremental doses of sufentanil (total dose 35 μg) for additional analgesia and light sedation during intubation. Endotracheal intubation was successful without distress or hypoxemic events. After induction of general

anesthesia (GA), direct laryngoscopy confirmed a Cormack Lehane 4 view. As alternate plan of securing the airway in case of failed AFOI or difficulties with ventilation, the attending surgeon remained in standby during induction to perform an awake tracheotomy in the spontaneously breathing patient.

Prior to skin incision, cisatracurium (10 mg) was administered once. GA was maintained by propofol (4-5 mg/kg/h) and sufentanil (50–70 μg/h) infusions titrated to bispectral indices between 40 and 60. A trigger-free anesthetic was chosen to mitigate the risk for malignant hyperthermia (MH) or anesthesia-induced rhabdomyolysis.

After uneventful replacement of his aortic valve with a 23 mm bioprosthesis (cross clamp time 56 min, cardiopulmonary bypass time 72 min) the patient was transferred to our intensive care unit sedated and intubated.

Sedation was stopped on postoperative day (POD) 1. The patient initially presented disoriented with weak muscular tone and only minimal movement. During a spontaneous breathing trial at that time his respiratory mechanics appeared insufficient and labored and he was lacking sufficient cough and appropriate swallowing reflexes. Subsequently, light sedation with propofol was continued (Richmond Agitation Sedation Score- (RASS-) 1). Six hours later, the patient's sensorium and muscular tone had recovered enough to allow for safe extubation.

During his postoperative course, creatine kinase levels were repeatedly measured and remained in low-normal range. Also, the patient never developed fever or acidemia.

The patient was discharged from the ICU on POD 4 and left the hospital to rehabilitation on POD 7.

4. Discussion

To our knowledge this is the first report on the anesthetic management of an adult FSS patient undergoing cardiac surgery.

While FSS remains a rare condition, the likelihood of perioperatively caring for adult patients with congenital pathologies will increase in the future. With an increasing life expectancy, ailments like cardiovascular disease become more prevalent and might require (surgical) interventions.

Managing orphan diseases and congenital syndromes remain challenging. Most available literature to guide decision-making stems from pediatric patients. The fundamental topics for perioperative clinicians caring for FSS patients are the management of a difficult airway and vascular access [5]. Moreover, pharmacologic choices in patients at risk for MH and additional perioperative complications require heightened vigilance within the care team.

Even though difficult airway anatomy is frequently encountered in patients undergoing thoracic surgery, patients with FSS almost invariably present with a challenging anatomy. Their small mouth opening and receding chin make oral intubation difficult and the limited nasopharyngeal space might render nasal placement of an adequately sized endotracheal tube impossible. A laryngeal mask airway can be a viable alternative in some patients without significant reflux disease or impaired gastrointestinal motility. AFOI is deemed best practice to secure these patients' airway.

However, AFOI in FSS frequently can present a significant challenge, even for experienced practitioners (Figure 1).

Establishing venous and arterial access can also be difficult in patients with contractures. The widespread utilization of ultrasound to visualize vessels has significantly improved success rates of vascular cannulation [6] (Figures 1 and 2).

While regional and local anesthesia are considered ideal in these patients and recommended where possible [7] they are not an option for cardiac surgery.

The choice of sedative and anesthetic drugs is still debated notwithstanding that detrimental side effects seem to be rare. Benzodiazepines have been safely used as premedication although their intrinsic potential for muscle relaxation must be taken into account [4, 8]. Ketamine or small doses of short-acting opioids might present viable alternatives. Given a shortage of remifentanil in Germany, we chose sufentanil as primary analgesic and sedative. In our patient benzodiazepines were omitted to avoid additional muscular weakness and prolonged postoperative mechanical ventilation and recovery. Muscle relaxation was, however, considered necessary by the surgical team to improve exposure. We chose a single dose of cisatracurium, which is degraded by Hofmann elimination independent of cholinesterase activity or metabolism and without metabolites with intrinsic relaxant activity. Nevertheless, our patient showed significantly slowed recovery and safe extubation was only possible with delay.

Several cases of hyperthermia possibly related to the use of anesthetics have been reported in FSS, and an inherent risk of MH cannot be safely confirmed or ruled out to date [9, 10]. Therefore, some authors recommend avoiding the use of potential triggers as best practice in FSS altogether. However, volatile agents as well as other known trigger substances have been used in pediatric patients: uneventful inhalational induction and maintenance of anesthesia have been described with sevoflurane [2, 8] whereas halothane has been linked to hyperpyrexia in several cases [5]. Muscular rigidity as an early sign of MH has been described using halothane plus succinylcholine [2]. However, in other cases, halothane has also been found not to be harmful [7, 11]. Importantly, all proven or suspected cases of MH were successfully treated with dantrolene. Given these nonuniform recommendations in the literature we used a trigger-free setup to avoid any risk of MH. For induction, maintenance, and postoperative sedation a combination of propofol and short-acting remifentanil would have been our preference. Unfortunately, remifentanil was not available in Germany at the time. We therefore decided on sufentanil as intraoperative opioid given its predictable context-sensitive half-life. Still, the prolonged weaning and muscular weakness in our patient highlight the need for increased perioperative vigilance despite careful titration of well-controllable anesthesia drugs. After extubation we preferentially used NSAIDS and carefully titrated piritramide, a selective μ-receptor agonist, based on the visualized analogue pain scale.

Metoclopramide has been linked to neuroleptic malignant hyperthermia in one patient with FSS, which was terminated by dantrolene [9]. Given several other case reports on neuroleptic malignant syndromes and hyperthermia we recommend avoidance of atypical neuroleptics altogether. For most indications prompting their use like postoperative nausea and vomiting (PONV), perioperative delirium, or postoperative delayed gastric emptying there are adequate alternatives. The use of alpha-2 agonists seems also a rational choice in these patients even though no validated studies are available to date.

5. Conclusions

Adult FSS patients undergoing cardiac surgery can be safely managed. Advance interdisciplinary planning and assignment of appropriate resources to the management of a potentially challenging airway and vascular access anatomy as well as planning for a prolonged ICU stay enable safe patient outcomes. A well-balanced, trigger-free anesthetic with short-acting opioids, limited use of muscle relaxants, and postoperative sedatives as well as neuroleptic drugs seem prudent in FSS.

Authors' Contributions

S. Viehmeyer and J. N. Hilberath helped collect data, analyze the data, and prepare the manuscript. P. Gabriel, K. Bauer, S. Bauer, and R. Sodian helped analyze the data and prepare the manuscript. All authors attest to having approved the final manuscript and the integrity of the original data reported in the manuscript.

Acknowledgments

Support for publication was provided solely from the Department of Anesthesiology and Critical Care Medicine, MediClin Heart Institute Lahr/Baden, Lahr, Germany.

References

[1] E. A. Freeman and J. H. Sheldon, "Cranio-carpo-tarsal dystrophy," *Archives of Disease in Childhood*, vol. 13, no. 75, pp. 277–283, 1938.

[2] D. A. Stevenson, J. C. Carey, J. Palumbos, A. Rutherford, J. Dolcourt, and M. J. Bamshad, "Clinical characteristics and natural history of Freeman-Sheldon syndrome," *Pediatrics*, vol. 117, no. 3, pp. 754–762, 2006.

[3] A. W. Racca, A. E. Beck, M. J. McMillin, F. Steven Korte, M. J. Bamshad, and M. Regnier, "The embryonic myosin R672C mutation that underlies Freeman-Sheldon syndrome impairs cross-bridge detachment and cycling in adult skeletal muscle," *Human Molecular Genetics*, vol. 24, no. 12, Article ID ddv084, pp. 3348–3358, 2015.

[4] S. Madi-Jebara, C. El-Hajj, D. Jawish, E. Ayoub, K. Kharrat, and M.-C. Antakly, "Anesthetic management of a patient with Freeman-Sheldon syndrome: case report," *Journal of Clinical Anesthesia*, vol. 19, no. 6, pp. 460–462, 2007.

[5] L. L. Ma, X. H. Zhang, Y. G. Huang, and Q. X. Zhang, "Anesthetic management of a patient with Freeman-Sheldon

syndrome: case report and literature review," *Chinese Medical Journal*, vol. 125, no. 2, pp. 390-391, 2012.

[6] K. Patel, A. Gursale, D. Chavan, and P. Sawant, "Anaesthesia challenges in Freeman-Sheldon syndrome," *Indian Journal of Anaesthesia*, vol. 57, no. 6, pp. 632-633, 2013.

[7] J. F. Mayhew, "Anesthesia for children with Freeman-Sheldon syndrome," *Anesthesiology*, vol. 78, no. 2, p. 408, 1993.

[8] A. Agritmis, O. Unlusoy, and S. Karaca, "Anesthetic management of a patient with Freeman-Sheldon syndrome," *Pediatric Anesthesia*, vol. 14, no. 10, pp. 874–877, 2004.

[9] M. H. Stein, M. Sorscher, and S. N. Caroff, "Neuroleptic malignant syndrome induced by metoclopramide in an infant with Freeman-Sheldon syndrome [22]," *Anesthesia & Analgesia*, vol. 103, no. 3, pp. 786-787, 2006.

[10] J. A. Katz and G. S. Murphy, "Anesthetic consideration for neuromuscular diseases," *Current Opinion in Anaesthesiology*, vol. 30, no. 3, pp. 435–440, 2017.

[11] L. Vas and P. Naregal, "Anaesthetic management of a patient with Freeman Sheldon syndrome," *Pediatric Anesthesia*, vol. 8, no. 2, pp. 175–177, 1998.

61

Hemodynamic Response to Massive Bleeding in a Patient with Congenital Insensitivity to Pain with Anhidrosis

Yuki Sugiyama ⓘ,[1] Sayako Gotoh,[1,2] Masatoshi Urasawa,[1,2] Mikito Kawamata,[1] and Koichi Nakajima[2]

[1]Department of Anesthesiology and Resuscitology, Shinshu University School of Medicine, Japan
[2]Division of Anesthesia, Shinonoi General Hospital, Japan

Correspondence should be addressed to Yuki Sugiyama; ysugiyama@shinshu-u.ac.jp

Academic Editor: Jian-jun Yang

A patient with congenital insensitivity to pain with anhidrosis (CIPA) underwent revision of total hip arthroplasty under general anesthesia with only propofol. During surgery, neither elevation of stress hormones nor hemodynamic changes associated with pain occurred; however, when blood was rapidly lost, compensatory tachycardia was observed. Although patients with CIPA are complicated with autonomic disturbance due to dysfunction of postganglionic sympathetic fibers, this compensatory response indicated that the adrenal glands in patients with CIPA secrete catecholamine as part of a compensatory response during bleeding under general anesthesia.

1. Introduction

Congenital insensitivity to pain with anhidrosis (CIPA) is a rare autosomal recessive disease that is characterized by unexplained fever, anhidrosis, and loss of pain sensation [1, 2]. Patients with CIPA frequently suffer recurrent episodes of wounds and bone fractures, which need surgical treatment. For the anesthetic management of patients with CIPA, the control of body temperature, analgesia, and treatment of dysfunction of the postganglionic sympathetic fibers are important. Massive bleeding occurred in a patient with CIPA who underwent revision of total hip arthroplasty under general anesthesia. Here, we discuss the compensatory hemodynamic change during massive bleeding and secretion of stress hormones associated with pain in the patient with CIPA.

2. Case Presentation

A 36-year-old woman (height, 147 cm; weight, 50 kg) with CIPA was scheduled for revision of left total hip arthroplasty. She was diagnosed as having CIPA because of recurrent episodes of unexplained fever, anhidrosis, burns, and bone fractures after birth. She had previously undergone 7 operations for spinal deformity and 1 operation of total hip arthroplasty in both the left and right sides. Although lack of general diaphoresis and thermal nociception were observed, the patient performed body surface cooling at her own discretion when she felt she was at a risk of hyperthermia, and her body temperature was kept approximately 36°C. No signs of mental retardation or orthostatic hypotension were observed. No abnormality was detected on chest radiographs and electrocardiograms. Blood biochemistry revealed no abnormality except mild anemia indicated by a hemoglobin level of 10.6 g/dl.

No premedication was administered. After the patient was brought into the operating room, routine monitoring and measurement of the bispectral index (BIS) were started. Body temperature was measured at 3 different sites (urinary bladder, esophagus, and precordial skin) and controlled by a hot-air-type heater. Propofol was administered at an effect-site concentration of 4 μg/ml by target-controlled infusion. After muscle relaxation had been achieved by administration of 50 mg of rocuronium, the trachea was intubated. Immediately after endotracheal intubation, systolic blood pressure increased from 130 to 145 mmHg, and heart rate increased from 60 to 95 beats per minute (bpm). Two minutes

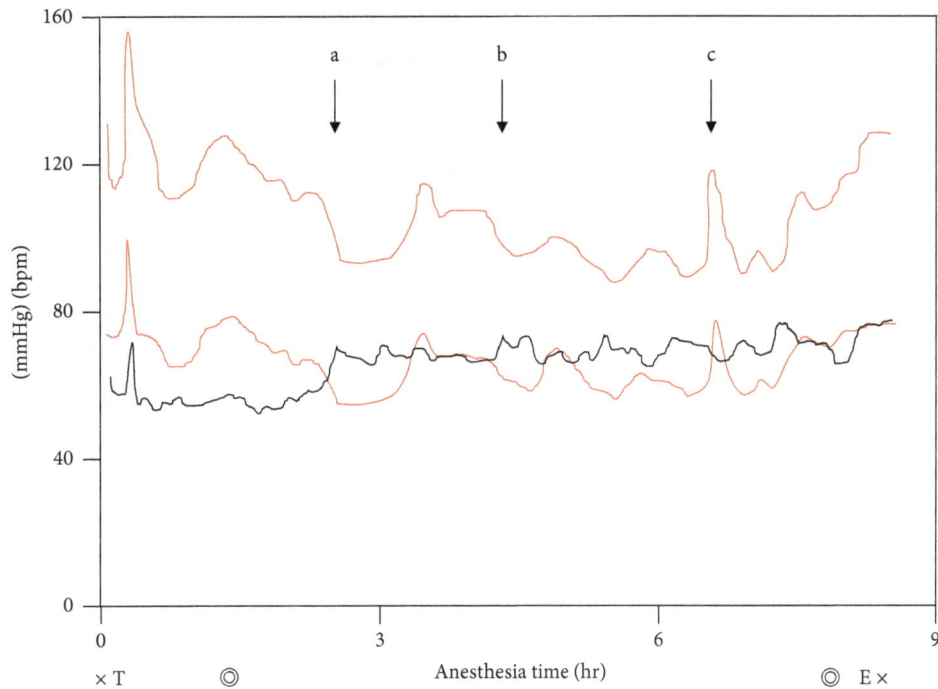

FIGURE 1: Anesthetic record. The black line indicates heart rate (HR) and the red lines indicate blood pressure (BP). a: six hundred mL of blood loss within 20 minutes, b: six hundred and fifty mL of blood loss within 30 minutes, c: administration of 0.1 mg phenylephrine, ×: start or end of anesthesia, ◎: start or end of the surgery, T: tracheal intubation, E: extubation, TCI: target-controlled infusion, and FFP: fresh frozen plasma.

later, systolic blood pressure had decreased to 125 mmHg. Propofol was continuously infused intravenously at a target concentration of 2 to 4 μg/ml (Figure 1) and BIS levels were maintained between 40 and 60. After an arterial catheter had been placed, her position was changed from the supine to right lateral position. Surgery was then started.

Since no circulatory change associated with pain occurred during surgery, opioids were not administered. Regarding hemodynamics, when 600 ml of blood was rapidly lost within 20 minutes, blood pressure decreased from 113/66 to 93/55 mmHg and heart rate increased from 55 to 70 bpm (Figure 1 a). Similarly, when 850 ml of blood was lost within 30 minutes, systolic blood pressure decreased from 108/65 to 95/60 mmHg and heart rate increased from 66 to 74 bpm (Figure 1 b). Administration of 0.1 mg of phenylephrine increased blood pressure from 87/55 to 117/76 mmHg and decreased heart rate from 70 to 65 bpm (Figure 1 c).

The operative time was 6 hours and 49 minutes, and the duration of anesthesia was 8 hours and 41 minutes. The volume of blood loss was 3350 ml. Blood transfusion was performed with 1600 ml of preoperatively donated autologous

blood, 900 ml of salvaged blood, and 720 ml of fresh frozen plasma. Intraoperative body temperature was controlled and kept between 36.0°C and 36.9°C at all 3 measurement points. After surgery had been completed, the patient was returned to the supine position and she was extubated. Since she did not complain of any pain after the surgery, no analgesic was administered. She was discharged at 6 weeks after the operation.

Blood samples were collected 3 times: before anesthesia induction, after the start of surgery, and at the end of surgery. The levels of catecholamine fractions and cortisol were measured. Norepinephrine levels were below the normal range at all time points, and the levels of epinephrine and cortisol were within the normal ranges at all time points (Table 1).

3. Discussion

CIPA is caused by a loss-of-function mutation of the TRKA gene, which encodes the receptor of the nerve growth factor (NGF) tyrosine kinase. Without this receptor, primary

TABLE 1: Levels of catecholamine fractions and cortisol.

	Before anesthesia	After the start of surgery	End of surgery	Normal range
Epinephrine	46	33	9	< 100 (pg/mL)
Norepinephrine	37	26	5	100 - 450 (pg/mL)
Cortisol	19	5.2	8.1	6.2 - 19.4 (mcg/dL)

afferent neurons and postganglionic sympathetic fibers, which are dependent on NGF for growth and survival, are lost, and their loss induces both autonomic disturbance and loss of pain sensation [1, 2]. In anesthetic management of patients with CIPA, attention should be paid to the use for analgesics, abnormal body temperatures due to abnormal sympathetic nervous activity, and their hemodynamics.

There have been some case reports on patients with CIPA who received general anesthesia without any analgesics [3–5] and in whom intraoperative levels of catecholamine and cortisol were measured [6]. In that previous study, levels of catecholamine and cortisol were not elevated by pain stimuli during surgery under general anesthesia. In our case, in which anesthesia was managed only with propofol, the levels of catecholamine and cortisol were also not elevated by pain stimuli (Table 1); however, it has been pointed out that catecholamine levels might not be elevated by stress induction because of the loss of postganglionic sympathetic fibers in patients with CIPA [7].

Recently, the ability of catecholamine secretion in patients with CIPA has been examined using a standing test [8]. In patients with CIPA, blood norepinephrine concentrations have been reported to be below the normal range [7, 8]. Normally, norepinephrine is mainly secreted by sympathetic nerve terminals and the brain, and epinephrine is mainly secreted by the adrenal medulla. When healthy volunteers were upright, normal blood pressure was maintained by norepinephrine. In contrast, when patients with CIPA were upright, blood pressure was maintained by epinephrine, not by norepinephrine [8]; therefore, this response is considered to be a compensatory response by the adrenal medulla in patients with CIPA. As for cortisol, it has been reported that cortisol secretion in patients with CIPA can be increased by stress from limited water intake [7]. The results of those studies suggest that patients with CIPA can secrete epinephrine and cortisol in response to stress.

In our case, a change in hemodynamics was not observed at the start of surgery (Figure 1), and both catecholamine and cortisol levels were low (Table 1), even though general anesthesia was maintained only by propofol. This indicated that the pain stimuli caused by incision did not induce catecholamine or cortisol secretion. In contrast, compensatory tachycardia was observed during bleeding (Figure 1a, b). Unfortunately, we could not obtain both a blood sample during massive bleeding and a control blood sample just before the bleeding, which was difficult to predict; however, this response was considered to be induced by epinephrine secreted from the adrenal grand, as mentioned above [8]. From these findings, we considered that our patient had the ability to secrete epinephrine from the adrenal grand under general anesthesia when the patient was exposed to some

stress, and the response after the start of surgery indicated that pain stimuli did not induce any stress in our patient.

Cortisol level usually increases continuously during surgery [9] and reaches a peak after extubation [10, 11]. In our case, cortisol level was within the normal range before anesthesia and decreased to less than the normal range after the start of surgery (Table 1). This decrease might have represented circadian rhythm or a decrease of mental stress after induction of general anesthesia. Although the cortisol level was slightly increased at the end of surgery, the level was close to the lower limit of the normal range and we thought that this small increase in cortisol level was not induced by strong stress but might have been due to the decreased administration of propofol at the end of surgery. These changes in hormones and the capability of hormone secretion suggested that pain stimuli during surgery did not induce any stress in our patient.

Hemodynamic changes in our case were observed at intubation and at administration of phenylephrine followed by bradycardia caused by baroreflex. The pharynx and larynx are innervated by glossopharyngeal and vagus nerves, and baroreflex is regulated by the vagus nerve [12]. These physiological responses occur because these cranial nerves are intact in patients with CIPA. A previous study showed that tachycardia within 10 minutes after induction occurred in 31% of CIPA patients and that the patients could respond to airway manipulation [13]. Intraoperative bradycardia was also observed in 2.8% of CIPA cases [13]. In pediatric patients, cardiovascular complications were reported to be common [3] and to sometimes induce hemodynamic change by an unpleasant sensation [3, 14]; therefore, attention should be paid to hemodynamics in patients with CIPA, even if a compensatory response is present.

Authors' Contributions

Yuki Sugiyama and Sayako Gotoh equally contributed to this study.

References

[1] Y. Indo, M. Tsuruta, Y. Hayashida et al., "Mutations in the TRKA/NGF receptor gene in patients with congenital insensitivity to pain with anhidrosis," *Nature Genetics*, vol. 13, no. 4, pp. 485–488, 1996.

[2] Y. Indo, "Nerve growth factor and the physiology of pain: lessons from congenital insensitivity to pain with anhidrosis," *Clinical Genetics*, vol. 82, no. 4, pp. 341–350, 2012.

[3] V. Rozentsveig, A. Katz, N. Weksler et al., "The anaesthetic management of patients with congenital insensitivity to pain with anhidrosis," *Pediatric Anesthesia*, vol. 14, no. 4, pp. 344–348, 2004.

[4] T. Tomioka, Y. Awaya, K. Nihei, H. Sekiyama, S. Sawamura, and K. Hanaoka, "Anesthesia for patients with congenital insensitivity to pain and anhidrosis: A questionnaire study in Japan," *Anesthesia & Analgesia*, vol. 94, no. 2, pp. 271–274, 2002.

[5] I. F. Brandes and E. A. E. Stuth, "Use of BIS monitor in a child with congenital insensitivity to pain with anhidrosis," *Pediatric Anesthesia*, vol. 16, no. 4, pp. 466–470, 2006.

[6] S. Yoshitake, K. Matsumoto, A. Miyagawa et al., "Anesthetic consideration of a patient with congenital insensitivity to pain with anhidrosis," *The Japanese Journal of Anesthesiology*, vol. 42, no. 8, pp. 1233–1236, 1993.

[7] N. Loewenthal, J. Levy, R. Schreiber et al., "Nerve growth factor-tyrosine kinase A pathway is involved in thermoregulation and adaptation to stress: Studies on patients with hereditary sensory and autonomic neuropathy type IV," *Pediatric Research*, vol. 57, no. 4, pp. 587–590, 2005.

[8] L. Norcliffe-Kaufmann, S. D. Katz, F. Axelrod, and H. Kaufmann, "Norepinephrine deficiency with normal blood pressure control in congenital insensitivity to pain with anhidrosis," *Annals of Neurology*, vol. 77, no. 5, pp. 743–752, 2015.

[9] T. Nishiyama, K. Yamashita, and T. Yokoyama, "Stress hormone changes in general anesthesia of long duration: Isoflurane-nitrous oxide vs sevoflurane-nitrous oxide anesthesia," *Journal of Clinical Anesthesia*, vol. 17, no. 8, pp. 586–591, 2005.

[10] R. Udelsman, J. A. Norton, S. E. Jelenich et al., "Responses of the hypothalamic-pituitary-adrenal and renin-angiotensin axes and the sympathetic system during controlled surgical and anesthetic stress," *The Journal of Clinical Endocrinology & Metabolism*, vol. 64, no. 5, pp. 986–994, 1987.

[11] K. Furuya, R. Shimizu, Y. Hirabayashi, R. Ishii, and H. Fukuda, "Stress hormone responses to major intra-abdominal surgery during and immediately after sevoflurane-nitrous oxide anaesthesia in elderly patients," *Canadian Journal of Anesthesia*, vol. 40, no. 5, pp. 435–439, 1993.

[12] K. T. Higa, E. Mori, F. F. Viana, M. Morris, and L. C. Michelini, "Baroreflex control of heart rate by oxytocin in the solitary-vagal complex," *American Journal of Physiology-Regulatory, Integrative and Comparative Physiology*, vol. 282, no. 2, pp. R537–R545, 2002.

[13] A. Zlotnik, D. Natanel, R. Kutz et al., "Anesthetic management of patients with congenital insensitivity to pain with anhidrosis: A retrospective analysis of 358 procedures performed under general anesthesia," *Anesthesia & Analgesia*, vol. 121, no. 5, pp. 1316–1320, 2015.

[14] C. Wang, X. Zhang, S. Guo, J. Sun, and N. Li, "Anesthetic management during adenotonsillectomy for twins with congenital insensitivity to pain with anhidrosis: two case reports," *Journal of Medical Case Reports*, vol. 11, no. 1, 2017.

62

The Anaesthesiologist and Palliative Care in a Newborn with the Adam "Sequence"

Alberto Vieira Pantoja,[1] Maria Emília Gonçalves Estevez,[2] Bruno Lima Pessoa,[1] Fernando de Paiva Araújo,[3] Bruno Mendonça Barcellos,[1] Ciro Augusto Floriani,[4] and Marco Antonio Cardoso de Resende[1]

[1]Fluminense Federal University (UFF), Niteroi, RJ, Brazil
[2]National Institute of Traumatology and Orthopaedics (INTO), Rio de Janeiro, RJ, Brazil
[3]Monte Sinai Hospital, Juiz de Fora, MG, Brazil
[4]National School of Public Health of the Osvaldo Cruz Foundation (ENSP-FOC), Rio de Janeiro, RJ, Brazil

Correspondence should be addressed to Marco Antonio Cardoso de Resende; macresende@gmail.com

Academic Editor: Renato Santiago Gomez

Reports focusing on biomedical principlism and the role of anaesthesiologists in palliative care are rare. We present the case of a newborn with multiple craniofacial anomalies and a diagnosis of ADAM "sequence," in which surgical removal of placental adhesions to the dura mater and the correction of meningocele was not indicated due to the very short life expectancy. After 48 hours, the odor from the placenta indicted a necrotic process, which prevented the parents from being close to the child and increased his isolation. Urgent surgery was performed, after which the newborn was transported to the ICU and intubated under controlled mechanical ventilation. The patient died a week later. The principles of beneficence, nonmaleficence, justice, and respect for autonomy are simultaneously an inspiratory and regulatory framework for clinical practice. Although only necessary procedures are defended, which suggests a position contrary to invasive interventions at the end of life, sometimes they are the best palliative measures that can be taken in cases like the one described here.

1. Introduction

The maintenance of life is historically the foundation of medical activity. However, scientific and technological developments lead to potential extremes that elicit questions concerning dignity at the end of life. Ethical decision-making cannot be conceived without propaedeutic and therapeutic details and the active and autonomous participation of the patient and/or their family. In this context, the doctor is inserted into a philosophical debate, which outperforms the technical possibilities, far from the protocols. Although dedicated to ethical values and practices, he is sometimes required to set limits on life support. Following the indication of surgical treatment, the anaesthesiologist's activity assumes the condition of intermediary, involving the patient and the surgeon, who eventually relates the patient to the hospital structure itself.

Reports that focus on biomedical principlism and the role of anaesthesiologists in palliative care in neonates are rare. We found it difficult to precisely define the boundary between what should be done and what could seem unnecessary. We report the case of a neonate with ADAM "sequence," showing frontal, temporal, and parietal cranial agenesis, facial cleft, encephalomeningocele, and placental adhesions to the dura mater, by which surgical removal was initially contraindicated due to the minimum duration of patient's survival.

2. Case Presentation

A two-day-old male newborn, weighing 3900 g, born by Caesarean section, Apgar score 6–9, Capurro assessment of 41 weeks and 6 days, presented with multiple craniofacial anomalies (hypertelorism, agenesis of eyelids, facial cleft, cleft lip, and palate), bilateral frontal parietal encephalocele, failed cerebral hemisphere separation and placental adhesions to the dura mater, and pseudosyndactyly on the right hand. The ultrasound exam at 20 weeks had already indicated possible brain malformation. At birth, he was diagnosed with a probable ADAM "sequence" and his prognosis was a life expectancy of fewer than 24 hours. Thus, removal of the placental adhesions from the dura mater and the correction of meningocele were not indicated. However, after 48 hours, the odour from the placenta indicated a necrotic process, preventing the parents from being close to the child and increasing his isolation, so an urgent surgery was requested. The newborn was eupneic without supplemental oxygen when he arrived at the operating room and hemodynamically stable without vasoactive amines. He was monitored with a precordial stethoscope, ECG in DII, noninvasive blood pressure, and rectal thermometer and actively heated by a thermal mattress. Preoxygenation was performed under a facial mask, and then pure inhalational induction with sevoflurane 5 vol% under spontaneous ventilation was used to achieve adequate anaesthesia. Venipuncture with a 22 G cannula in the left forearm and tracheal intubation tube with 3.5 MMDI were performed. Anaesthesia was maintained with 0.4 FiO$_2$ and 2-3 vol% sevoflurane and titrated fentanyl up to a total dose of 15 μg, under controlled ventilation, in PCV (15 cm H$_2$O) with PEEP (5 cm H$_2$O) in a CO$_2$ absorber system. He was hydrated with 130 mL of 0.9% NaCl. During the procedure, no hemodynamic instability or other significant complications were observed. After surgery had ended (95 min), the intubated newborn was transferred to the ICU, under controlled ventilation, and died a week later. Importantly, his parents signed a term of free, informed consent.

3. Discussion

ADAM sequence is an uncommon congenital disorder with highly variable spectrum. It comprises a series of craniofacial, thoracic, abdominal, and limb malformations in different proportions in association with amniotic bands [1, 2]. In the literature, this condition is also known as ADAM complex, amniotic band sequence, Streeter's dysplasia, congenital constriction bands, and pseudoainhum [3]. ADAM is an acronym for amniotic deformities, adhesions, and mutilations. It remains as a causal and pathogenetic enigma. Among the major diagnostic criteria are amniotic adhesions anywhere on body usually with associated disruptions of limb(s) and/or trunk and /or head; pseudosyndactyly; ring constrictions of limbs; apparent amputations; variable internal primary malformations [4].

The ADAM sequence occurs in 1 in 1,200–15,000 in live births [1, 5, 6] and 1 : 70 in stillbirths [7]. It affects both genders in the same proportion. Clinically it may present as a minor digital abnormality or limb malformation, with syndactyly or clubfoot, but also as autoamputation and catastrophic craniofacial deformities [8, 9]. Importantly, often times are incompatible with life, as in our case here reported.

Craniofacial anomalies and brain deformities are a challenge for the anaesthesiologist. The known risks include difficult airway management, undiagnosed malformations

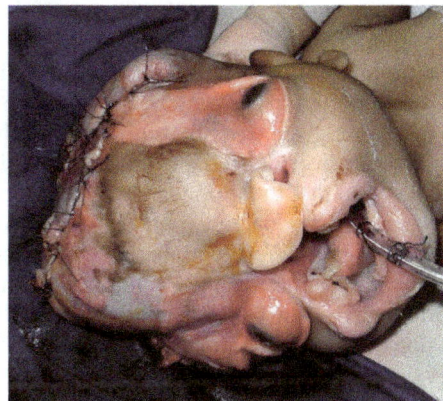

FIGURE 1: After surgical intervention.

(particularly in the cardiovascular system), significant hypovolemia disproportional to intraoperative bleeding, and prolonged brain exposure. Hypothermia and secondary complications when handling vital brain structures may be exacerbated. In this case, the facial anomaly (Figure 1) prevented from mask ventilation, so inhalational induction was the chosen approach to preserving spontaneous ventilation. The main demands the team faced were the desires of the family, the commitment to life, and the dignity of death in children with poor prognosis. Understanding the relationship between patients and physicians as the core of medical ethics, Truog sets out the evolution of the same in three interrelated spheres—clinical care, research, and society [10]. The behaviour of anaesthesiologists, indeed any medical professional, should value the biomedical principialist approach, despite its potential deficiencies, in which the principles of beneficence, nonmaleficence, justice, and respect for autonomy are simultaneously an inspiratory and regulatory framework for clinical practice [11].

Nonmaleficence, the oldest of the four principles of biomedical ethics—*primum non nocere*—, was observed through the desire of not leaving the placental material attached to the newborn during the process of necrosis. This fact mobilized the parents and pediatrician to request urgent surgery and facilitated some decisions. Beneficence was acted on when preparing the newborn with the most appropriate anaesthesia and proceeding to clean the necrotic area. The surgery was also useful measure for others since it enabled the parents to be close to the newborn and resolved the isolation caused by the strong odor. The principle of justice can also be observed in this case, since the hospital structure was placed at the service of a profoundly vulnerable human being in their nascence and, paradoxically, at the end of life. This ensured equitable access to resources, that is, providing the best conditions available to those with limited access. Although the principle of autonomy cannot be directly applied to the newborn, the parents' wishes were addressed. In other words, all the decisions that the team had made were what the parents expected to be done.

In Brazil, unilateral decisions taken by the physicians, regarding not to interfere, can be registered in the medical records without the permission or notification of the family. However, it should be clear that such measures are not intended to prolong patient suffering before the inevitable outcome. In paediatrics, in particular, this approach implies the risk of not having the parents' approval, and that such decisions may result in errors in the survival prognosis [12]. It should be addressed that the team was attentive to the plight of the newborn and his parents, with no error occurring concerning his prognosis. Yet the mobilizing force was driven by the understanding that caring for this newborn should have been done according to the reconsideration about the initial decision of not to operate him on. In the end, all the conditions needed for the team to care for him until his death were reached.

One important aspect that permitted the care provided in this case is that there was no contradiction between the practice of care and the use of high technology. Our understanding is that, even when defending necessary procedures only, which suggests a position contrary to invasive interventions at the end of life, sometimes they are the best palliative measures that might be taken in cases like the one described here. Importantly, the understanding between the family and the medical team was established, with the outcome showing that the approach of surgical intervention—initially discarded—was the most appropriate. Thus, we argue that before and after birth and when the outcome is uncertain, all available options and detailed information should be fully explained to the family members.

The role of anaesthesiologists goes beyond of relieving pain, and it is important to invite them to participate in decisions like the case in question, actively. The foundations of such cases must be established based on the best available reasoning and not on individual emotions and valuations [13]. Altogether, our approach for the case represented all the principles mentioned earlier.

Competing Interests

The authors declare that there is no conflict of interests regarding the publication of this paper.

References

[1] J. W. Seeds, R. C. Cefalo, and W. N. P. Herbert, "Amniotic band syndrome," *American Journal of Obstetrics and Gynecology*, vol. 144, no. 3, pp. 243–248, 1982.

[2] A. G. W. Hunter and B. F. Carpenter, "Implications of malformations not due to amniotic bands in the amniotic band sequence," *American Journal of Medical Genetics*, vol. 24, no. 4, pp. 691–700, 1986.

[3] P. Shetty, L. T. Menezes, L. F. Tauro, and K. A. Diddigi, "Amniotic band syndrome," *Indian Journal of Surgery*, vol. 75, no. 5, pp. 401–402, 2013.

[4] J. M. Opitz, D. R. Johnson, and E. F. Gilbert-Barness, "ADAM "sequence" part II: hypothesis and speculation," *American Journal of Medical Genetics. A*, vol. 167, no. 3, pp. 478–503, 2015.

[5] J. K. Muraskas, J. F. McDonnell, R. J. Chudik, K. E. Salyer, and L. Glynn, "Amniotic band syndrome with significant orofacial clefts and disruptions and distortions of craniofacial structures," *Journal of Pediatric Surgery*, vol. 38, no. 4, pp. 635–638, 2003.

[6] C. G. Morovic, F. Berwart, and J. Varas, "Craniofacial anomalies of the amniotic band syndrome in serial clinical cases," *Plastic and Reconstructive Surgery*, vol. 113, no. 6, pp. 1556–1562, 2004.

[7] D. K. Kalousek and S. Bamforth, "Amnion rupture sequence in previable fetuses," *American Journal of Medical Genetics*, vol. 31, no. 1, pp. 63–73, 1988.

[8] J. H. Walter Jr., L. R. Goss, and A. T. Lazzara, "Amniotic band syndrome," *Journal of Foot and Ankle Surgery*, vol. 37, no. 4, pp. 325–333, 1998.

[9] G. Menekse, M. K. Mert, B. Olmaz, T. Celik, U. S. Celik, and A. I. Okten, "Placento-cranial adhesions in amniotic band syndrome and the role of surgery in their management: an unusual case presentation and systematic literature review," *Pediatric Neurosurgery*, vol. 50, no. 4, pp. 204–209, 2015.

[10] R. D. Truog, "Patients and doctors—the evolution of a relationship," *New England Journal of Medicine*, vol. 366, no. 7, pp. 581–585, 2012.

[11] A. Udelsmann, "Bioethics—issues regarding the anesthesiologist," *Revista Brasileira de Anestesiologia*, vol. 56, no. 3, pp. 325–333, 2006.

[12] M. R. Mercurio, P. D. Murray, and I. Gross, "Unilateral pediatric "do not attempt resuscitation" orders: the pros, the cons, and a proposed approach," *Pediatrics*, vol. 133, supplement 1, pp. S37–S43, 2014.

[13] A. Janvier, K. Barrington, and B. Farlow, "Communication with parents concerning withholding or withdrawing of life-sustaining interventions in neonatology," *Seminars in Perinatology*, vol. 38, no. 1, pp. 38–46, 2014.

63

Takotsubo Cardiomyopathy after Spinal Anesthesia for a Minimally Invasive Urologic Procedure

Emmanuel Lilitsis,[1] **Despina Dermitzaki,**[1] **Georgios Avgenakis,**[2] **Ioannis Heretis,**[2] **Charalampos Mpelantis,**[2] **and Charalampos Mamoulakis**[2]

[1]*Department of Anesthesiology, University General Hospital of Heraklion, University of Crete, Medical School, Heraklion, Crete, Greece*
[2]*Department of Urology, University General Hospital of Heraklion, University of Crete, Medical School, Heraklion, Crete, Greece*

Correspondence should be addressed to Emmanuel Lilitsis; mlilitsis@yahoo.gr

Academic Editor: Anjan Trikha

We present the case of a patient who suffered from Takotsubo cardiomyopathy (TCM) immediately after the initiation of subarachnoid anesthesia for a minimally invasive urologic procedure (tension-free vaginal tape (TVT) surgery for stress urine incontinence). TCM mimics acute coronary syndrome and is caused by an exaggerated sympathetic reaction to significant emotional or physical stress. Our patient suffered from chest pain, palpitations, dyspnea, and hemodynamic instability immediately following subarachnoid anesthesia and later in the postanesthesia care unit. Blood troponin was elevated and new electrocardiographic changes appeared indicative of cardiac ischemia. Cardiac ultrasound indicated left ventricular apical akinesia and ballooning with severely affected contractility. The patient was admitted to coronary intensive care for the proper care and finally was discharged. TCM was attributed to high emotional preoperative stress for which no premedication had been administered to the patient. In conclusion, adequate premedication and anxiety management are not only a measure to alleviate psychological stress of surgical patients, but, more importantly, an imperative mean to suppress sympathetic nerve system response and its cardiovascular consequences.

1. Introduction

Takotsubo cardiomyopathy (TCM) or stress-induced cardiomyopathy or "broken heart syndrome" is a transient cardiac syndrome that was first described in Japan in 1990 by Sato et al. [1]. The Japanese word *Takotsubo* translates to "octopus trap," a pot with a wide base and narrow top, which left ventricle resembles during systole. Although considered rare diagnosis, TCM has been identified in 2% of patients presenting with acute coronary syndrome [2]. Patients at high risk to develop the syndrome are considered to be postmenopausal women under severe emotional or psychological stress. TCM mimics acute coronary syndrome and is usually presented with chest pain, ST-segment elevation on electrocardiogram (ECG), and elevated cardiac enzyme levels consistent with a myocardial infarction. However, when the patient undergoes cardiac angiography, left ventricular apical ballooning is present and there is no significant coronary artery stenosis. At time of presentation, cardiogenic shock and malignant arrhythmias may be present [3]. Although the exact etiology is still unknown, the syndrome appears to result from an exaggerated sympathetic "crisis" triggered by significant emotional or physical stress, leading to catecholaminergic storm and myocardial stunning [4]. There are numerous cases published reporting perioperative cardiomyopathy, mostly related either to surgery under general anesthesia or to administration of vasoactive drugs, such as epinephrine, ephedrine, or dobutamine [5]. Preoperative anxiety and anticipation of surgery are also included in the so-called stress response to anesthesia and surgery [6]. We present the case of a patient who suffered from stress-induced cardiomyopathy with severe left ventricular dysfunction immediately after the initiation of subarachnoid anesthesia for a minimally invasive urologic procedure.

2. Case Presentation

A 46-year-old, premenopausal Caucasian woman with body mass index of $24 \, kg/m^2$ was scheduled for a minimally invasive urologic procedure (tension-free vaginal tape (TVT) surgery for stress urine incontinence). Preoperative evaluation revealed an unusually nervous patient quoting very unpleasant experience regarding prior uneventful operations (appendectomy in childhood; caesarian section twice) and postulating not to be admitted before the day of surgery. Her medical history included Hashimoto's disease adequately controlled by thyroxine replacement therapy (ASA class II). Cardiovascular and respiratory clinical examination was normal on admission (blood pressure (BP): 116/57 mmHg, heart rate (HR): 58 beats per minute, and SpO_2 99%). Preoperative 12-lead ECG, chest X-ray, and routine laboratory tests were normal. Informed consent was obtained for subarachnoid anesthesia, the standard for TVT surgery. The patient asked to be discharged the same day, if possible. Premedication, although routinely used for ASA II patients, was withheld because there was a concern about delay from hospital discharge, which was the patient's primary wish.

Upon arrival to the operating room, vital signs recordings were BP: 110/65 mmHg, HR: 75 bpm, and SpO_2 98% (room air). Although anxious, she was cooperative. Successful subarachnoid anesthesia was performed with 10 mg bupivacaine heavy 5% and 20 μg fentanyl. Immediately after the subarachnoid injection, the patient complained of chest pain, palpitations, dyspnea, and nausea. BP dropped to 65/43 mmHg and HR increased to 94 bpm, while several supraventricular ectopic beats appeared. SpO_2 was 98% on O_2 nasal cannula 2 L/min. A bolus of 10 mg of ephedrine was administered along with a 250 ml bolus crystalloid fluids and BP increased slightly to 75/50 mmHg. The patient continued to complain of dyspnea and chest pain. A second bolus of 15 mg of ephedrine was administered along with 2 mg of midazolam for anxiety relief. BP and HR reached 103/68 mmHg and 110 bpm, respectively. She stopped complaining and remained calm and stable thereafter. Nevertheless, persistent hypotension was recorded throughout the operation (systolic BP: 90–100 mmHg, HR: 90–110 bpm), which was attributed to the anesthetic technique and the procedure was uneventfully completed within 30 minutes.

After surgery, the patient was transferred to the postanesthesia care unit for complete recovery from motor and sensory blockade. Five minutes later, she complained of chest pain again and she became hypotensive (BP: 72/59 mmHg), dyspneic, and tachypneic (SpO_2 88% on nasal cannula). Phenylephrine infusion was started at 400 $\mu g/h$ and nasal cannula was switched to a 50% Venturi mask with normalization of BP and SpO_2. Auscultation of lungs and heart revealed no pathologic sounds. A new 12-lead ECG indicated sinus rhythm with no ST elevation or depression and—not preexisting—poor progress of R waves on precordial leads and negative T wave on leads I and AVL. The new chest X-ray was normal. Arterial blood gases showed PO_2 78 mmHg, PCO_2 27 mmHg, and pH 7.43 on 50% Venturi mask. Biochemical tests were normal apart from troponin which was elevated 9.407 ng/ml (normal < 0.04) and D-dimmers

1245 ng/ml (probably expected postoperatively). Since there was no residual motor or sensory blockade but the patient was still on phenylephrine, a spiral computed tomography was performed. The possibility of pulmonary embolism was excluded but a suspicion of interstitial/alveolar edema was set. A cardiac ultrasound detected left ventricular apical akinesia and ballooning with severely affected contractility sparing basic parts and ejection fraction ~20%. The patient was transferred to the coronary intensive care unit for further assessment. Emergency coronary angiography revealed no indication of stenosis. On left ventriculography, there were decreased apical contractility and balloon shape with contraction of basic parts. Ejection fraction was approximately 25%.

A diagnosis of Takotsubo cardiomyopathy was made according to Mayo Clinic diagnostic criteria [7]. For the next day, she remained severely dyspneic and unable to sustain normal SpO_2 with supplemental O_2. New chest X-ray was compatible with acute pulmonary edema. She received noninvasive mechanical ventilation in order to decrease preload and afterload of the left ventricle and to alleviate work of breathing. Drug therapy was initiated (furosemide 10 mg × 3, carvedilol 6,25 mg × 2, and bromazepam 1.5 mg × 3). A rhythm Holter was applied with no complex ventricular arrhythmogenesis. Within the following six days, troponin levels normalized as well as left ventricular systolic performance (ejection fraction reached 50%) on consecutive ultrasounds. The patient was transferred to the cardiology department and was discharged in good physical status seven days later with follow-up instructions.

3. Discussion

A case of TCM immediately after initiation of subarachnoid anesthesia for a minimally invasive urologic procedure is presented. Stress-induced cardiomyopathy has been previously reported to happen throughout the perioperative period as a result of an exaggerated adrenergic response to increased perioperative physical and emotional stress. Both increased circulating catecholamines and sympathetic outflow in cardiac nerve endings result in impaired myocardial perfusion, myocyte injury, and left ventricular outflow tract obstruction [3]. Regarding perioperative period, TCM has been identified immediately prior or during the induction of general anesthesia [8, 9], as well as intra- and postoperatively [10–14]. Perioperative pain and anxiety, light depth of anesthesia, and increased stress response to surgery have been identified as factors responsible for stress-induced cardiomyopathy. Regarding regional anesthesia, TCM has already been reported 15 min following subarachnoid anesthesia for caesarean section and our case is the second one in series [15].

These two case reports shed light on regional anesthesia as not "stress-free" anesthetic since an awake patient cannot always tolerate the emotional stress. Takotsubo cardiomyopathy in our patient was attributed to exaggerated preoperative anxiety. The latter should not be regarded as an innocent emotional state of surgical patients with minimal effect on actual physical status. Possibly, deteriorating mechanisms for the development of cardiomyopathy were the acute decrease of pre- and afterload of left ventricle and the stressful feeling of rapid ascending level of paralysis, in combination with the psychological background of the patient.

Premedication is no longer considered to prolong hospitalization for one-day adult surgery and such patients should not be denied anxiolytics [16]. It is well known that preoperative anxiety and catastrophizing are well correlated not only with the intensity of acute postsurgical pain but also with the development of chronic pain [17, 18]. Emotional stress consists also of an independent factor for arrhythmias and has been implicated for stress-related sudden cardiac death [19, 20]. Proper anxiolytic premedication before surgery also results in lower incidence of surgical site infection even up to 30 days after surgery due to decreased stress response [21]. The application of a proper protocol preoperatively, both pharmacological and nonpharmacological, including patient's training and behaviour modification, could affect outcome and even hospital length of stay [22]. There is no consensus regarding the most appropriate anesthetic management for patients with a prior history of stress-induced cardiomyopathy. Although relied on weak evidence, regional anesthesia is considered as the safest and most appropriate anesthetic technique for those patients [23].

4. Conclusion

A case of a patient who suffered stress-induced cardiomyopathy following subarachnoid anesthesia was presented. It is assumed that exaggerated preoperative anxiety, for which no premedication was given, caused a catecholaminergic storm state to the patient. Regional anesthesia, under certain circumstances, can be a quite harmful situation inducing an even higher adrenergic response. Management of preoperative anxiety, as an integral part of anesthetic practice, should target not only the patient's psychological comfort, but, most importantly, the prevention of possible cardiovascular and other complications related to it.

Acknowledgments

The authors would like to thank Mrs. D. Pantartzi, Scientific Secretary of the Clinical Trial Office of the Department of Urology, University of Crete, Medical School, Heraklion, Crete, Greece, for the administrative and technical support.

References

[1] H. Sato, H. Tateishi, and T. Uchida, *Clinical Aspect of Myocardial Injury: From Ischaemia to Heart Failure*, Kagakuhyouronsya, Tokyo, Japan, 1990.

[2] G. Parodi, S. Del Pace, N. Carrabba et al., "Incidence, Clinical Findings, and Outcome of Women With Left Ventricular Apical Ballooning Syndrome," *American Journal of Cardiology*, vol. 99, no. 2, pp. 182–185, 2007.

[3] E. A. Hessel and M. J. London, "Takotsubo (stress) cardiomyopathy and the anesthesiologist: Enough case reports. Let's try to answer some specific questions!," *Anesthesia and Analgesia*, vol. 110, no. 3, pp. 674–679, 2010.

[4] S. Liu and M. S. Dhamee, "Perioperative transient left ventricular apical ballooning syndrome: Takotsubo cardiomyopathy: a review," *Journal of Clinical Anesthesia*, vol. 22, no. 1, pp. 64–70, 2010.

[5] K. Komamura, M. Fukui, T. Iwasaku, S. Hirotani, and T. Masuyama, "Takotsubo cardiomyopathy: pathophysiology, diagnosis and treatment," *World Journal of Cardiology*, vol. 6, no. 7, pp. 602–609, 2014.

[6] J. P. Desborough, "The stress response to trauma and surgery," *British Journal of Anaesthesia*, vol. 85, no. 1, pp. 109–117, 2000.

[7] S. Kawai, A. Kitabatake, H. Tomoike et al., "Guidelines for diagnosis of takotsubo (Ampulla) cardiomyopathy," *Circulation Journal*, vol. 71, no. 6, pp. 990–992, 2007.

[8] A. K. Wong, W. J. Vernick, S. E. Wiegers, J. A. Howell, and A. C. Sinha, "Preoperative takotsubo cardiomyopathy identified in the operating room before induction of anesthesia," *Anesthesia and Analgesia*, vol. 110, no. 3, pp. 712–715, 2010.

[9] M. Jabaudon, M. Bonnin, F. Bolandard, S. Chanseaume, C. Dauphin, and J. E. Bazin, "Takotsubo syndrome during induction of general anaesthesia," *Anaesthesia*, vol. 62, no. 5, pp. 519–523, 2007.

[10] A. K. Tiwari and N. D'Attellis, "Intraoperative Left Ventricular Apical Ballooning: Transient Takotsubo Cardiomyopathy During Orthotopic Liver Transplantation," *Journal of Cardiothoracic and Vascular Anesthesia*, vol. 22, no. 3, pp. 442–445, 2008.

[11] F. Artukoglu, A. Owen, and T. M. Hemmerling, "Tako-Tsubo syndrome in an anaesthetised patient undergoing arthroscopic knee surgery," *Annals of cardiac anaesthesia*, vol. 11, no. 1, pp. 38–41, 2008.

[12] H. Itoh, Y. Miyake, I. Hioki, S. Tanaka, and M. Okabe, "Report of takotsubo cardiomyopathy occurring during cardiopulmonary bypass," *Journal of Extra-Corporeal Technology*, vol. 39, no. 2, pp. 109–111, 2007.

[13] M. Ide, Y. Esaki, K. Yamazaki, and H. Kato, "Newly developed T-wave inversion with cardiac wall-motion abnormality predominantly occurs in middle-aged or elderly women after noncardiac surgery," *Journal of Anesthesia*, vol. 17, no. 2, pp. 79–83, 2003.

[14] J. B. Jensen and J. F. Malouf, "Takotsubo cardiomyopathy following cholecystectomy: a poorly recognized cause of acute reversible left ventricular dysfunction," *International Journal of Cardiology*, vol. 106, no. 3, pp. 390-391, 2006.

[15] E. Crimi, A. Baggish, L. Leffert, M. C. M. Pian-Smith, J. L. Januzzi, and Y. Jiang, "Acute reversible stress-induced cardiomyopathy associated with cesarean delivery under spinal anesthesia," *Circulation*, vol. 117, no. 23, pp. 3052-3053, 2008.

[16] K. J. Walker and A. F. Smith, "Premedication for anxiety in adult day surgery," *Cochrane Database of Systematic Reviews*, vol. 7, no. 4, Article ID CD002192, 2009.

[17] M. Sobol-Kwapinska, P. Bąbel, W. Plotek, and B. Stelcer, "Psychological correlates of acute postsurgical pain: A systematic review and meta-analysis," *European Journal of Pain (United Kingdom)*, vol. 20, no. 10, pp. 1573–1586, 2016.

[18] M. Theunissen, M. L. Peters, J. Bruce, H.-F. Gramke, and M. A. Marcus, "Preoperative anxiety and catastrophizing: a systematic review and meta-analysis of the association with chronic postsurgical pain," *Clinical Journal of Pain*, vol. 28, no. 9, pp. 819–841, 2012.

[19] R. C. Ziegelstein, "Acute emotional stress and cardiac arrhythmias," *The Journal of the American Medical Association*, vol. 298, no. 3, pp. 324–329, 2007.

[20] S. Graff, M. Fenger-Grøn, B. Christensen et al., "Long-term risk of atrial fibrillation after the death of a partner," *Open Heart*, vol. 3, no. 1, Article ID e000367, 2016.

[21] R. Levandovski, M. B. Cardoso Ferreira, M. P. Loayza Hidalgo, C. A. Konrath, D. Lemons da Silva, and W. Caumo, "Impact of preoperative anxiolytic on surgical site infection in patients undergoing abdominal hysterectomy," *American Journal of Infection Control*, vol. 36, no. 10, pp. 718–726, 2008.

[22] C. J. Wilson, A. J. Mitchelson, T. H. Tzeng et al., "Caring for the surgically anxious patient: a review of the interventions and a guide to optimizing surgical outcomes," *American Journal of Surgery*, vol. 212, no. 1, pp. 151–159, 2016.

[23] S. Liu, C. Bravo-Fernandez, C. Riedl, M. Antapli, and M. S. Dhamee, "Anesthetic Management of Takotsubo Cardiomyopathy: General Versus Regional Anesthesia," *Journal of Cardiothoracic and Vascular Anesthesia*, vol. 22, no. 3, pp. 438–441, 2008.

64

Pulmonary Edema and Diastolic Heart Failure in the Perioperative Period

Galen Royce-Nagel[1] and Kunal Karamchandani ⓘ [2]

[1]*Department of Anesthesia, Critical Care and Pain Medicine, Massachusetts General Hospital, Boston, MA, USA*
[2]*Department of Anesthesiology and Perioperative Medicine, Penn State Health Milton S. Hershey Medical Center, Hershey, PA, USA*

Correspondence should be addressed to Kunal Karamchandani; kkaramchandani@pennstatehealth.psu.edu

Academic Editor: Latha Hebbar

Heart failure with preserved ejection fraction (HFPEF) is a diagnosis encountered with increasing frequency in the aging population. We present a case of postoperative pulmonary edema in 63-year-old male with HFPEF. This patient highlights the gap in risk stratification with respect to diastolic heart failure.

1. Introduction

Heart failure with preserved ejection fraction (HFPEF), or diastolic heart failure (HF), refers to the clinical syndrome of HF coupled with evidence of diastolic dysfunction and is associated with significant mortality and morbidity [1]. The incidence of HFPEF has been variably described between 30 and 50% among patients with heart failure [2]. The goals of care for perioperative management of these patients include maintenance of adequate preload, slower heart rate to accommodate for adequate diastolic filling time, and avoidance of hypertension to decrease the afterload to the left ventricle. The association of acute myocardial infarction with perioperative HFPEF is rare but can have disastrous consequences. We describe the case of acute HFPEF presenting as a harbinger of myocardial infarction in the perioperative period.

2. Case Description

A 63-year-old male, weighing 82 kg (BMI 28), was scheduled for abdominoperineal resection (APR) and right partial hepatectomy for metastatic colon cancer. His past medical history was significant for hypertension, recently diagnosed non-insulin dependent diabetes, a cerebral vascular accident 9

years prior to surgery, an 80-pack year smoking history (quit 20 years prior to surgery), and an episode of acute congestive heart failure with preserved ejection fraction approximately one year before surgery.

At preoperative evaluation, the patient described his functional capacity as excellent (able to climb 2 flights of stairs multiple times a day with no symptoms; worked more than 60 hrs. a week as a mechanic) and denied any symptoms of HF. The physical examination did not reveal any signs of congestive heart failure. Transthoracic echocardiogram (TTE) showed normal left ventricular (LV) size and function (EF of 55%) and no significant valvular pathology. Since the patient was scheduled for an intermediate risk surgery, had no active cardiac conditions, and had good functional capacity, a decision was made to proceed with surgery without further work-up based on guidelines established by the American College of Cardiology and the American Heart association (ACC/AHA).

General anesthesia was induced with propofol and maintained with isoflurane plus an air-oxygen mixture of equal parts. Standard ASA monitors were applied along with invasive hemodynamic monitoring using a right radial arterial line. Patient had a preexisting tunneled central venous catheter that was accessed and 2 large bore IVs were inserted for intravenous access. He received muscle relaxation with intermittent doses of intravenous (i.v.) rocuronium titrated to keep the train of four to less than 2 twitches. He received a total of 2 mg i.v. hydromorphone in divided doses and 1000 mg of i.v. acetaminophen for analgesia.

The surgery lasted approximately eight hours. His estimated blood loss was 400 ml and urine output was 300 ml. He received 7 liters of crystalloid and 1 liter of albumin. His intraoperative fluid management was guided by measurement of stroke volume variation (SVV) via Vigileo™, serum lactate levels, and urine output. He received fluid boluses to keep the SVV less than 13, lactate levels less than 2 mg dl^{-1}, and urine output greater than 0.5 ml kg^{-1} per hour. He remained hemodynamically stable throughout the surgery. He did not have any significant electrolyte abnormalities as determined by hourly arterial blood gases (ABGs) during the surgery. The patient's trachea was extubated at the end of the procedure after ensuring adequate reversal of neuromuscular blockade and responsiveness to commands.

Immediately after extubation, he developed hypertension and tachycardia with a high blood pressure of 273/100 mm Hg and heart rate ranging between 120 and 130 beats/minute. His oxygen saturation declined to a low of 89% despite supplemental oxygen and airway recruitment maneuvers. He progressively became agitated and less responsive. Pink frothy sputum was noted upon suctioning of his oropharynx. The patient's trachea was promptly reintubated, and 20 mg of i.v. furosemide was given. He was then transferred to the surgical intensive care unit for further management.

The immediate postoperative chest X-ray revealed bilateral vascular congestion. The electrocardiograph (ECG) showed nonspecific inferior lead changes without ST elevations. The serial troponin I levels were obtained and peaked at 0.5 ng ml^{-1} (normal < 0.12). He received an additional dose of i.v. furosemide and over the next 12 hours his respiratory status improved. After meeting all the necessary criteria, his trachea was extubated. His home doses of aspirin, atorvastatin, and metoprolol were restarted. A repeat TTE done on postoperative day 1 (POD 1) showed an ejection fraction of 60% without any wall motion abnormalities. Despite this, he had another episode of acute pulmonary edema on POD 1 followed by atrial fibrillation (AF) with rapid ventricular response (RVR). He was successfully treated with noninvasive continuous positive airway pressure (CPAP) of 5 cm H$_2$O and a dose i.v. furosemide for acute pulmonary edema. For his AF with RVR, he received intermittent doses of i.v. metoprolol to achieve rate control with a target heart rate of <100 beats/minute. His dose of oral metoprolol was also increased from 25 mg every 12 hours to 50 mg every 12 hours.

On POD 4, he developed a third episode of respiratory distress with minimal response to diuretics and antihypertensives. His ECG now showed ST elevations in anterior and inferior leads and his troponin I level was 0.74. He underwent emergent cardiac catheterization with placement of two bare metal stents in the mid-left anterior descending and left circumflex vessels for 80% and 85% occlusion, respectively. The remainder of his hospital course was uneventful and he was discharged home on POD 12.

3. Discussion

Our patient with postoperative pulmonary edema due to HFPEF serves to highlight a gap in preoperative risk stratification. He attended our preoperative clinic but due to his excellent functional status and resolved HF did not meet criteria for further work-up. The combination of significant fluid shifts and the hyperadrenergic state associated with perioperative stress unmasked his true cardiac deficit with resultant episodes of pulmonary edema. In reflection, is there anything more that could have been done to recognize his increased risk for cardiac complications?

HFPEF is a well-described entity with prevalence ranging from 1.1 to 1.5% [3]. Studies have reported mixed results for perioperative risk in patients with HF and preserved LVEF [4]. In a recent meta-analysis, patients with HFPEF had a lower all-cause mortality rate than did those with HF and reduced LVEF [5]. However, the absolute mortality rate was still high in patients with HF and preserved LVEF as compared with patients without HF. There is limited data on perioperative risk stratification related to diastolic dysfunction and perioperative HFPEF has traditionally been underestimated and not well described in literature.

The American College of Cardiology and the American Heart association (ACC/AHA) as well as the European Society of Cardiology and European Society of Anesthesiology (ESC/ESA) guidelines recommend the use of risk indices for preoperative cardiac evaluation for noncardiac surgery [4, 6]. The commonly used indices, Goldman, Detsky, and Revised Cardiac Risk Index (RCRI), all include HF as an independent prognostic variable [7–9]. Although a history of HF is considered a significant risk for perioperative complications, there is no recommendation for further cardiac testing in patients who are asymptomatic with good functional status [4]. When patients with a prior episode of decompensated HF who improve both symptomatically and functionally on medical therapy present for elective surgery several months later, as our patient did, the perioperative risk calculated comes out markedly low and does not warrant further testing.

Although a goal directed fluid management strategy was chosen for our patient, we believe that the fluid administration was slightly excessive and in hindsight should have been curtailed. The significant fluid shifts associated with such a major surgical procedure along with the mild tachycardia and hypertension experienced during emergence from anesthesia may have contributed to his initial episode of acute pulmonary edema. Conditions unique to the immediate postoperative period such as pain-induced sympathetic activation, shivering, anemia, hypovolemia, and hypoxia may alter the myocardial oxygen balance [10] and further predispose patients with diastolic dysfunction to an episode of acute diastolic HF.

The cardiac catheterization findings in our patient were quite significant despite a seemingly normal TTE. Coronary artery disease is present in 40–55% of patients with diastolic HF [11]. The first abnormality induced by epicardial ischemia is reduced ventricular compliance, not wall motion abnormality, ECG changes, or chest pain [12]. Therefore, patients presenting with acute diastolic HF without clinical or ECG evidence of myocardial ischemia may still have significant angiographic ischemic heart disease [13]. Delay to diagnosis of coronary artery disease for our patient was likely due to his normal preoperative exercise tolerance, a clinical picture of postoperative fluid overload, the mild increase in troponin I levels, and a normal postoperative ECG and TTE.

HFPEF is a category of heart failure that is poorly defined and therefore poorly understood. Development of validated preoperative risk indices that focus on this entity would be valuable in the management of our increasingly at risk population. Our patient's clinical course highlights the importance of keeping diastolic dysfunction high on the differential despite preoperative presentation. It also stresses the possibility of perioperative HFPEF presenting as a harbinger of acute myocardial infarction.

References

[1] A. Kovacs, Z. Papp, and L. Nagy, "Causes and pathophysiology of heart failure with preserved ejection fraction," *Heart Failure Clinics*, vol. 10, no. 3, pp. 389–398, 2014.

[2] C. S. P. Lam, E. Donal, E. Kraigher-Krainer, and R. S. Vasan, "Epidemiology and clinical course of heart failure with preserved ejection fraction," *European Journal of Heart Failure*, vol. 13, no. 1, pp. 18–28, 2011.

[3] T. A. Gelzinis, "New insights into diastolic dysfunction and heart failure with preserved ejection fraction," *Seminars in Cardiothoracic and Vascular Anesthesia*, vol. 18, no. 2, pp. 208–217, 2014.

[4] L. A. Fleisher, K. E. Fleischmann, A. D. Auerbach et al., "ACC/AHA guideline on perioperative cardiovascular evaluation and management of patients undergoing noncardiac surgery: a report of the American College of Cardiology/American Heart Association Task Force on practice guidelines," *Journal of the American College of Cardiology*, vol. 64, no. 22, pp. e77–137, 2014.

[5] Meta-analysis Global Group in Chronic Heart Failure (MAG-GIC), "The survival of patients with heart failure with preserved or reduced left ventricular ejection fraction: an individual patient data meta-analysis," *European Heart Journal*, vol. 33, no. 14, pp. 1750–1757, 2012.

[6] Task Force for Preoperative Cardiac Risk A, Perioperative Cardiac Management in Non-cardiac S, European Society of C et al., "Guidelines for pre-operative cardiac risk assessment and perioperative cardiac management in non-cardiac surgery," *European Heart Journal*, vol. 30, no. 22, pp. 2769–2812, 2009.

[7] A. S. Detsky, H. B. Abrams, J. R. McLaughlin et al., "Predicting cardiac complications in patients undergoing non-cardiac surgery," *Journal of General Internal Medicine*, vol. 1, no. 4, pp. 211–219, 1986.

[8] L. Goldman, D. L. Caldera, S. R. Nussbaum et al., "Multifactorial index of cardiac risk in noncardiac surgical procedures," *The New England Journal of Medicine*, vol. 297, no. 16, pp. 845–850, 1977.

[9] T. H. Lee, E. R. Marcantonio, C. M. Mangione et al., "Derivation and prospective validation of a simple index for prediction of cardiac risk of major noncardiac surgery," *Circulation*, vol. 100, no. 10, pp. 1043–1049, 1999.

[10] R. Pirracchio, B. Cholley, S. De Hert, A. C. Solal, and A. Mebazaa, "Diastolic heart failure in anaesthesia and critical care," *British Journal of Anaesthesia*, vol. 98, no. 6, pp. 707–721, 2007.

[11] T. E. Vanhecke, R. Kim, S. Z. Raheem, and P. A. McCullough, "Myocardial ischemia in patients with diastolic dysfunction and heart failure," *Current Cardiology Reports*, vol. 12, no. 3, pp. 216–222, 2010.

[12] R. Maharaj, "Diastolic dysfunction and heart failure with a preserved ejection fraction: Relevance in critical illness and anaesthesia," *Journal of the Saudi Heart Association*, vol. 24, no. 2, pp. 99–121, 2012.

[13] S. Arques, P. Ambrosi, R. Gelisse, E. Roux, M. Lambert, and G. Habib, "Prevalence of angiographic coronary artery disease in patients hospitalized for acute diastolic heart failure without clinical and electrocardiographic evidence of myocardial ischemia on admission," *American Journal of Cardiology*, vol. 94, no. 1, pp. 133–135, 2004.

65

Management of Anesthesia under Extracorporeal Cardiopulmonary Support in an Infant with Severe Subglottic Stenosis

Rie Soeda,[1] Fumika Taniguchi,[1] Maiko Sawada,[1] Saeko Hamaoka,[1] Masayuki Shibasaki,[1] Yasufumi Nakajima,[2] Satoru Hashimoto,[3] Teiji Sawa,[1] and Yoshinobu Nakayama[1]

[1]Department of Anesthesiology, Kyoto Prefectural University of Medicine, 465 Kajii-cho, Kamigyo, Kyoto 602-8566, Japan
[2]Department of Anesthesiology, Kansai Medical University, 2-5-1 Shin-machi, Hirakata, Osaka 573-1010, Japan
[3]Division of Critical Care, Kyoto Prefectural University of Medicine Hospital, 465 Kajii-cho, Kamigyo, Kyoto 602-8566, Japan

Correspondence should be addressed to Teiji Sawa; anesth@koto.kpu-m.ac.jp

Academic Editor: Ilok Lee

A 4-month-old female infant who weighed 3.57 kg with severe subglottic stenosis underwent tracheostomy under extracorporeal cardiopulmonary support. First, we set up extracorporeal cardiopulmonary support to the infant and then successfully intubated an endotracheal tube with a 2.5 mm inner diameter before tracheostomy by otolaryngologists. Extracorporeal cardiopulmonary support is an alternative for maintenance of oxygenation in difficult airway management in infants.

1. Introduction

We experienced difficult airway management under extracorporeal cardiopulmonary support in an infant with severe subglottic stenosis. An algorithm of difficult airway management for infants with subglottic stenosis should effectively include extracorporeal cardiopulmonary support. This support includes cardiopulmonary bypass (CPB) and/or extracorporeal membrane oxygenation (ECMO) to maintain blood gas exchange during insecure tracheal intubation and difficult tracheostomy in infants with subglottic airway stenosis.

2. Case Presentation

A 4-month-old female infant, who weighed 3.57 kg and was 54.6 cm in height, was hospitalized because of the diagnosis of severe subglottic stenosis. At birth, she was diagnosed with 22q11.2 deletion syndrome with multiple anomalies, including thymic aplasia, aortic arch interruption, ventricular septal defect, atrial septal defect, and subvalvular aortic stenosis. Eight days after birth, when she weighed 2.77 kg and was 46 cm in height, she had surgery of the right pulmonary artery banding under general anesthesia. This anesthesia management allowed easy intubation (Cormack-Lehane Grade I) with a cuffed endotracheal tube (3.0 mm inner diameter (ID)). She was extubated at the pediatric intensive care unit (PICU) without any complications the next day after surgery. Three weeks later, she had secondary radical surgery of the aortic arch and intracardiac repair under general anesthesia with intubation with a cuffed endotracheal tube (3.0 mm ID) without any problems. After the second surgery, she was under artificial ventilation in the PICU. On the 5th postsurgical day, she was extubated and placed under bubble continuous positive airway pressure (bCPAP). However, after extubation, she had stridor in her respiration and had difficulty weaning from bCPAP for the next 3 days. At the 7th postsurgical day, an otolaryngologist performed nasolaryngeal optical fiberscopy, and she was diagnosed with right vocal cord paralysis. Six weeks after surgery, she was discharged from the hospital and was placed at home care. However, 6 weeks after discharge, at 4 months old, she was rehospitalized because of respiratory distress with the constriction situation at the time of crying and reduced suckling force at breastfeeding. Blood arterial gas analysis showed hyper apnea and metabolic alkalosis as

(a)

(b)

Subglottic stenosis

(c)

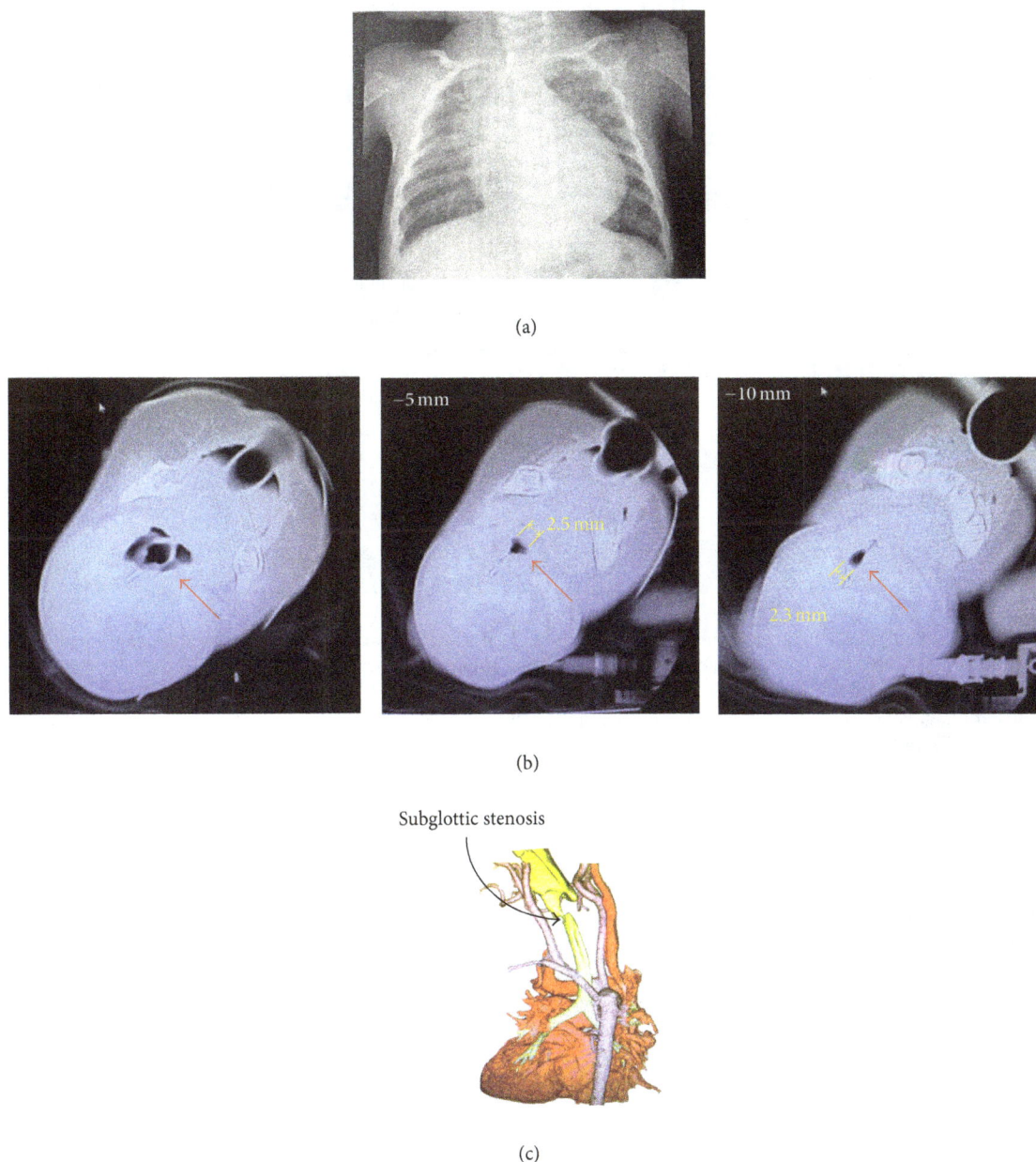

FIGURE 1: Chest X-ray posterior-anterior view and computed tomographic images. (a) Chest X-ray posterior-anterior (PA) view. (b) Computed tomographic (CT) images of the neck region (every 5 mm). Left panel: level of the larynx. Center panel: −5 mm from the level of the larynx. Right panel: −10 mm from the level of the larynx. (c) Three-dimensional CT reconstruction image of the larynx and vessels. The arrow shows subglottic stenosis.

follows: pH, 7.45; PaO_2, 67.8 mmHg; $PaCO_2$, 54.9 mmHg; base excess, 11.7; lactate level, 1.0 mEq/L; and SaO_2, 95.4% at room air. Severe subglottic stenosis with an estimated diameter of 2.3–2.5 mm in the narrowest portion of her larynx was diagnosed by computed tomography (Figure 1). Emergent tracheostomy was then planned under general anesthesia, and the method of induction of anesthesia was discussed.

Because the patient just maintained spontaneous ventilation with depression of epigastric intercostal, there was a high risk of "cannot intubate cannot ventilate" during induction of anesthesia under the method of being either awake or anesthetized during induction. Therefore, in advance of the procedure of tracheal intubation, we decided to keep her under spontaneous ventilation and performed extracorporeal cardiopulmonary support under regional anesthesia with light sedation (Figure 2). Venoarterial extracorporeal cardiopulmonary support with cannulation by the open cut method was performed by cardiac surgeons in case of resuscitation with cardiac support. She was sedated with dexmedetomidine (0.7 μg/kg/h), ketamine 1.0 mg (0.5 mg, 2 shots), and midazolam 0.2 mg (0.1 mg, twice). Total heparinization followed

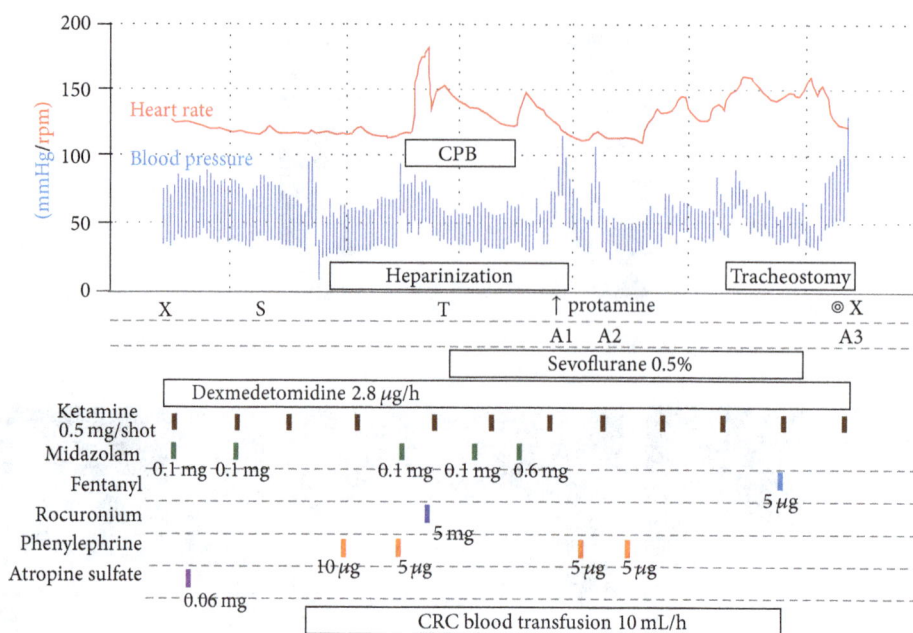

FIGURE 2: Time course of anesthesia management under extracorporeal cardiopulmonary support and the following tracheostomy. X: start and end of anesthesia management. S: start of surgery for extracorporeal cardiopulmonary support. T: tracheal intubation. Arterial blood gas data were measured at A1, A2, and A3. A1: pH, 7.46; $PaCO_2$, 36.8 mmHg; PaO_2, 240 mmHg; base excess, 2.4 mmol/L; and SaO_2, 100%. A2: pH, 7.39; $PaCO_2$, 46.8 mmHg; PaO_2, 118 mmHg; base excess, 2.8 mmol/L; and SaO_2, 99%. A3: pH, 7.49; $PaCO_2$, 33.3 mmHg; PaO_2, 509 mmHg; base excess, 2.9 mmol/L; and SaO_2, 100%.

by arterial and venous cannulation of the extracorporeal circuit to the right femoral artery and right femoral vein was then performed under local anesthesia with 1% lidocaine (1.7 mL). Additional administration of ketamine (0.5 mg, 2 shots) and midazolam (0.1 mg, once) was performed after the extracorporeal circuit was started and oxygenation of arterial blood was attained by evaluation using pulse oximetry. Semi-awake tracheal intubation was carried out with an uncuffed endotracheal tube (2.5 mm ID). Although slight resistance was felt at the time the tip of the endotracheal tube passed through the narrowest region of the subglottis, the tube was successfully placed in an appropriate position with a depth of 8.5 cm from the infant's mouth. A total of 5 mg rocuronium bromide was administered intravenously and respiration of the patient was under the control of positive airway pressure ventilation. Ten minutes after tracheal intubation, extracorporeal cardiopulmonary support was stopped and decannulation and neutralization of heparin with protamine were carried out. Tracheostomy was successfully performed by an otolaryngologist in the next 20 min. The anesthesia time was 3 hours and 8 minutes and the extracorporeal cardiopulmonary support time was 19 minutes. The patient was admitted to the PICU for postoperative management.

3. Discussion

For more than 50 years, anesthesia management of an infant who has subglottic stenosis has been discussed [1–3]. Although subglottic stenosis can occur in all age groups, pediatric cases can be pathophysiologically divided into two categories, which are congenital and acquired. Our patient was diagnosed with 22q11.2 deletion syndrome (22q11.2DS), which is also known as DiGeorge syndrome, DiGeorge anomaly, and velocardiofacial syndrome. This syndrome is caused by deletion of a small piece of chromosome 22 with five typical symptoms, such as cardiac defects, abnormal facies, thymic hypoplasia, cleft palate, and hypocalcemia [4, 5]. In our case, radical repair of aortic arch interruption probably caused right vocal cord paralysis due to recurrent nerve injury, which was eventually associated with the occurrence of acquired subglottic stenosis.

Various research groups have proposed guidelines or an algorithm for difficult airway management in pediatrics [6–9]. Among them, the pediatric difficult airway guidelines by the Guidelines Group, which is supported by the Association of Paediatric Anaesthetists, the Difficult Airway Society, are the most popular [7–9]. Three guidelines relate to the management of a difficult airway in children aged 1 to 8 years as follows: APA1 is difficult mask ventilation during routine induction of anesthesia; APA2 is unanticipated difficult tracheal intubation during routine induction of anesthesia; and APA3 is cannot intubate cannot ventilate in paralyzed, anesthetized patients. However, these guidelines are for patients aged older than 1 year, and difficult airway cases in pediatrics frequently occur under 1 year of age. Recently, we experienced three different infant cases with difficult airway management, including this case. One case was a newborn who had large tumors extruding out of his mouth and mask ventilation was difficult to perform in induction of anesthesia [10]. Another case was a girl with a malignant rhabdoid tumor in her oral

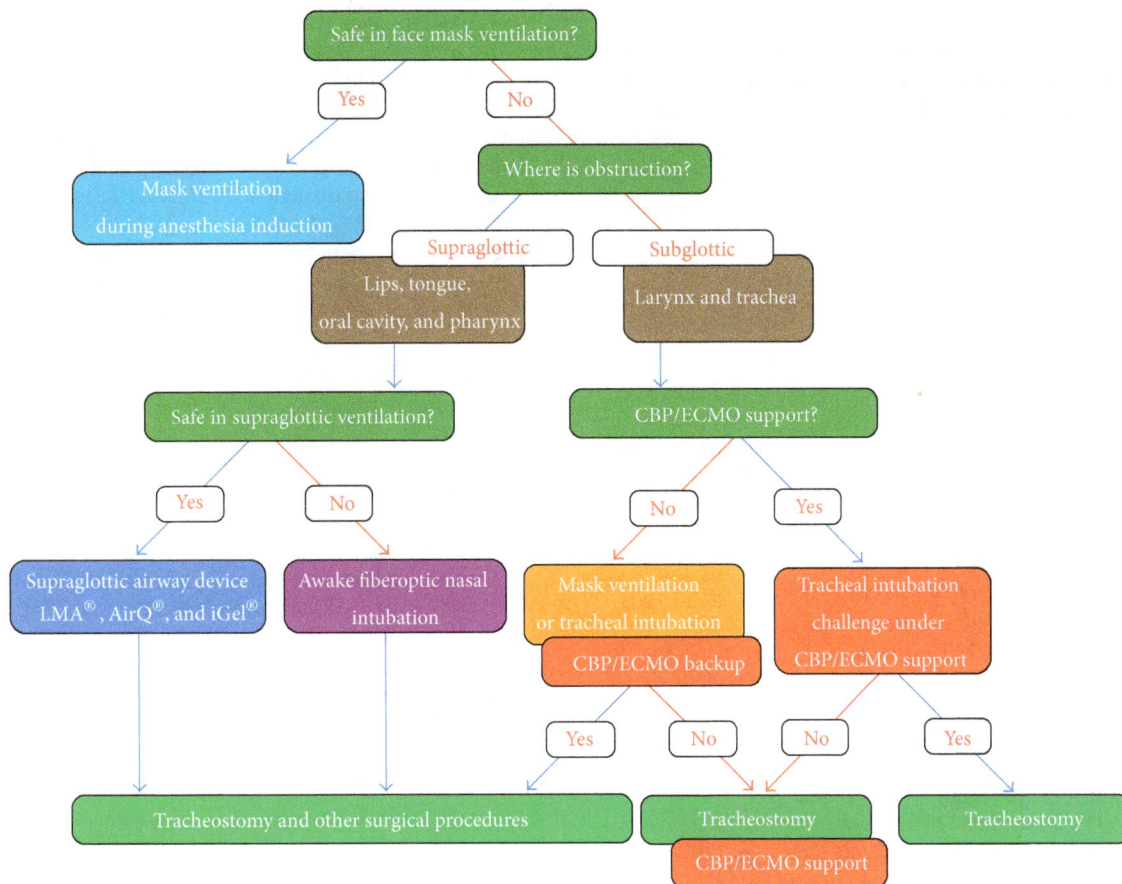

FIGURE 3: Algorithm for anticipated difficult airway management for infants. Supraglottic airway devices and awake nasal fiberoptic intubation, as well as extracorporeal cardiopulmonary support or extracorporeal cardiopulmonary backup support, are incorporated into the algorithm.

cavity and she was difficult to intubate through oral access [11]. Therefore, guidance or an algorithm for management of a difficult airway in children aged younger than 1 year is required separately from the currently available guidelines for patients who are aged older than 1 year.

During induction of anesthesia for tracheostomy in a pediatric subglottic stenosis patient, gas exchange can be maintained in one of five ways [12]: (1) jet ventilation, (2) distal tracheal intubation and intermittent positive pressure ventilation, (3) spontaneous ventilation, (4) mask ventilation (and tracheal intubation) under backup support of extracorporeal cardiopulmonary, including CPB and ECMO, and (5) intubation challenge (and tracheostomy) under CPB or ECMO support. CPB and ECMO, both of which can be a life-saving maneuver for near or total occlusion of the airway, have been used for tracheal surgery [13–16]. Tracheostomy in infants with subglottic stenosis is a challenging approach, even for experienced otolaryngologists [17, 18]. In addition, because there is a potential risk of excessive bleeding due to anticoagulation requirements, tracheostomy should be performed only after establishment of an airway on induction under the support (or the backup support)

of these devices. In our case, tracheal intubation was safely carried out under the support of CPB. After CPB was terminated and anticoagulation was neutralized, tracheostomy was performed under safe conditions to avoid the risk of bleeding at the surgical site. Instead of tracheal intubation challenge under the direct support of CPB, mask ventilation or tracheal intubation challenge under backup support of CPB for emergent oxygenation was an alternative choice in the airway management of this case. However, in this case, we chose a safer oxygenation strategy because the good support of an experienced pediatric cardiac surgery team was available in our facility. We think that, regardless of direct support or backup support, CPB and/or ECMO should be incorporated into the algorithm of anticipated difficult airway management for infants as an alternative procedure (Figure 3).

In conclusion, under extracorporeal cardiopulmonary support, we successfully managed anesthesia for tracheostomy in an infant with severe subglottic stenosis. CPB and/or ECMO should be incorporated into the algorithm of anticipated difficult airway management for infants.

Acknowledgments

The authors would like to thank Drs. Yoichiro Sugiyama and Ryuichi Hirota, Assistant Professors, Department of Otolaryngology, and Dr. Masaaki Yamagishi, Hospital Professor, Department of Pediatric Cardiovascular Surgery, Kyoto Prefectural University of Medicine, for their technical assistance with tracheostomy.

References

[1] F. J. Colgan and A. S. Keats, "Subglottic stenosis: a cause of difficult intubation," *Anesthesiology*, vol. 18, no. 2, pp. 265–269, 1957.

[2] K. Sato, T. Horiguchi, and T. Nishikawa, "Unsuspected subglottic stenosis in a 5-year-old scheduled for elective surgery," *Journal of Clinical Anesthesia*, vol. 17, no. 6, pp. 470–472, 2005.

[3] J. Belanger and M. Kossick, "Methods of identifying and managing the difficult airway in the pediatric population," *Journal of the American Association of Nurse Anesthetists*, vol. 83, no. 1, pp. 35–41, 2015.

[4] A. Swillen, A. Vogels, K. Devriendt, and J. P. Fryns, "Chromosome 22q11 deletion syndrome: update and review of the clinical features, cognitive-behavioral spectrum, and psychiatric complications," *American Journal of Medical Genetics*, vol. 97, no. 2, pp. 128–135, 2000.

[5] D. M. McDonald-Mcginn and K. E. Sullivan, "Chromosome 22q11.2 deletion syndrome (DiGeorge syndrome/velocardiofacial syndrome)," *Medicine*, vol. 90, no. 1, pp. 1–18, 2011.

[6] P. C. E. Marin and T. Engelhardt, "Algorithm for difficult airway management in pediatrics," *Colombian Journal of Anesthesiology*, vol. 42, no. 4, pp. 325–324, 2014.

[7] The Guidelines Group, The Association of Paediatric Anaesthetists, and The Difficult Airway Society, "Difficult mask ventilation during routine induction of anaesthesia in a child aged 1 to 8 years," September 2015, https://www.das.uk.com/guidelines/paediatric-difficult-airway-guidelines.

[8] The Guidelines Group, the Association of Paediatric Anaesthetists, the Difficult Airway Society, "Unanticipated difficult tracheal intubation during routine induction of anaesthesia in a child aged 1 to 8 years", 2015, https://www.das.uk.com/guidelines/paediatric-difficult-airway-guidelines.

[9] The Guidelines Group, The Association of Paediatric Anaesthetists, and The Difficult Airway Society, "Cannot intubate and cannot ventilate (CICV) in a paralysed anaesthetised child aged 1 to 8 years," 2015, https://www.das.uk.com/guidelines/paediatric-difficult-airway-guidelines.

[10] C. Hasegawa, S. Maeda, K. Kageyama, M. Shibasaki, Y. Nakajima, and T. Sawa, "Anesthesia induction using the Air-Q™ supraglottic airway device in a neonate with suspected difficulty of facemask ventilation due to large oral tumor masses," *EC Anaesthesia*, vol. 2, no. 1, pp. 52–55, 2015.

[11] A. Tatsuno, H. Katoh, F. Taniguchi et al., "Awake fiberoptic nasal intubation in an infant with a malignant rhabdoid tumor occupying the oral cavity: a case report," *Journal of Anesthesiology and Clinical Science*, vol. 4, no. 3, pp. 52–55, 2015.

[12] J. George III and D. J. Doyle, "Anesthesia for the management of subglottic stenosis and tracheal resection," in *Anesthesia for Otolaryngologic Surgery*, B. Abdelmalak and D. J. Doyle, Eds., pp. 263–270, Cambridge University Press, Cambridge, UK, 2nd edition, 2012.

[13] C. L. Chiu, B. T. Teh, and C. Y. Wang, "Temporary cardiopulmonary bypass and isolated lung ventilation for tracheal stenosis and reconstruction," *British Journal of Anaesthesia*, vol. 91, no. 5, pp. 742–744, 2003.

[14] R. C. DeWitt and C. H. Hallman, "Use of cardiopulmonary bypass for tracheal resection: a case report," *Texas Heart Institute Journal*, vol. 31, no. 2, pp. 188–190, 2004.

[15] D. Valencia, D. Overman, R. Tibesar, T. Lander, F. Moga, and J. Sidman, "Surgical management of distal tracheal stenosis in children," *Laryngoscope*, vol. 121, no. 12, pp. 2665–2671, 2011.

[16] H. Gao, B. Zhu, J. Yi, T.-H. Ye, and Y.-G. Huang, "Urgent tracheal resection and reconstruction assisted by temporary cardiopulmonary bypass: a case report," *Chinese Medical Sciences Journal*, vol. 28, no. 1, pp. 55–57, 2013.

[17] R. T. Cotton and C. M. Myer III, "Contemporary surgical management of laryngeal stenosis in children," *American Journal of Otolaryngology—Head and Neck Medicine and Surgery*, vol. 5, no. 5, pp. 360–368, 1984.

[18] D. C. Brodner and J. L. Guarisco, "Subglottic stenosis: evaluation and management," *The Journal of the Louisiana State Medical Society*, vol. 151, no. 4, pp. 159–164, 1999.

In-Flight Hypoxemia in a Tracheostomy-Dependent Infant

Jason Quevreaux and Christopher Cropsey

Department of Anesthesiology, Educational Affairs, Vanderbilt University Medical Center, 2301 VUH, Nashville, TN 37232-7237, USA

Correspondence should be addressed to Jason Quevreaux; jason.m.quevreaux@vanderbilt.edu

Academic Editor: Richard Riley

Millions of passengers board commercial flights every year. Healthcare providers are often called upon to treat other passengers during in-flight emergencies. The case presented involves an anesthesia resident treating a tracheostomy-dependent infant who developed hypoxemia on a domestic flight. The patient had an underlying congenital muscular disorder and was mechanically ventilated while at altitude. Although pressurized, cabin barometric pressure while at altitude is less than at sea level. Due to this environment patients with underlying pulmonary or cardiac pathology might not be able to tolerate commercial flight. The Federal Aviation Administration (FAA) has mandated a specific set of medical supplies be present on all domestic flights in addition to legislature protecting "Good Samaritan" providers.

1. Introduction

According to the US Department of Transportation, domestic airlines transported 696 million passengers in 2015 [1]. This represented a 5% increase in passengers from 2014. Peterson et al., using flight data taken from 7 million domestic and international flights, found that in-flight medical emergencies resulting in a call to ground-based health providers occurred in 1 in 604 flights [2]. As passenger load is projected to increase in the near future it is reasonable to assume the number of in-flight emergencies will increase as well. The most common causes of in-flight emergency were presyncope/syncope followed by respiratory compromise [2]. Often passengers who are in health-related fields are called upon to render care during these emergencies. The process of flying can be very physically challenging to patients with prior health problems. Passengers often have long walks between terminals or from ground transport, and they frequently have heavy luggage to carry. In addition, they may have limited access to their prescription medicines in-flight. The Aerospace Medical Association recommends preflight assessment of passengers for whom flight might exacerbate underlying pathology. This includes recognizing unstable cardiac, pulmonary, or other disease processes [3]. This however does not preclude the incidence of an acute event.

2. Case Report

While traveling as a passenger at a cruising altitude of 36,000 ft, an overhead page went out calling for medical personnel. The author responded to this call. The patient was a 12-month-old male with a tracheostomy tube attached to the portable ventilator his mother had brought on the plane. Also present were a portable suction device, a portable nebulizer, and a portable monitor showing a pulse oximetry reading of 80%. The resident quickly assessed the situation and introduced himself and his qualifications to both the flight attendants present and the patient's family.

A history was gathered from the mother and was significant for an unknown congenital muscular dystrophy rendering poor resting tone and difficulty with self-ventilation. The patient had no known congenital heart issues and no known allergies as per the mother. The child was tracheostomy-dependent and was regularly seen by a pulmonologist. Of note the child was seen by the pulmonologist recently and deemed fit-to-fly. As per the family, because of the muscular disorder the child's lungs were not well functioning, but no additional details could be provided. At home the patient largely tolerated room air without the need for ventilator support. He primarily needed to be mechanically ventilated during nighttime hours or while asleep. His mother reported normal resting oxygen saturations ($SpO_2 > 96\%$)

at baseline. The child was initially on room air unsupported when boarding the plane, but as the plane reached terminal altitude the patient's saturation had deteriorated. The mother placed the child on a pressure support mode without oxygen supplementation. Another responder had attempted to fit one of the airline's portable oxygen cylinders to the machine without success. The mother had attempted an albuterol nebulizer and tracheal suctioning; however, there were no secretions and the oxygen saturation remained low.

Although required to be present on all domestic flights in the United States a stethoscope was unable to be found by the cabin staff; ear-to-chest auscultation and thoracic palpation revealed a symmetrically expanding chest without evidence of obstruction to air movement. The oxygen inflow for the ventilator did not match the outflow from the portable oxygen tanks provided by the airline. Additionally there was not a way to use the auxiliary oxygen supply (the supply providing oxygen to the emergency drop down masks). By utilizing a makeshift design of tape, supplemental oxygen was able to be delivered to the ventilator which resulted in improvement of the SpO_2 to >90%. As the author was unfamiliar with the type of ventilator the mother had brought, and there was no display to show volumes delivered or returned, he asked the mother to continue to utilize only the settings that she used at home. This was done to minimize the risk of either barotrauma or volutrauma; the mother had been educated by the child's pulmonologist on this specific ventilator and thus had training in its operation.

While initially stabilized, the child began to have desaturation again on descent of the aircraft. The resident checked the tracheostomy tube and realized that the cuff had not been inflated on boarding the flight or on initiation of mechanical support. At this time it was also noted that the child was ventilating with a fair amount of air from his mouth. The cuff was inflated with a few milliliters of air that resulted in an increase in oxygen saturation. However, concordantly with this, palpable crackles began on thoracic excursion. The tracheostomy tube was again suctioned with mild increase in secretions. Oxygen saturations remained >90% throughout this time. The plane landed shortly after and the child was taken to a waiting, on-ground EMS team. The team was informed of the situation and the child was taken to a local hospital for further workup and treatment.

The differential generated included ventilator deficit such as patient fatigue or mucus plugging, negative pressure pulmonary edema, oxygenation deficit due to intrinsic lung disease, resorption atelectasis from high F_iO_2 (during the second desaturation event), intracardiac shunting, thrombotic or embolic event, and malfunctioning equipment. An additional concern would be the decreased partial pressure of oxygen present in a pressurized cabin. The only evidence of poor ventilation came on the final descent so it seemed unlikely that airway obstruction was the primary pathology. More likely it is the hypobaric environment leading to hypoxemia. As stated, thromboembolic events could not be ruled out in this environment. The equipment did not appear to be giving false reading, and the low pulse oximetry reading corresponded to patient's activity level and cyanosis. Because the author was unfamiliar with the particular ventilator he

was unable to conclusively determine whether or not it was functioning appropriately.

3. Discussion

Hypoxemia occurs at altitude because of decreases in barometric pressure resulting in reduction of partial pressure of oxygen. According to the alveolar gas equation (1), the reduction in the partial pressure of oxygen results in the loss of diffusional capacity of oxygen across the alveolar membrane and endothelium. Internal cabin altitude is the result of cabin pressurization to counteract the flight altitude, that is, the environmental altitude outside of the airplane. The FAA mandates that commercial flights maintain a cabin pressurization equivalent to no more than 8000 ft [4]. This limit allows for a minimum environmental pressure of 564 mmHg, a significant decrease from the 760 mmHg pressure at sea level. The cabin pressurization limit was initially derived based on weight and longevity of pressurization systems, fuel economy, and patient comfort [5]. One study revealed that average cabin altitude across 207 commercial flights was 6341 ft with longer flights resulting in higher average altitudes [6]. Another study revealed an average pressure of 634 mmHg across 45 commercial flights and three airlines in Boeing 747 airplanes [7]. This represents a decrease in the partial pressure of oxygen of greater than 15% from that of sea level.

Alveolar gas equation:

$$p_AO_2 = F_iO_2 (P_{ATM} - pH_2O)$$
$$- \frac{p_aCO_2 (1 - F_iO_2 [1 - RER])}{RER}, \quad (1)$$

where p_AO_2 is the alveolar partial pressure of oxygen, F_iO_2 is the fraction of inspired oxygen, P_{ATM} is the atmospheric pressure, pH_2O is the vapor pressure of water, p_aCO_2 is the arterial partial pressure of CO_2, and RER is the respiratory exchange ratio.

Arterial oxygen tension has been shown to decrease in simulated hypobaric environments more than 20 mmHg in patients with chronic obstructive lung disease [8]. Patients with normal physiology tend to tolerate a hypobaric airplane environment well [9, 10]; however concern exists for patients with existing pulmonary or cardiac or hematological disease and decompensation in this environment [11–15]. Normal respiratory changes to increasing altitude include increased minute ventilation through hyperventilation [16]. Hypoxic pulmonary vasoconstriction increases the resistance through the pulmonary arteriolar and capillary bed with a concordant increase in pulmonary artery pressures [17]. Increased wall tension in the pulmonary vasculature causes an increase in extravascular fluid in the lung parenchyma [18]. Acutely an increase in cardiac output occurs at altitude due to increased sympathetic activity and is largely mediated through increased heart rate [16, 19]. Mixed venous oxygen is expected to drop due to a decrease in oxygen delivery which also drives the increase in cardiac output.

Regarding the patient presented, although not stated by the family, it is likely that the child had underlying pulmonary disease that prevented compensation for the hypobaric environment. It is felt that the hypoxemia originated from decreased diffusional capacity. Due to the decreased arterial saturation resistance in the pulmonary vasculature increased. The tachycardia is likely a response to acute altitude exposure and now decreased right heart output due to increasing pulmonary vascular resistance. This caused or exacerbated right to left shunting resulting in decreasing delivery of oxygen to the tissues. Supplemental oxygen along with mechanical ventilation helped compensate for the hypobaric environment leading to increased arterial oxygen saturations, decreased cyanosis, reduction of heart rate, and increased activity of the child. The second desaturation event on descent of the aircraft is thought to be attributable to developing pulmonary edema. The evidence for this lies in increasing rales in the child's lungs and increasing secretions suctioned from the tracheotomy tube concordant with desaturations on pulse oximetry. Development of pulmonary edema at altitude is secondary to compensatory pulmonary vascular changes [18].

Commercial flights in the United States and international flights with airline agencies originating in the US are federally mandated to have an in-flight emergency medical kit [20] (Table 1). These kits offer a basic first aid kit including supplies for wound dressing as well as more advanced cardiopulmonary resuscitation supplies such as oropharyngeal airways and an automated external defibrillator. The cabin staff are required to have basic CPR certification with recertification every two years [21]. Additionally, some arguments have been raised as to the suitability of both FAA kits for pediatric emergencies [22]. Some airlines have contracted with on-ground medical provider for in-flight emergency advice, even including the use of in-flight telemetry [23–25]. Thus, although every flight should have basic medical equipment available, one of the key initial steps in response to an in-flight medical emergency should be to evaluate the resources at hand. This is especially true for pediatric patients.

One survey taken from physicians in the United Kingdom revealed that the vast majority of survey responders had been called upon to treat patients outside of the clinical setting [26]. Other studies have shown mixed evidence as to the response rate, that is, to treat or not treat, when healthcare providers are placed in this type of situation [26–30]. DiMaggio et al. (1994) found that the two most influential factors associated with healthcare providers responding to a call was distance to the nearest medical facility and familiarity with the type of patient presented [27]. Other concerns were unknown infectious disease or nonwillingness to engage in mouth-to-mouth resuscitation on a stranger [29]. One survey noted a significant increase in response rate when the provider had stronger knowledge of the legal aspects of providing care [30]. Of note on this last point congress passed the FAA Aviation Medical Assistance Act (AMAA) on April 24th, 1998, to protect Good Samaritans on US commercial flight [31]. This law is designed to mitigate legal liability of medically trained persons who respond to in-flight emergencies. The AMAA does not suspend liability if the responder is thought to be in "gross negligence" of care.

TABLE 1: FAA mandated medical supplies on commercial flights [34].

Item	Quantity
Diagnostic tools	
Sphygmomanometer	1
Stethoscope	1
Airway supplies	
Oropharyngeal airways (various sizes including pediatric)	3
CPR masks (various sizes including pediatric)	3
Self-inflating manual resuscitation device with various mask sizes including pediatric	1
Basic wound supplies	
Alcohol sponges	2
1-inch adhesive tape roll	1
Tape scissors pair	1
Tourniquet	1
Nonpermeable gloves pair	1
IV equipment	
IV start kit with Y-connector	1
Needles (various gauges)	6
Syringes (various volumes)	4
Medicine	
Saline solution 500 cc	1
Analgesic tablet (nonopiate) 325 mg	4
Antihistamine tablet, 25 mg	4
Antihistamine injectable 50 mg ampule	2
Atropine 0.5 mg ampule	2
Aspirin tablet 325 mg	4
Bronchodilator metered dose inhaler	1
Dextrose 50%/50 cc ampule injectable	1
Epinephrine 1 : 1000 1 cc ampule Injectable	2
Epinephrine 1 : 10,000 2 cc ampule injectable	2
Lidocaine 5 cc 20 mg/ml ampule injectable	2
Nitroglycerine tablet 0.4 mg	10
Instructions for use of kit drugs	1

4. Recommendations

Moving forward several recommendations can be made based on this case and through literature review. The authors of this paper will first echo some broad recommendations of prior articles. Gendreau and Dejohn (2002) published a suggested response to being called to act in the extraclinical setting [23] including introducing oneself to the patient/family, stating qualifications, asking for permission to treat, taking a patient history and physical, and always working within one's qualifications [23]. Chandra and Conry (2013) recommend that seeking input from other healthcare providers present might also facilitate better patient care [32]. Another recommendation from that article is to obtain a personal copy of any forms documenting the incident [32].

The Aerospace Medical Association has published more comprehensive guide for responding providers [33] and would be beneficial to any medical provider with plans for travel. A final generalized recommendation is to gather and evaluate all medical resources available. This includes surveying the in-flight medical kit and discussing with the airline staff supplemental resources such as the ground based telemetry discussed above.

More specifically to the case presented it is recommended that patients with preexisting cardiac and pulmonary conditions be seen by their physicians and discuss fitness-to-fly prior to traveling. If the patient's treating physician is unfamiliar with air travel then consultation with an aviation medicine colleague is advised, specifically if the patient is traveling with medical devices or equipment. Patients with medical devices are recommended to have all the needed components of that device prior to traveling. It is also recommended that the patient or the physician discuss with the manufacturer of the device concerns regarding functionality during flight. The airline should be made aware in advance of the device and all components needed to utilize. This includes discussion regarding supplemental oxygen for O_2 dependent patients or mechanically supported patients. Also it is important to note, in patients with an endotracheal tube or tracheostomy tube in place, the incidence of mucosal trauma/ischemia secondary to increased cuff pressures. As the barometric pressure drops the air within the cuff expands and increases pressure against the tracheal mucosa. Use of saline in the cuff prior to takeoff has been proposed to mitigate this risk [34–37]. There are drawbacks to this method that should be recognized; saline in the cuff has been associated with elevated cuff pressures at sea level [37] and inflation/deflation with saline increases procedural time versus use of air [34]. Overpressurization of the cuff can be avoided with the use of a manometer [38]. It is also important to recognize that endotracheal tube manufacturers have advocated against this practice [37].

5. Summary

Responding to in-flight medical emergencies can be extremely challenging for healthcare workers. In additional to unfamiliarity with the patient and equipment, there are unique physiologic implications due to a decrease in atmospheric pressure. However, this should not serve as an absolute barrier to involvement. In addition, providers should not be dissuaded by concerns for legal ramifications as current law provides a fair amount of protection for those who deliver care in good faith.

Competing Interests

The authors of this paper have neither financial disclosures nor conflict of interests to disclose.

References

[1] 2015 U.S.-Based Airline Traffic Data — Bureau of Transportation Statistics, http://www.rita.dot.gov/bts/press_releases/bts018_16.

[2] D. C. Peterson, C. Martin-Gill, F. X. Guyette et al., "Outcomes of medical emergencies on commercial airline flights," *New England Journal of Medicine*, vol. 368, no. 22, pp. 2075–2083, 2013.

[3] C. Thibeault, A. D. Evans, and N. P. Dowdall, "AsMA medical guidelines for air travel: fitness to fly and medical clearances," *Aerospace Medicine and Human Performance*, vol. 86, no. 7, p. 656, 2015.

[4] Federal Aviation Administration, "Pressurized Cabins. Federal Aviation Regulations Title 14 Part 25 Section 841," Federal Aviation Administration.

[5] R. A. McFarland, "Human factors in relation to the development of pressurized cabins," *Aerospace Medicine*, vol. 42, no. 12, pp. 1303–1318, 1971.

[6] N. B. Hampson, D. A. Kregenow, A. M. Mahoney et al., "Altitude exposures during commercial flight: a reappraisal," *Aviation Space and Environmental Medicine*, vol. 84, no. 1, pp. 27–31, 2013.

[7] P. T. Kelly, L. M. Seccombe, P. G. Rogers, and M. J. Peters, "Directly measured cabin pressure conditions during Boeing 747-400 commercial aircraft flights," *Respirology*, vol. 12, no. 4, pp. 511–515, 2007.

[8] T. A. Dillard, B. W. Berg, K. R. Rajagopal, J. W. Dooley, and W. J. Mehm, "Hypoxemia during air travel in patients with chronic obstructive pulmonary disease," *Annals of Internal Medicine*, vol. 111, no. 5, pp. 362–367, 1989.

[9] J. M. Muhm, P. B. Rock, D. L. McMullin et al., "Effect of aircraft-cabin altitude on passenger discomfort," *New England Journal of Medicine*, vol. 357, no. 1, pp. 18–27, 2007.

[10] W. D. Toff, C. I. Jones, I. Ford et al., "Effect of hypobaric hypoxia, simulating conditions during long-haul air travel, on coagulation, fibrinolysis, platelet function, and endothelial activation," *Journal of the American Medical Association*, vol. 295, no. 19, pp. 2251–2261, 2006.

[11] M. E. Spoorenberg, M. H. A. H. van den Oord, T. Meeuwsen, and T. Takken, "Fitness to fly testing in patients with congenital heart and lung disease," *Aerospace Medicine and Human Performance*, vol. 87, no. 1, pp. 54–60, 2016.

[12] T. T. Nicholson and J. I. Sznajder, "Fitness to fly in patients with lung disease," *Annals of the American Thoracic Society*, vol. 11, no. 10, pp. 1614–1622, 2014.

[13] A. M. Luks, "Do lung disease patients need supplemental oxygen at high altitude?" *High Altitude Medicine and Biology*, vol. 10, no. 4, pp. 321–327, 2009.

[14] T. Goto, M. Sato, A. Yamazaki et al., "The effect of atmospheric pressure on ventricular assist device output," *Journal of Artificial Organs*, vol. 15, no. 1, pp. 104–108, 2012.

[15] Aerospace Medical Association, Aviation Safety Committee, and Civil Aviation Subcommittee, "Cabin cruising altitudes for regular transport aircraft," *Aviation, Space, and Environmental Medicine*, vol. 79, no. 4, pp. 433–439, 2008.

[16] J. P. Brown and M. P. Grocott, "Humans at altitude: physiology and pathophysiology," *Continuing Education in Anaesthesia, Critical Care & Pain*, vol. 13, no. 1, pp. 17–22, 2013.

[17] S. Huez, V. Faoro, H. Guénard, J.-B. Martinot, and R. Naeije, "Echocardiographic and tissue doppler imaging of cardiac adaptation to high altitude in native highlanders versus acclimatized lowlanders," *American Journal of Cardiology*, vol. 103, no. 11, pp. 1605–1609, 2009.

[18] A. M. Luks and E. R. Swenson, "Travel to high altitude with preexisting lung disease," *European Respiratory Journal*, vol. 29, no. 4, pp. 770–792, 2007.

[19] J. P. Higgins, T. Tuttle, and J. A. Higgins, "Altitude and the heart: is going high safe for your cardiac patient?" *American Heart Journal*, vol. 159, no. 1, pp. 25–32, 2010.

[20] Federal Aviation Administration, *First-Aid Kits and Emergency Medical Kits. Federal Aviation Regulations Title 14 Part 121 Appendix-A*, Federal Aviation Administration, 2012.

[21] Federal Aviation Administration, *Advisory Circular: Emergency Medical Equipment Training. AC No. 121-34B*, Federal Aviation Administration, Washington, DC, USA, 2006.

[22] S. M. Badawy, A. A. Thompson, and M. Sand, "In-flight emergencies: medical kits are not good enough for kids," *Journal of Paediatrics and Child Health*, vol. 52, no. 4, pp. 363–365, 2016.

[23] M. A. Gendreau and C. Dejohn, "Responding to medical events during commercial airline flights," *New England Journal of Medicine*, vol. 346, no. 14, pp. 1067–1073, 2002.

[24] International Air Transport Association (IATA), *Medical Manual Montreal*, IATA, 2006.

[25] T. Bashir, "Patients crash more than airlines: a medical emergency at 35,000 ft," *Journal of Community Hospital Internal Medicine Perspectives*, vol. 4, no. 3, Article ID 24730, 2017.

[26] K. Williams, "Doctors as good samaritans: some empirical evidence concerning emergency medical treatment in Britain," *Journal of Law and Society*, vol. 30, no. 2, pp. 258–282, 2003.

[27] L. A. DiMaggio, S. E. Rubino, and R. V. Lee, "Good samaritans or reticent bystanders?" *Journal of Travel Medicine*, vol. 1, no. 3, pp. 143–146, 1994.

[28] R. J. Gray and G. S. Sharpe, "Doctors, Samaritans and the accident victim," 1972, http://wbldb.lievers.net/10104908.html.

[29] C. P. Gross, A. B. Reisman, and M. D. Schwartz, "The physician as ambivalent samaritan: will internists resuscitate victims of out-of-hospital emergencies?" *Journal of General Internal Medicine*, vol. 13, no. 7, pp. 491–494, 1998.

[30] W. M. Garneau, D. M. Harris, and A. J. Viera, "Cross-sectional survey of Good Samaritan behaviour by physicians in North Carolina," *BMJ Open*, vol. 6, no. 3, Article ID e010720, 2016.

[31] "Aviation Medical Assistance Act of 1998, Pub. L. No. 105–170," Washington, DC, USA: National Archives and Records Administration.

[32] A. Chandra and S. Conry, "In-flight medical emergencies," *Western Journal of Emergency Medicine*, vol. 14, no. 5, pp. 499–504, 2013.

[33] Aerospace Medical Association, *Medical Emergencies: Managing In-Flight Medical Events (Guidance Material for Health Professionals)*, Aerospace Medical Association, 2016.

[34] J. Orsborn, J. Graham, M. Moss, M. Melguizo, T. Nick, and M. Stroud, "Pediatric endotracheal tube cuff pressures during aeromedical transport," *Pediatric Emergency Care*, vol. 32, no. 1, pp. 20–22, 2016.

[35] J. Henning, P. Sharley, and R. Young, "Pressures within air-filled tracheal cuffs at altitude—an in vivo study," *Anaesthesia*, vol. 59, no. 3, pp. 252–254, 2004.

[36] C. Mann, N. Parkinson, and A. Bleetman, "Endotracheal tube and laryngeal mask airway cuff volume changes with altitude: a rule of thumb for aeromedical transport," *Emergency Medicine Journal*, vol. 24, no. 3, pp. 165–167, 2007.

[37] T. Britton, T. C. Blakeman, J. Eggert, D. Rodriquez, H. Ortiz, and R. D. Branson, "Managing endotracheal tube cuff pressure at altitude: a comparison of four methods," *Journal of Trauma and Acute Care Surgery*, vol. 77, no. 3, pp. S240–S244, 2014.

[38] P. Brendt, M. Schnekenburger, K. Paxton, A. Brown, and K. Mendis, "Endotracheal tube cuff pressure before, during, and after fixed-wing air medical retrieval," *Prehospital Emergency Care*, vol. 17, no. 2, pp. 177–180, 2013.

Permissions

All chapters in this book were first published in CRA, by Hindawi Publishing Corporation; hereby published with permission under the Creative Commons Attribution License or equivalent. Every chapter published in this book has been scrutinized by our experts. Their significance has been extensively debated. The topics covered herein carry significant findings which will fuel the growth of the discipline. They may even be implemented as practical applications or may be referred to as a beginning point for another development.

The contributors of this book come from diverse backgrounds, making this book a truly international effort. This book will bring forth new frontiers with its revolutionizing research information and detailed analysis of the nascent developments around the world.

We would like to thank all the contributing authors for lending their expertise to make the book truly unique. They have played a crucial role in the development of this book. Without their invaluable contributions this book wouldn't have been possible. They have made vital efforts to compile up to date information on the varied aspects of this subject to make this book a valuable addition to the collection of many professionals and students.

This book was conceptualized with the vision of imparting up-to-date information and advanced data in this field. To ensure the same, a matchless editorial board was set up. Every individual on the board went through rigorous rounds of assessment to prove their worth. After which they invested a large part of their time researching and compiling the most relevant data for our readers.

The editorial board has been involved in producing this book since its inception. They have spent rigorous hours researching and exploring the diverse topics which have resulted in the successful publishing of this book. They have passed on their knowledge of decades through this book. To expedite this challenging task, the publisher supported the team at every step. A small team of assistant editors was also appointed to further simplify the editing procedure and attain best results for the readers.

Apart from the editorial board, the designing team has also invested a significant amount of their time in understanding the subject and creating the most relevant covers. They scrutinized every image to scout for the most suitable representation of the subject and create an appropriate cover for the book.

The publishing team has been an ardent support to the editorial, designing and production team. Their endless efforts to recruit the best for this project, has resulted in the accomplishment of this book. They are a veteran in the field of academics and their pool of knowledge is as vast as their experience in printing. Their expertise and guidance has proved useful at every step. Their uncompromising quality standards have made this book an exceptional effort. Their encouragement from time to time has been an inspiration for everyone.

The publisher and the editorial board hope that this book will prove to be a valuable piece of knowledge for researchers, students, practitioners and scholars across the globe.

List of Contributors

Pragati Ganjoo, Vijay K. Pandey and Monica S. Tandon
Department of Anaesthesiology and Intensive Care, GB Pant Hospital, Maulana Azad Medical College, New Delhi 110002, India

Hukum Singh and Daljit Singh
Department of Neurosurgery, GB Pant Hospital, Maulana Azad Medical College, New Delhi 110002, India

Michel Casanova and Wolfgang Ummenhofer
Department for Anesthesia, Surgical Intensive Care, Prehospital Emergency Medicine and Pain Therapy, University Hospital of Basel, Spitalstrasse 21, 4031 Basel, Switzerland

Jasmina Kurdija and Jan G. Jakobsson
Department of Anaesthesia and Intensive Care, Institution for Clinical Science, Karolinska Institutet, Danderyds Hospital, 182 88 Stockholm, Sweden

Hesham A. Elsharkawy and Ursula Galway
Department of General Anesthesiology and Outcomes Research, Anesthesiology Institute, Cleveland Clinic, 9500 Euclid Avenue, Cleveland, OH 44195, USA

Pietro Paolo Martorano
Head of Neuroanesthesia Unit, Ospedali Riuniti, Via Conca 71 - 60126 Ancona, Italy

Edoardo Barboni
Clinic of Anesthesia and Intensive Care Unit, Department of Emergency, Ospedali Riuniti, Via Conca 71 - 60126 Ancona, Italy

Giovanni Buscema
Anesthesia and Intensive Care Unit, AOUG. Rodolico, Via S. Sofia 78 - 95123 Catania, Italy

Alessandro Di Rienzo
Department of Neurosurgery, Università Politecnica delle Marche, Ospedali Riuniti, Via Conca 71 - 60126 Ancona, Italy

Ayse B. Ozer, Omer L. Erhan, Cevdet Sumer and Ozden Yildizhan
Anaesthesiology and Reanimation Department, Faculty of Medicine, Firat University, 23119 Elazig, Turkey

Jeremy Kaplowitz and Paul Bigeleisen
Department of Anesthesiology, University of Maryland School of Medicine, 22 S. Greene Street S11C00, Baltimore, MD 21201, USA

Jahan Porhomayon
VA Western New York Healthcare System, Division of Critical Care and Pain Medicine, Department of Anesthesiology, School of Medicine and Biomedical Sciences, State University of New York at Buffalo, Buffalo, NY, USA
VA Medical Center, Rm 203C, 3495 Bailey Ave, Buffalo, NY 14215, USA

Gino Zadeii
Mason City Cardiology Clinic, University of Iowa, Mason City, IA 50401, USA

Alireza Yarahamadi
Mason City Neurology Clinic, University of Iowa, Mason City, IA 50401, USA

Nader D. Nader
VA Western New York Healthcare System, Division of Cardiothoracic Anesthesia and Pain Medicine, Department of Anesthesiology, School of Medicine and Biomedical Sciences, State University of New York at Buffalo, Buffalo, NY 14215, USA

Stephan Klumpp and Lydia M. Jorge
Department of Clinical Anesthesia, Jackson Memorial Hospital, University of Miami, Miami, FL 33136, USA

Mohammed Ali Aziz-Sultan
Department of Clinical Neurologic Surgery, 201 Pope Life Center, University of Miami, Miami, FL 33136, USA

Collin Sprenker and Devanand Mangar
Florida Gulf to Bay Anesthesiology Associates, LLC, Tampa, FL 33606, USA

John Schweiger, Rachel Karlnoski and Enrico M. Camporesi
Florida Gulf to Bay Anesthesiology Associates, LLC, Tampa, FL 33606, USA
University of South Florida, Department of Surgery, Tampa, FL 33606, USA

Naga Pullakhandam
Florida Hospital, Orlando, FL 32804, USA

Akihiro Kashiwai, Takahiro Suzuki and Setsuro Ogawa
Department of Anesthesiology, Nihon University School of Medicine, 30-1 Oyaguchi Kamimachi, Itabashi-ku, Tokyo 173-8610, Japan

Vittorio Pavoni, Valentina Froio, Alessandra Nella, Martina Simonelli, Lara Gianesello and Massimo Micaglio
Department of Anesthesia and Intensive Care, University-Hospital Careggi, Largo Brambilla 3, 50134 Firenze, Italy

Andrew Horton
Faculty Practice Group, University of California, Los Angeles, CA 90095, USA

Luca Malino
Ambu Srl, Via Paracelso 18, Agrate Brianza, 20041 Milano, Italy

Scott C. Watkins, Lewis McCarver, Alicia VanBebber and David P. Bichell
Monroe Carell Jr. Children's Hospital at Vanderbilt, Vanderbilt University Medical Center, Nashville, N 37232, USA

Conor Skerritt and Stephen Mannion
Department of Anaesthesia, South Infirmary, Victoria University Hospital, Old Blackrock Road, Cork, Ireland

Jianguo Cheng
Department of Pain Management, Cleveland Clinic, 9500 Euclid Avenue, Cleveland, OH 44195, USA

Anuj Daftari
Department of Physical Medicine and Rehabilitation, Metro health Medical Center, 2500 Metro health Drive, Cleveland, OH 44109, USA

Lan Zhou
Department of Neurology, Cleveland Clinic, 9500 Euclid Avenue, Cleveland, OH 44195, USA

Manzo Suzuki, Toshiichiro Inagi and Hiroyasu Bito
Department of Anesthesiology, Musashikosugi Hospital, Nippon Medical School, 1-396 Kosugi-cho, Nakahara-ku, Kanagawa 211-8533, Japan

Takehiko Kikutani
Department of Anesthesiology, Higashitotuka Memorial Hospital, 548-7 Shinano-cho, Totsuka-ku, Yokohama-shi, Kanagawa 244-0801, Japan

Takuya Mishima
Department of Surgery, Higashitotuka Memorial Hospital, 548-7 Shinano-cho, Totuka-ku, Yokohama-shi, Kanagawa 244-0801, Japan

Vianey Q. Casarez, Acsa M. Zavala, Pascal Owusu-Agyemang and Katherine Hagan
Department of Anesthesiology and Perioperative Medicine, The University of Texas MD Anderson Cancer Center, 1515 Holcombe Boulevard, Unit 409, Houston, TX 77030, USA

Rajeev Puri, Arpita Saxena, Zia Arshad, Yogita Dwivedi, Trilok Chand, Apurva Mittal, Archna Agrawal, Jay Prakash and Sathiyanarayanan Pilendran
Department of Anaesthesia and Critical Care, S. N. Medical College, Agra, India

Awak Mittal
Department of Orthopaedics, S. N. Medical College, Agra, India

Nicolas J. Mouawad and Michael R. Go
Department of Surgery, The Ohio State University Wexner Medical Center, 410West 10th Avenue, Columbus, OH 43210, USA

Erica J. Stein, Kenneth R. Moran and Thomas J. Papadimos
Department of Anesthesiology, The Ohio State University Wexner Medical Center, 410West 10th Avenue, Columbus, OH 43210, USA

R. Ketelaars and A. P. Wolff
Department of Anaesthesia, Radboud University Nijmegen Medical Centre, P.O. Box 9101, 6500 HB Nijmegen, The Netherlands

Ahmed Abdelgawwad Wefki Abdelgawwad Shousha, Maria Sanfilippo, Antonio Sabba and Paolo Pinchera
Department of Anesthesiology and Intensive Care, Sapienza University, Viale del policlinico 155, 00161 Rome, Italy

Ihab Kamel, Gaurav Trehan and Rodger Barnette
Temple University School of Medicine, 3401 N. Broad Street, 3rd Floor Outpatient Building, Zone B, Philadelphia, PA 19140, USA

Qingfu Zhang, Wei Jiang, Quanhong Zhou, Guangyan Wang and Linlin Zhao
Department of Anesthesiology, Shanghai Jiao Tong University Affiliated Shanghai Sixth People's Hospital, 600 Yishan Road, Shanghai 200233, China

I. J. J. Dons-Sinke, M. Dirckx and G. P. Scoones
Department of Anesthesiology, Erasmus MC-Sophia, Postbus 2060, 3000 CB Rotterdam, The Netherlands

Christian Seefelder and Navil F. Sethna1
Department of Anesthesiology, Perioperative and Pain Medicine, Children's Hospital Boston, Boston, MA 02115, USA

Rosalie F. Tassone
Department of Anesthesiology, Perioperative and Pain Medicine, Children's Hospital Boston, Boston, MA 02115, USA

Division of Pediatric Anesthesiology, Department of Anesthesiology, University of Illinois Medical Center, 1740 West Taylor Street, Chicago, IL 60612, USA

Johnathan Gardes and Tracey Straker
Department of Anesthesiology, Montefiore Medical Center, Bronx, New York City, NY 10467, USA

Vijay Krishnamoorthy and Sumidtra Prathep
Department of Anesthesiology and Pain Medicine, University of Washington, WA 98104, USA

Deepak Sharma
Departments of Anesthesiology and Pain Medicine, Neurological Surgery (Adj.), University of Washington, WA 98104, USA

Monica S. Vavilala
Departments of Anesthesiology and Pain Medicine, Neurological Surgery (Adj.), Pediatrics (Adj.), and Radiology (Adj.), University of Washington, WA 98104, USA

Maria Sanfilippo, Ahmed Abdelgawwad Wefki Abdelgawwad Shousha and Antonella Paparazzo
Department of Anesthesiology and Intensive Care, Sapienza University, Viale del policlinico 155, 00161 Rome, Italy

Manila Singh
Department of Anesthesia and Intensive Care, G.B. Pant Hospital, E-269, East of Kailash, New Delhi, India

Saket Singh
Department of Anesthesia and Intensive Care, G.B. Pant Hospital, E-269, East of Kailash, New Delhi, India
Department of C.V.T.S, G.B. Pant Hospital, New Delhi, India

Nune Matinyan, Alexander Saltanov, Leonid Martynov and Anatolij Kazantsev
N. N. Blokhin Cancer Research Center, Pediatric Oncology and Hematology Research Institute, Moscow 115478, Russia

K. Sanem Cakar Turhan, Yeşim Batislam and Oya Özatamer
Department of Anaesthesiology and Reanimation, Ankara University Medical School, Ankara, Turkey

Volkan Baytaş
Department of Anaesthesiology and Reanimation, Ankara Güven Hospital, Ankara, Turkey

Clark K. Choi and Kalpana Tyagaraj
Department of Anesthesiology, Maimonides Medical Center, 4802 10th Avenue, Brooklyn, NY 11219, USA

Arjun Desai, Brendan Carvalho, Jenna Hansen and Jonay Hill
Department of Anesthesia, H3580, Stanford University School of Medicine, Stanford, CA 94305, USA

Huili Lim, Chuen Jye Yeoh, Jerry Tan, Harikrishnan Kothandan and May U. S. Mok
Department of Anesthesia and Intensive Care, Singapore General Hospital, Singapore

José Raul Soberón
Department of Anesthesiology, Ochsner Clinic Foundation, 1514 Jefferson Highway, New Orleans, LA 70121, USA

Scott F. Duncan
Department of Orthopedic Surgery, Ochsner Clinic Foundation, 1514 Jefferson Highway, New Orleans, LA 70121, USA

W. Charles Sternbergh
Vascular and Endovascular Surgery, Ochsner Clinic Foundation, 1514 Jefferson Highway, New Orleans, LA 70121, USA

Sankalp Sehgal and Joshua C. Chance
Department of Anesthesiology and Pain Medicine, University of Arkansas for Medical Sciences, Little Rock, AR 72205, USA

Matthew A. Steliga
Department of Cardiothoracic Surgery, University of Arkansas for Medical Sciences, Little Rock, AR 72205, USA

Jeffrey M. Carness
Department of Anesthesiology, United States Naval Hospital Yokosuka, Yokosuka, Japan

Mark J. Lenart
Department of Anesthesiology, Naval Medical Center Portsmouth, Portsmouth, VA, USA

Madhu Gupta, Shalini Subramanian and Preeti Adlakha
Department of Anaesthesiology, ESI-PGIMSR, Basaidara Pur, New Delhi, India

Ali Movafegh, Alireza Saliminia, Reza Atef-Yekta and Omid Azimaraghi
Department of Anesthesiology and Critical Care, Dr. Ali Shariati Hospital, Tehran University of Medical Sciences, Tehran, Iran

Federico Boncagni
Clinica di Rianimazione Generale, Respiratoria e del Trauma Maggiore, Azienda Ospedaliero-Universitaria "Ospedali Riuniti Umberto I-G. M. Lancisi-G. Salesi", 60126 Ancona, Italy

Luca Pecora
Anestesia e Rianimazione dei Trapianti e della Chirurgia Maggiore, Azienda Ospedaliero-Universitaria "Ospedali Riuniti Umberto I-G. M. Lancisi-G. Salesi", 60126 Ancona, Italy

Vasco Durazzi
Clinica di Neurologia, AziendaOspedaliero-Universitaria "Ospedali Riuniti Umberto I-G. M. Lancisi-G. Salesi", 60126Ancona, Italy

Francesco Ventrella
Anestesia e Rianimazione Pediatrica, Azienda Ospedaliero-Universitaria "Ospedali Riuniti Umberto I-G. M. Lancisi-G. Salesi", 60126 Ancona, Italy

John C. Coffman, Kasey Fiorini, Meghan Cook and Robert H. Small
Department of Anesthesiology, The Ohio State University Wexner Medical Center, Columbus, OH 43210, USA

Benjamin B. Bruins
Department of Anesthesiology and Critical Care, Hospital of the University of Pennsylvania, Philadelphia, PA 19104, USA

Natasha Mirza
Department of Otorhinolaryngology, Head and Neck Surgery, Perelman School of Medicine, The University of Pennsylvania, Philadelphia, PA 19104, USA

Ernest Gomez
Department of Otorhinolaryngology, Head and Neck Surgery, Hospital of the University of Pennsylvania, Philadelphia, PA 19104, USA

Joshua H. Atkins
Department of Anesthesiology and Critical Care, Department of Otorhinolaryngology, Head and Neck Surgery, Perelman School of Medicine, The University of Pennsylvania, PA 19104, USA

S. E. Verstraeten, A. H. M. van Straten and E. Berreklouw
Department of Cardiothoracic Surgery, Catharina Hospital Eindhoven, Michelangelolaan 2, 5623 EJ Eindhoven, The Netherlands

H. H. M. Korsten and E. W. G. Weber
Department of Anesthesiology, Catharina Hospital Eindhoven, Michelangelolaan 2, 5623 EJ Eindhoven, The Netherlands

P. L. M. L. Wielders
Department of Pulmonary Disease, Catharina Hospital Eindhoven, Michelangelolaan 2, 5623 EJ Eindhoven, The Netherlands

Menekse Oksar and Selim Turhanoglu
Department of Anesthesiology and Reanimation, Mustafa Kemal University Faculty of Medicine, 31100 Hatay, Turkey

Alper Kilicaslan, Ahmet Topal, Atilla Erol, Hale Borazan and Seref Otelcioglu1
Department of Anaesthesiology, Meram Medical Faculty, Necmettin Erbakan University, 42080 Konya, Turkey

Onur Bilge
Department of Orthopaedic Surgery, Meram Medical Faculty, Necmettin Erbakan University, 42080 Konya, Turkey

Rashmi Vandse and Thomas J. Papadimos
Department of Anesthesiology, Wexner Medical Center, Ohio State University, Columbus, OH 43210, USA

Benjamin Kloesel
Department of Anesthesia, Perioperative and Pain Medicine, Boston Children's Hospital, Boston, MA 02115, USA
Department of Anesthesia, Perioperative and Pain Medicine, Brigham and Women's Hospital, Boston, MA 02115, USA

Robert W. Lekowski
Department of Anesthesia, Perioperative and Pain Medicine, Brigham and Women's Hospital, Boston, MA 02115, USA

Christopher Allen-John Webb, Shara Cohn and Jennifer Lee1
Department of Anesthesiology, Perioperative and Pain Medicine, Stanford University School of Medicine, Stanford, CA, USA

Paul David Weyker
Department of Anesthesia and Perioperative Care, San Francisco School of Medicine, University of California, San Francisco, CA, USA

Amanda Wheeler
Department of Surgery, Stanford University School of Medicine, Stanford, CA, USA

Serkan Tulgar and Onur Selvi
Department of Anesthesiology and Reanimation, Maltepe University Faculty of Medicine, Istanbul, Turkey

Mahmut Sertan Kapakli
Department of General Surgery, Maltepe University Faculty of Medicine, Istanbul, Turkey

Howard D. Palte, Don P. Hoa and Aldo Pavon Canseco
Department of Anesthesiology, Miller School of Medicine, University of Miami, Miami, FL, USA

Sasima Dusitkasem, Blair H. Herndon, Dalton Paluzzi, Joseph Kuhn, Robert H. Small and John C. Coffman
Department of Anesthesiology, The Ohio State University Wexner Medical Center, Columbus, OH, USA

Nicholas L. Giordano and Noud van Helmond
Spine and Pain Institute of New York, New York City, NY, USA

Kenneth B. Chapman
Spine and Pain Institute of New York, New York City, NY, USA
Department of Anesthesiology, New York University Langone Medical Center, New York City, NY, USA
Northwell Health, New York City, NY, USA

Anis Dizdarevic and Anthony Fernandes
Anesthesiology and Pain Management, Columbia University Medical Center, 622 West 168th Street, PH 5, New York, NY 10032, USA

Talal W. Khan
Department of Anesthesiology and Pain Medicine, University of Kansas Medical Center, Kansas City, KS, USA

Abdulraheem Yacoub
Division of Medical Oncology, Department of Internal Medicine, University of Kansas Medical Center, Kansas City, KS, USA

Eric Kamenetsky, Mark C. Kendall, Antoun Nader and Jessica J. Weeks
Department of Anesthesiology, Feinberg School of Medicine, Northwestern University, Chicago, IL, USA

Rahul Reddy
Department of Anesthesiology, McGaw Medical Center, Northwestern University, Chicago, IL, USA

Michael S. Green, Archana Gundigi Venkatesh and Ranjani Venkataramani
Department of Anesthesiology and Perioperative Medicine, Drexel University College of Medicine, 245 N. 15th Street, Suite 7502, MS 310, Philadelphia, PA 19102, USA

Roman Dudaryk, Julio Benitez Lopez and Jack Louro
Department of Anesthesiology, Perioperative Medicine, and Pain Management, University of Miami Miller School of Medicine, Miami, FL, USA

Andrew T. Koogler and Michael Kushelev
Department of Anesthesiology, The Ohio State University Wexner Medical Center, 410W. 10th Ave., Columbus, OH 43210, USA

Hiroyuki Nakao
Department of Emergency and Critical Care Medicine, Hyogo College of Medicine, Hyōgo Prefecture, Japan

Nobue Terabe
Department of Anesthesiology, University of Tsukuba Hospital, Tsukuba, Japan

Soichiro Yamashita and Makoto Tanaka
Department of Anesthesiology, Faculty of Medicine, University of Tsukuba, Tsukuba, Japan

Ramon Go, David Wang and Danielle Ludwin
Department of Anesthesiology, New York-Presbyterian, Columbia University Medical Center, New York, NY, USA

S. Viehmeyer, P. Gabriel and J. N. Hilberath
Department of Anesthesiology and Critical Care Medicine, MediClin Heart Institute Lahr/Baden, Lahr, Germany

K. Bauer, S. Bauer and R. Sodian
Department of Cardiac Surgery, MediClin Heart Institute Lahr/Baden, Lahr, Germany

Yuki Sugiyama and Mikito Kawamata
Department of Anesthesiology and Resuscitology, Shinshu University School of Medicine, Japan

Sayako Gotoh and Masatoshi Urasawa
Department of Anesthesiology and Resuscitology, Shinshu University School of Medicine, Japan
Division of Anesthesia, Shinonoi General Hospital, Japan

Koichi Nakajima
Division of Anesthesia, Shinonoi General Hospital, Japan

Alberto Vieira Pantoja, Bruno Lima Pessoa, Bruno Mendonça Barcellos and Marco Antonio Cardoso de Resende
Fluminense Federal University (UFF), Niteroi, RJ, Brazil

Maria Emília Gonçalves Estevez
National Institute of Traumatology and Orthopaedics (INTO), Rio de Janeiro, RJ, Brazil

Fernando de Paiva Araújo
Monte Sinai Hospital, Juiz de Fora, MG, Brazil

Ciro Augusto Floriani
National School of Public Health of the Osvaldo Cruz Foundation (ENSP-FOC), Rio de Janeiro, RJ, Brazil

Emmanuel Lilitsis and Despina Dermitzaki
Department of Anesthesiology, University General Hospital of Heraklion, University of Crete, Medical School, Heraklion, Crete, Greece

Georgios Avgenakis, Ioannis Heretis, Charalampos Mpelantis and Charalampos Mamoulakis
Department of Urology, University General Hospital of Heraklion, University of Crete, Medical School, Heraklion, Crete, Greece

Galen Royce-Nagel
Department of Anesthesia, Critical Care and Pain Medicine, Massachusetts General Hospital, Boston, MA, USA

Kunal Karamchandani
Department of Anesthesiology and Perioperative Medicine, Penn State Health Milton S. Hershey Medical Center, Hershey, PA, USA

Rie Soeda, Fumika Taniguchi, Maiko Sawada, Saeko Hamaoka, Masayuki Shibasaki, Teiji Sawa and Yoshinobu Nakayama
Department of Anesthesiology, Kyoto Prefectural University of Medicine, 465 Kajii-cho, Kamigyo, Kyoto 602-8566, Japan

Yasufumi Nakajima
Department of Anesthesiology, Kansai Medical University, 2-5-1 Shin-machi, Hirakata, Osaka 573-1010, Japan

Satoru Hashimoto
Division of Critical Care, Kyoto Prefectural University of Medicine Hospital, 465 Kajii-cho, Kamigyo, Kyoto 602-8566, Japan

Jason Quevreaux and Christopher Cropsey
Department of Anesthesiology, Educational Affairs, Vanderbilt University Medical Center, 2301 VUH, Nashville, TN 37232-7237, USA

Index